Devoured

Devoured

From Chicken Wings to Kale Smoothies—
How What We Eat Defines Who We Are

SOPHIE EGAN

WM

WILLIAM MORROW
An Imprint of HarperCollinsPublishers

HarperCollins books may be purchased for educational, business, or sales promotional use. For information please e-mail the Special Markets Department at SPsales@harpercollins.com.

FIRST EDITION

Illustrations by Ciara Gay

Library of Congress Cataloging-in-Publication Data has been applied for.

ISBN 978-0-06-239098-1

16 17 18 19 20   OV/RRD   10 9 8 7 6 5 4 3 2 1

For Sam, who always knew

Contents

How convenience has always been part of our national heritage, and yet today, with the plague of overwork, we have taken that value to new extremes—snacking more than ever and overhauling the very definition of the American meal.

TELLING FACTS: Between 1978 and 1996, calories consumed from dinner decreased 37 percent, and increased 16 percent from breakfast, 21 percent from lunch, and 101 percent from snacks. More than half of Americans now snack two to three times daily.

The range of workplace food experiences, and why the social mores of office dining are unlike anywhere else.

TELLING FACTS: Americans work 200 more hours per year compared with 1970. Forty percent of North American workers eat lunch at their desks.

Why we love customizing our orders for everything from burritos to bicycles. Rather than participating in some time-tested tradition or sharing with a broader collective, Americans are hard-wired to individualize our eating experiences.

TELLING FACT: There are eighty-seven thousand different drink combinations at Starbucks.

Why we buy foods like nonfat milk, gluten-free pastries, GMO-free cereal, and air-popped chips on the basis of what they lack.

TELLING FACTS: We attribute a range of health benefits to foods labeled low-fat, in a phenomenon called "health halos": We believe they are lower in calories, higher in quality, and more natural. And we will eat far more of a food if it is labeled low-fat.

What's different about weekends, the psychology of waiting in line, and why so many Americans spend half their Sunday in pursuit of eggs Benedict. Spoiler alert: When it comes to work, solo dining, and food as fuel, brunch just might be our saving grace.

TELLING FACT: Nearly 40 percent of Americans say they skip breakfast because of lack of time.

What fad diets—and preaching the gospel of those diets—reveal about who we are. Plus, what finding God and dieting have in common.

TELLING FACT: The inventors of Soylent, peddling a new meal-replacement drink, hoped to raise $100,000 through a month of crowdfunding. They got it in two hours.

How America welcomed wine into its drinking culture, and what's unique about our relationship to vino.

TELLING FACTS: Today, Americans drink over three times as much wine per person as we did in 1951. In 2010, for the first time ever, America beat out France as the number one wine market in the world. (They still beat us per capita, but used to outpace us in total consumption, too.)

Why we are such suckers for stunts.

TELLING FACTS: The Doritos Locos Taco quickly became Taco Bell's most popular menu item of all time, hitting the 100-million mark in an unprecedented ten weeks. (Granted, times were different, but it took McDonald's ten years to sell its 100-millionth burger during the 1950s.)

The marketing secrets behind limited time offers, seasonal specials, and the annual "shortages" of Super Bowl foods.

TELLING FACT: Super Bowl Sunday is our nation's second-highest day of food consumption—trailing only Thanksgiving.

How the melting pot mentality helped transform Italian food from an intact cultural import to a fusion cuisine—distinctly Italian *American*—so deeply embedded in daily life we can hardly define American food without it.

TELLING FACT: Two-thirds of Americans now eat a greater variety of cuisines from around the world than they did just five years ago.

The American Food Psyche

Wednesday, 7:00 A.M.

An alarm clock blares, and a guy we'll call Josh bolts out of bed. The noise is definitely alarming because he has the alarm set to the one that sounds like bad things are happening on a submarine. Ambling into the kitchen, Josh finds his neatly lined rows of Keurig K-Cup coffee pods and goes for the southern pecan flavor. Fall has just begun, and at that particular moment, he's in the mood for something comforting.

Josh is a thirty-one-year-old hardware operations quality engineer at Google. At six feet tall with pale, freckled skin, brown hair, and blue eyes, he's got somewhere between a cross-country runner's build and a "dad bod"—the latter thanks to a slight paunch that's developed since taking the Google position three years earlier (surely a small price to pay for finally having landed his dream job at the best company to work for *in the country*).

Like people in more than one in four American households, Josh lives alone. He rents a one-bedroom apartment in the Old Fourth Ward (O4W) neighborhood of Atlanta. With a great park, art and music festivals, and historical warehouses turned into cool lofts and retail spaces, O4W was the clear choice when he moved there.

7:08 A.M.

Josh opens his laptop and plunges deep into the Internet. With seven different windows open, his screen flashes with a whirl of activity. The number of e-mails waiting for him this morning is massive. It's not so much that the deluge has already begun, but that it never really ends. Every minute he sleeps, the more behind he gets at work. So now he takes a sip of coffee and starts firing e-mails back.

Josh is a member of the millennial generation, the largest in the United States and about a third of the total population. A graduate of the University of Michigan, he's among the 61 percent of his cohort with a college degree, 15 percent higher than his parents'. He's among the 62 percent who prefer to live in mixed-use urban areas, according to consumer insights firm Nielsen. Work, nightlife, shopping—all at their doorsteps. Also like other millennials, he was raised on cereal, computers, and a congratulations every time he put his socks on straight.

Josh scrolls through his Facebook feed and sees that his flame from a summer internship in Austin a few years back is on a two-week liquid diet. She has posted a photo of herself sipping a kale smoothie at Starbucks. Josh also sees that his sister in Portland made homemade pizza last night with arugula, burrata, and gluten-free dough, topped with poached eggs from the chickens in her backyard. And Josh's former college roommate has posted from a CrossFit box in New York, bragging about his WOD, which means "workout of the day." He's eating a strawberry coconut Paleo breakfast bar he got from the gym.

7:55 A.M.

Josh has an 8:30 A.M. meeting, so he grabs a Kind brand roasted jalapeño almond protein bar because it is non-GMO and gluten-free and has 10 grams of protein. He takes the keys with his other hand and heads out the door.

While driving to work—which he does because he can leave when he wants and listen to his favorite NFL podcast as loudly as he wants, because it takes five minutes longer by bus, and, well, because every minute counts these days—he remembers he's out of toilet paper, Sriracha, and plain, nonfat Greek yogurt. When he doesn't have an early meeting, he eats Greek yogurt at home before work because one time at the airport he read in *Men's Fitness* that Greek yogurt is one of those foods that "Fill You Up While You Trim Down."

Given his hectic schedule that day, he doesn't know when he'll have time to get groceries. So, at a stoplight, he takes out his phone (even though he promised his sister he'd stop doing that), opens his Instacart app, and quickly places an order. Before checkout, the page reminds him about grocery items he has purchased in the past, so he throws in some sour cream and onion Popchips, which he eats a few times a week because the label says "all the flavor. half the fat." Their absence of evil means it's totally fine to eat the whole bag after dinner.

8:20 A.M.

Josh arrives at his desk, puts his stuff down, and tosses the Kind bar wrapper in the garbage. He quickly walks to the micro-kitchen to grab a bottle of kombucha, a fermented tea, on his way to his meeting. He drinks one each morning because his uncle died of pancreatic cancer, and he'd like to live a long and healthy life. He's convinced himself that what the marketing gurus say about the beverage is true, that it's the "elixir of life" and that it boosts energy and immunity and helps digestion. *Everyone* seems to be talking about gut health these days.

9:36 A.M.

Is that his stomach growling? Just in case, he tears open a 100-calorie bag of Trader Joe's oatmeal chocolate chip cookies from his desk drawer. They contain oatmeal, which means you're obviously supposed to eat them for breakfast. It's like grapefruit: If you don't eat oats in the morning, let's face it, you're having an oats-free day. The portion control will keep his sweet tooth in check, and since it says 0 grams trans fat on the box, he can eat them guilt-free.

Josh is watching his calories because after his thirtieth birthday, he noticed that all the Mellow Mushroom pizza started going straight to his abs—fine, *stomach*—more than it used to. (He eats pizza on a regular basis because he is a human, and all humans like pizza.) In the spring, he managed to lose five pounds, but with all the Halloween candy floating around the office lately, he's gained it all back.

11:03 A.M.

In the conference room for yet another meeting, someone has put out bowls of almonds, dried mangos, and banana chips. He's not *hungry*, per se, but he has back-to-back meetings until at least early afternoon, and he's already forgotten the three slivers of homemade snickerdoodle scone he carved out from the tray on his colleague's desk an hour earlier. So . . . why not? He takes a few scoops from each bowl.

1:25 P.M.

Josh sees that he has thirty-five minutes until a conference call. Although he could eat any number of lunch options for free from Google's top-notch cafés, it's faster to order a Chipotle burrito that Postmates will deliver straight to his office. Plus, he's free to tailor his order exactly how he likes it. He'll eat the burrito over his keyboard as he evaluates product designs. Some might call this Sad Desk Lunch, but Josh calls it efficiency.

His team is responsible for the reliability of Google's data centers, and I mean, honestly, what single invention better captures the very meaning of progress in the world than the *Google search function*!? You don't prove you understand that responsibility by taking an effing siesta. Dine? Ha! He hardly has time to chew.

1:35 P.M.

As Josh types away while waiting for his lunch, he thinks about dinner that night. He's meeting friends at Marlow's Tavern at 7:15 P.M. They've made it a weekly Hump Day tradition. Normally he wouldn't decide his dinner plans until he gets off work, since typically he eats by himself. For tonight, Marlow's is just two blocks from his office, which is good because he could never leave before 7:00 P.M.

Last week at Marlow's, he ordered the Crispy Snapper with udon noodles, shiitake mushroom, Thai basil leaf, and miso soy broth. But he remembers eyeing his friend's Grilled Chicken Panini, which comes with fried green tomato and basil aioli on crisp Cuban bread (a fusion dish if there ever was one, and never mind that "panini" actually means "sandwiches" *plural* in Italian).

His panini thoughts are interrupted by a text message: "Your burrito has landed." He notices that the Postmates delivery woman is wearing a Pebbles Flintstone T-shirt, which reminds him of those Flintstones Push-Ups he loved to get from the ice cream truck as a kid. *Whoa, fifth-grade flashback! Hey, whatever happened to WarHeads?* His mom always had those on hand at his birthday parties so he could beat his friends at the game of who-can-handle-the-sour-candy-the-longest. *Aw, what a nice mom I have. I wonder how she's doing . . . I should probably call her some time. Anyway, enough day-dreaming. Back to work.*

3:48 P.M.
He'd never admit it, but by this time in the afternoon, Josh is dragging. Sure, he hasn't had a break all day and he only got six hours of sleep last night, but there's no time to recharge. Caffeine is the answer! He makes a quick run to the Starbucks around the corner, where he orders a Pumpkin Spice Latte, because, hello, it's only October once a year—carpe diem!

6:30 P.M.
Ugh, what an afternoon. No chance of making it to the restaurant in time. Too many fires to put out, and he's not even through the worst of it. He texts his friends that he's running late, suggesting they order an appetizer and start without him. (They decide on the Hot & Sweet Wings, classic buffalo style, because they're good for sharing, and because, what kind of person *doesn't* like chicken wings?)

7:43 P.M.
Josh finally arrives at Marlow's and orders a local craft beer, Terrapin Hi-5 IPA. He looks around the table. These people are the first friends he made when he moved to Atlanta. Two live in his apartment building, and soon after they met, they had taken Josh to Sunday brunch in the neighborhood, where they all bonded over cornmeal pancakes and eggs Benedict with

fried chicken. Of course, waiting forty-five minutes on the sidewalk for a table helped kickstart all the bonding.

Three of the four female friends have ordered wine—one Argentinian Malbec, one Merlot from Washington State, and one German Riesling (but only because Marlow's doesn't have Moscato, a shock they're still getting over). The fourth woman picked a cocktail with wildflower honey and Belle Meade craft bourbon because, well, men aren't the only ones keeping the coopers of Kentucky working overtime. The one male friend in the group went with a dry Manhattan.

Marlow's serves "the 'Best of the Best' in American tavern fare," which means no fewer than a dozen different cultural influences from around the country and around the globe: Asian ahi tuna salad, hummus and pita, nachos, shrimp and grits, Hawaiian-style poke, and chicken queso soup. The tavern's offerings are rounded out by some American standbys like burgers and Caesar salad, except the latter is made with kale, because at least for now, kale is still enjoying its trendy-veggie status on menus nationwide.

9:07 P.M.

One of the two Jennys in the group pulls up an Instagram photo from Sonic Drive-In. The photo is announcing their new Oreo & Cake Shake: pieces of Oreo cookie and vanilla cake swirled together with cake batter frosting and vanilla ice cream, available for a limited time only! If they don't act now, they risk missing out on this experience for*ever*. So they quickly decide they just have to go try it.

10:22 P.M.

Josh is now full of cookie-cake ice cream and beer, as well as a much-needed night of fun with some friends. But he still has a few dozen e-mails to take care of before bed. So he calls it a night and heads home.

There is no real Josh, but this sketch of his day shows how our lives drive how we eat, and how the ways we eat fit with the ways we think about our days and our lives. I wanted to write a book that looks at what and how we eat because I had a hunch it would say a lot about who we are.

This fascination with food as a mirror for our mind-sets began at an early age for me.

I was in fourth grade, and my family was living above two tenant farmers in a tiny village in Italy. One morning I woke to a whacking sound and Sergio's rapid-fire Italian coming from the apartment below.

Sun streamed in my second-floor window, and I hopped out of bed to peer down at the courtyard. Streaks of blood stained the pavement, and there, on a clothesline, was a dripping, filleted rabbit. It was Easter Sunday 1997, and I would never think of the Easter bunny in the same way again.

This image stayed with me throughout the morning until Rina and Sergio knocked on our door around noon and presented my younger brother and me with the traditional Easter gift: a foot-tall chocolate egg with a small toy inside.

I suppose I forgave Sergio after that.

In all seriousness, it was the moment I was made to realize that killing the rabbit did not make Sergio a ruthless murderer. Rather, it was a consecrated act. More likely than not, his rabbit was organic and cage-free, and for all I know had had a blissful life. (It was definitely locally sourced.) Butchering his own bunny probably made Sergio a more ethical eater, not less.

When it comes to food today, we've got *a lot* on our minds. We've always been concerned about the price of food, but today we're concerned about the price to the planet, too. Eating "ethically" in America can mean caring about everything from whether your waitress gets paid sick leave to the square footage of a chicken coop, from the carbon footprint of a sandwich to what type of fishing gear was used to catch your tuna.

In the daily game of food decisions, convenience and health are veterans on our mental rosters, though now they're getting more play time than ever before. Ditto for novelty and personalization, while rookies like water footprint and antibiotic use have gained attention.

For me, it's never been enough to ask, What do we think about when we think about food? The bigger question is: *Why* do we think about what we think about when we think about food?

How do our shared values as Americans shape our eating habits, for better and for worse? In short: *Why do we eat what we eat?*

I don't study consumer behavior for a living, but I know some people who do.

Meet Hank Cardello, author of *Stuffed*, senior fellow and director of the Obesity Solutions Initiative at the Hudson Institute, former president of Sunkist Soft Drinks, former director of marketing for Coca-Cola USA, and former brand manager for Anheuser-Busch and General Mills. He breaks American consumers into five buckets with respect to how they view food and health. Based on research he's involved with at the Natural Marketing Institute, each category of consumers makes up roughly 20 percent of the U.S. population, plus or minus a few percentage points. Here are his buckets:

"Well Beings" are the most proactive group regarding healthy eating, seeking complete purity and transparency to nourish their bodies as optimally as possible. "Food Actives" see through BS health claims and generally don't trust food companies, yet they're a bit more mainstream about their approach to healthy eating, not quite as hard-core as the Well Beings.

On the far opposite end of the spectrum are the people Cardello calls the "Eat, Drink & Be Merrys," the consumers he says simply don't care about health. "What they care about is taste taste taste—squared," Cardello says. This is the group where, he adds, "If you tell me it's healthy, I'll order a second monster cheeseburger just to spite you." Maybe they've never cared, and never will, or maybe they just don't care at this point in their lives. (Read: teenagers.)

The second-least health-conscious group is the largest of his groups, called "Magic Bullets." Give them the easy way or they're not interested. They want to take vitamins instead of eating fruits and vegetables. "This is the group that's allergic to exercise," Cardello says. "They break out in hives just at the *discussion* of exercise."

That leaves everybody else. The rest of the population in the middle. Called "Fence Sitters," they may want to be healthy but don't have, or feel they have, the time to figure out *how*. Fence Sitters are the most diverse with regard to income and race and ethnicity, and many are young families juggling jobs and parenting. If a food or food product tastes great, is prepackaged and convenient, they're all over it.

So essentially what Cardello is telling us is that there are really *three* buckets: For some people, healthy eating is a constant on their radar screens, for others it's nowhere to be seen, and for the vast majority of us it comes and goes amid a flurry of twenty-seven other things we have to worry about on a given day.

————

Clearly we're hardwired in some different ways. At the same time, depending on various personal goals or life events that crop up, we might fall on different spots on the healthy eating spectrum one month or one year or even one-half of our lives. And you could present an infinite number of spectrums to represent other consumer preferences and behaviors, like spice tolerance, willingness to spend money on food, likelihood to take pictures of one's food, likelihood to eat insects, and so on.

Without question, our diversity as Americans is cause for celebration. But I can't kick the idea that, collectively, we share a certain psyche about food. It's hard to pin down because it's constantly changing and evolving. For another, every person has a different take. I don't have all the answers. This is not the final word, and it's not an encyclopedia. It's an invitation to a conversation about what our eating habits reveal about who we are.

I'm here to take on the idea that we don't even *have* a national food culture, and find out what connects us.

Our industrial food system is responsible for one level of unity— the baked goods at my Starbucks in Seattle are the same as at yours in Memphis, and the products lining the shelves in my Safeway are the same as those in yours. But a food culture is about much more than identical processed foods. I'm interested in our common habits and tendencies. The things we do because . . . we just do. From DC to Missoula, Americans wait in long lines for brunch on weekends. Why do we do that?

In March 2015, for the first time ever, we spent more money at restaurants and bars than at grocery stores. The Commerce Department has been tracking American spending habits on food since 1992, and the trend lines have been gradually converging. But this milestone is a huge deal. It means that, more and more, we aren't a nation that cooks. What's behind this?

And we're united by food events. One Sunday a year, from Indianapolis to Oakland, we gather with friends and sit down to our second-biggest meal of the year. Why did we pick the Super Bowl for this honor? Why not, say, the World Series? Or the Fourth of July? Or were we the ones who picked it at all?

I'm also fascinated by our contradictions. If we're all eating healthier than ever, and we've turned into such a nation of foodies—with artisan this and small-batch that—why do we eat about as much fast food as we did a decade ago, and why have products like Taco Bell's Doritos Locos Tacos sold in record-breaking numbers? After years of buying large quantities of nonfat, gluten-free, low-carb, and air-based products, why have we been eating *more* calories over time? Our definition of a "meal" is something plated that we enjoy at a table with family or friends, but increasingly we're consuming snack bars in the car and lunch at our desks. What does that say about who we have become?

During my research, I learned about a guy named Harry Balzer, the former chief industry analyst at the NPD Group, who is now a semi-retired consumer researcher. He's had his ear to the ground for thirty-seven years and can explain every peculiar nuance of your habits in the ice cream aisle and why you love Five Guys burgers. He arguably understands American eaters better than anyone. Each year, he has authored the NPD Group's *Annual Report on Eating Patterns in America,* which is the food industry equivalent to the Dead Man's Chest in *Pirates of the Caribbean.* Total jackpot.

NPD Group charges thousands of dollars for access to the report. So I gave Balzer a call and asked what he could offer from his padlocked 750-pager. He asked me to pick a random number. I went with 176. He purported, on the other end of the phone, to open the report (which he keeps on his desk) to page 176 and read me the graph from it. It revealed four of the twenty foods that have grown the fastest in the American diet over the last thirty years, and four that have decreased the most. Four that have increased were bottled water, snack bars, frozen sandwiches, and frozen entrées; four that have decreased were carbonated soft drinks, beef, salads, and bread. I was enthralled. I wanted to know the stories behind the stats. These stats and so many others that shed light on what unites us.

But before we get to all that—and it's juicy, I promise—let's pull over for a pit stop at Merriam-Webster.

What is a "food culture" anyway?

The dictionary defines culture as "a way of thinking, behaving, or working that exists in a place or organization." Our culture is made up of specific modes of thinking and acting. These are called mores—that's *MOH-rays*—"the customs, values, and behaviors that are accepted by a particular group, culture, etc." Often mores are so automatic, so embedded in the fabric of daily life, that we mistake them for human nature.

Now, if you're like me, abstract concepts like these feel a little fuzzy until you put some examples in front of me. Here are a few.

► Women wear bikinis all over the world. In France, they wear only the bottom. In Brazil, the bottom covers only the front.

► In India, some women use creams to lighten their skin color. In America, some women use creams to darken theirs. Maybe we should just swap countries.

► In certain parts of the American South, people have a special term used to convey that they haven't quite gotten around to a task, but they're in the process of thinking about getting around to it. That term is "fixin' to." For instance, "I'm fixin' to make us some breakfast." You can insert it into a sentence when describing just about any activity. The rest of us just have to own up to whether or not we've actually produced breakfast yet.

► Let's say you're in Seattle or Portland, dining at a fancy restaurant. Gentle mood music plays in the background.

Then: flash flood! Mixed with . . . a cougar on the loose! But wait: You're wearing your trusty moisture-wicking Capilene synthetic base layer from Patagonia. Ready to spring into action for a quick paddle or a trail run at a moment's notice. If you showed up looking like that in, perhaps, Washington, DC, or Charleston, South Carolina, you would be kindly barred from entering the restaurant.

So culture is made up of a bunch of mores—customs, values, and behaviors.

American *food culture* is the set of customs, values, and behaviors related to eating and drinking. These form the scaffolding of daily life.

Here are some examples of American food culture:

▶ Fast food. This is arguably the best-known feature of our food culture, and the one we've exported most widely around the globe. Not just the food but the way it's consumed, at drive-thrus or taking it to go.

▶ When we watch movies, we eat popcorn.

▶ At state fairs, food is fried. Foods you didn't even know could be fried are fried.

▶ In the summer, we invite friends over for barbecues.

▶ Unlike in Britain, Canada, or Ireland, in the United States, bacon is supposed to be crispy.

▶ Don't eat anything when riding the subway.

▶ Eat pizza. All kinds. Any time.

   ▶ When eating pizza, adhere to some very important rules regarding the delivery of the slice into your mouth: New York style=fold it. Chicago deep dish=fork and knife. Otherwise, no utensils involved. Unless, of course, you want to look like an Italian, in which case: Pinkies up.

Traveling to a foreign country, just like traveling to different parts of the United States, holds up a mirror to our ways. Whenever I visit a new city, the first thing I do is head to the nearest grocery store. Granted, I'm the type of person who views grocery shopping as a form of recreation. But still, you can learn a lot about a place. What it grows, what it subsidizes, what it does or doesn't value.

And much of this perspective can be gained without traveling far at all; your own nearest grocery store will do the trick if you give it time. Typically, you're trying to get in and out as quickly as possible. You're dodging promos and seasonal items, bright signs and hungry people. But slow down next time. You may notice things that make you see yourself and your culture differently. You may find yourself thinking, *Waiiit a minute— Weight Watchers has its own line of ice cream novelties!?* Or *If there are whole-wheat Fig Newtons in the cookie aisle, and chocolate "breakfast biscuits" in the cereal aisle, then what, exactly, is the difference between dessert and breakfast?* These are some of the conversations I've been having with myself lately. Because, along with the countless fast-food and restaurant dishes populating our modern eating landscape, there are 42,214 items in the average American supermarket. Every one of them has its own story—and the story is usually about us.

Michael Pollan, author of *The Omnivore's Dilemma: A Natural History of Four Meals* and many other books about food, has said that, given Americans' multiethnic makeup and our relatively new status as a nation, we have never had a stable food culture—as in passing on customs of eating from one generation to the next. This leaves us vulnerable to marketing and the latest nutrition study, "willing to throw it all out every few years," as he once said in an interview.

In other words, without an enduring set of social norms around eating, we are constantly reinventing them. The support for this idea is in strong supply, but there is an untapped layer that deserves inspecting: how this unstable food culture is shaped by our core values as a country. As we know from Merriam-Webster, these are one of the three key types of mores. They help explain why we eat the things we eat and the ways we eat them—and they equip us to understand how we might eat in the future.

At every step of my research, this is what I have found: We don't put food first. We put three main values above all: *work, freedom,* and *progress.* They drive what we strive for and cringe at, what we do without even realizing. Through all the churn, these three values thread across our history as a people.

These are also the very values that are (sorry, folks!) hurting us. They're taking years off our lives and depriving us of some of life's simple moments of happiness. The kicker? We didn't do this on purpose. We never set out to have the craziest food system on the planet, or crushing rates of obesity and type 2 diabetes. We never intended to be so guilt ridden and confused about food.

As a way of understanding the American Way of Eating, I have zeroed in on ten phenomena that illustrate what our food shows about who we are. Some food trends come and go, but the cultural patterns I focus on speak to these three abiding values of the American character. To help us along the way, you'll meet culinary historians, consumer behavior experts, food psychologists, even a woman who identifies as a "cultural scientist."

We're going to start by exposing the "Muddle of the Modern Meal." We will see how blurred the lines are between snacks and meals. And why, in prioritizing convenience and efficiency, we're missing out on some pretty nice things in life. Things like how satisfying it feels to cook a meal from scratch.

About 700 years ago, the first mechanical clocks were installed in public squares in Germany. They signaled the start and end of the workday, and when to break for lunch. Today, for salaried employees and those holding down multiple jobs, the American work clock is all out of whack—the starting and stopping of work is far less clear than it used to be. Partly because of greater flexibility, but mostly because technology tethers us to work like never before. Long known for our work ethic, today we are out-working even ourselves: Americans now work 200 more hours per year than they did in 1970. From the realization that "sitting is the new smoking" to the chronic stress and the brunt we bear with our food, our workaholic culture is killing us.

As a result of longer hours, we've had to bring food into the workplace. Forty percent of us dine at our desks, partic-ipating in the national pastime known as multitasking. We make a point of minimizing the time spent obtaining, prepar-ing, and consuming food—to maximize the time spent, yes, taking BuzzFeed personality tests and binge-watching *Game of Thrones*, but mostly working. Ironically, though, many of us will gladly spend half our Sunday in pursuit of brunch. That may involve waiting in line at a brunch spot or actually cook-ing, as pancakes and French toast are among the most-searched of all recipes online. Making a day of the weekend meal sug-gests a silent protest against our workaholic society. It also sug-gests a rejection of all the solo dining and of the idea that food is fuel. That's the notion promoted by some nutrition and fit-ness pros that our bodies are machines and food the gas in our tanks. It reduces food to a balance of energy in and energy out.

In the United States everyone is free to make their own choices, from carrying a weapon to eating a Doritos Locos Taco for breakfast. Individualism is at the heart of how we think about everything from health and disease to the economy and free enterprise.

As a result, we customize our eating experiences. I'm looking at you, Starbucks, Chipotle, and Cold Stone Creamery, to name a few. These popular eateries cater to our birthright as Americans.

Individual rights also make it socially acceptable to dine alone. Even families who sit down together are increasingly eating different meals, tailored to different preferences and sensitivities. But most of the time, we eat exactly what we want, where we want, when we want, as fast as we want. And again, it's our loss. But it's so second nature not to share tastes or conversation anymore that we may not even fully understand what a loss they are. We'll look at why and how we insist on having it our way.

In America, we also share a fundamental belief in the idea that we can always find a better way to do something. The idea that today is better than yesterday, and tomorrow will be better than today. Progress, ladies and gentlemen.

Pew polls consistently reflect Americans' confidence that science and technology can solve just about everything. We've put men on the moon, vaccines in clinics, and personalized computing in the pocket of every tween from Cupertino to Cairo. We've had good reason to pride ourselves on progress, and I can't imagine my life without traffic lights, Tupperware, or texting. And thank God for lint rollers. But we don't often stop and think about whether it's such a good idea to apply that same faith in innovation to our food.

Rather than trust our intuition or common sense, we look to scientific solutions or sexy new strategies. We put *nutrients* first. Tallies of grams and percentages.

Our nutrient-centric environment often makes us buy foods not because they contain worthwhile ingredients, but for the crazy reason that they omit something (fat, calories, etc.). And it's not only that our lack of a stable food culture leaves us jumping from one fad diet to the next. Our faith in progress gives us the unshakable assurance that the holy grail of healthy eating is just around the corner—or rather, awaiting us in a lab somewhere. I'm talking about the antioxidant pills, the dietary supplements, the meal-replacement bars, the juice cleanses.

Consider one extreme, Soylent, a meal-replacement drink whose producers argue that food is inefficient, and Soylent makes you feel *amaaaazing.* Promising whiter teeth and a stronger physique, Soylent will—wait for it—completely change your life! Just a few daily doses of the beige, gooey cocktail (which claims to contain all the key nutrients), and you can forgo food altogether. We'll see that converts to each new fad share a common habit: proselytizing about having found that holy grail, once and for all.

More and more, we look to food *products* to provide nutrients in inventive ways. From fortified cereals to air-popped snacks, the number of new food products introduced each year has been increasing over the last decade. Each year we are hit with over 20,000 new items. When I get to "stunt foods," you'll be dazzled by novelty.

By extension, our deference to science and new food products means deference to food scien*tists,* which means—whether we intend it or not—deference to food companies. We take cues on what to eat not from, say, our parents, but from the marketing magicians of the food industry. They are behind the fabricated food shortages on Super Bowl Sunday, which are just one example of how food companies create both the chaos and the supposed solutions.

A melting pot is defined as "a place where a variety of races, cultures, or individuals assimilate into a cohesive whole." Americans take immense pride in this notion. How this concept influences our eating relates to the term's second definition: "a process of blending that often results in invigoration or novelty." This means that the hope for the future of food in America sits on the positive side of the coin of reinvention. It's why we are willing to embrace new norms around dining, like wine for the masses, food trucks, Tex-Mex, and Italian food that is really a distinct Italian *American* genre, without which there would be no "American" food to speak of.

Harried Americans want to know why our lifestyles are making us sick. Why, along the path to chronic illness, we often sap the small pleasures out of life. We'll see how our values shape our eating habits, who and what we allow to influence us, and the upside of that very instability.

If we can laugh at ourselves, it might be the first step to saving ourselves. We might add years to our lives—or at least joy to our years.

CHAPTER 1

The Muddle of the Modern Meal

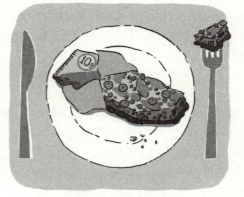

We have always had a tendency to eat and run. Even as early as the 1800s, a European traveler remarked that the U.S. national motto might as well have been "Gobble, gulp, and go." Convenience is part of our national heritage. Yet today we have taken that value to new extremes—snacking more than ever, and overhauling the very definition of the American meal.

The latest market research shows that ease of preparation and consumption are the driving forces of twenty-first-century food product development. Sales of Keurig machines—the speedy, single-serving coffee maker even a five-year-old can operate—have soared. We now have individual-size Keurig K-Cup pods of Campbell's soup. Surely *phở* is next.

Prepared-foods sections at grocery stores are going gang-busters, and we're dining out more than any time in our history. Not coincidentally, the percentage of single-person households ·is at an all-time high. (Who likes cooking for one?) We'll do whatever it takes to finish the eating to move on to just about any other activity.

What is it about Americans that makes us view food consumption this way? Why have we always been like this? Why have we really *never* put food first?

Harry Balzer, the expert on eating and drinking patterns from the market research firm NPD Group, argues that "one of the core tenets of human evolution is: Find someone else to do the cooking."

To survive, we need food. Yet we also need things like shelter, clothes, and high-speed Internet. In order to pay for things like shelter, clothes, and high-speed Internet, one must have money. To make money, one must (at least theoretically) work. Therefore, evolutionarily speaking, time working cannot be threatened by time feeding ourselves. So what to do?

"You'd have to hire someone," Balzer says. Or better yet, "You'd have to get married." But today, with most women also working, they are no longer the "someone else to do the cooking," and both men and women are looking for someone, or some*thing,* to prepare food for us.

Enter the food industry.

This means a greater reliance on food in restaurants (sit-down or take-out) and on processed foods (high and low quality and everything in between).

Our American work ethic undermines our eating. And being this busy has brought two major changes to our food culture: how we define *what* is a meal and *when* is a meal.

Today, a mere 20 percent of snacking happens outside the home. When we think snacks, we think dashboard dining or keyboard munching. But that's not how we mostly snack. When we think snacks, we also think cuddling a bowl of chips while watching TV. This kind of snacking and the term "couch potato" are still apt. But there is a stunning new development: "The snack food is becoming the meal," Balzer says.

Food and Work

Among the thirty-four developed countries in the Organisation for Economic Co-operation and Development (OECD), the United States ranks around twelfth each year for annual hours worked per person, and we always beat the average across the countries. We work more than Japan and pretty much all the European countries but less than some, including Russia and Mexico.

In Danish, there is a word that I can't begin to pronounce: *arbejdsglæde*. It means "happiness at work." Swedish, Norwegian, Finnish, and Icelandic also have words for this. There is no English word for it.

On the flipside, Japanese has a special word of its own: *karoshi*. It means "death from overwork." *Washington Post* reporter Blaine Harden reported in 2008: "For decades, the Japanese government has been trying, and largely failing, to set limits on work and overtime. The problem of *karoshi* became prevalent enough to warrant its own word in the boom years of the late 1970s, as the number of Japanese men working more than 60 hours a week soared." In 2007, the single-greatest cause of suicides there related to work? Too much of it.

So it could be worse, but the United States still has it pretty bad.

Work and time constraints affect both how we eat at the workplace and how we eat in the hours outside of work. We can't understand American food culture without understanding American work culture. It's all interconnected.

When asked how important working hard is to getting ahead in life, 73 percent of Americans rate it a ten or "very important," compared to the median of just 50 percent among forty-four countries worldwide.

When you're a salaried employee, does time belong to you or to your employer? The latter is true for the vast majority of workers—because their natural eagerness to work hard runs smack into their employers not being required to pay them overtime. The thinking by both parties is that if you're earning a salary over a certain threshold, working beyond forty hours a week is merely a trade-off you accept.

"As a nation, we work harder and longer than almost all of our competitors, and much of that work is uncompensated," writes Fran Sussner Rodgers, a work and family consultant, in a *New York Times* op-ed. "We accept that that is the way it has to be, without much questioning."

But there is something of a rejectionist group brewing, and they're challenging the going norm that time is not your own but your employer's, that the best you can do is eke out the occasional happy hour or be among the 59 percent of Americans who actually take all their paid vacation time.

They're asking us to ask ourselves: Are we really okay signing up for a lifetime of blurred lines between work and home?

Many outside the United States have heeded similar calls. For example, at Volkswagen, e-mail for some employees is shut down from thirty minutes after the end of their shift until thirty minutes before the next day's shift starts. If you work at Daimler, you can opt to have all the e-mails you receive while you're on vacation automatically deleted. The program resulted from work done by psychologists at the University of Heidelberg, and nearly every worker at Daimler has enthusiastically embraced it. (The sender is kindly notified their e-mail has been deleted and provided with a colleague to contact in the meantime.) That leaves the vacationer no reason—other than e-mail junkie disorder—to check work e-mail from the beach.

So why the desperate measures? The desperate times, of course!

Workers are burned out, and mental health is suffering. If you work at our country's most valuable retailer, Amazon, you can expect to receive e-mails past midnight followed by text messages asking why you haven't responded quickly enough. Americans today are taking less vacation time than at any point in nearly forty years, according to a recent analysis conducted by Oxford Economics for the U.S. Travel Association. The top reasons for not taking vacation are fear of losing one's job (being replaced) and fear of returning to a mountain of backlogged work. *The New York Times* editorial board endorsed programs like those at Volkswagen and Daimler, lamenting the "babbling brook of email" and our "relentless digital age."

As clichéd as it is to wax lyrical about the sultry Spanish siesta, or the ambrosial French bistro lunch, we can learn a thing or two from the Europeans. Even countries like Bulgaria, South Korea, and Mexico are ahead of us in some respects: Of all thirty-four OECD nations, the United States ranks last for time off provided to new parents. Employers vary widely in their beneficence regarding paid parental leave, but any stabs at how many weeks are federally mandated? A quick calculation, carry the two, ah yes . . . none.

We can't fathom that there is anything but a direct correlation between productivity and number of hours worked. In fact, workers who are simply seen in the office—called "passive" face time—are viewed as dependable and reliable, even more favorably if they are seen before or after regular work hours. So you could be cranking out reports left and right from your home office, or raking in clients while walking your dog in your PJs, but it won't do squat for your image compared to parking your butt in that office chair.

On the flip side, workers who take all their vacation time are viewed as less dedicated by at least 15 percent of senior managers (the portion honest enough to admit it in a recent survey).

The American work ethic is second to none. But we're in a quantity-versus-quality pickle. Because there's just one hitch: We have a limit. We aren't infinity pools. Like the bottomless chips and salsa at Chili's, there does exist a point at which more is actually *not* better.

For those of you who like your sweeping generalizations served with a side of data: A study by *Business Roundtable* found that, for the average team, there is such a sharp drop in productivity after working sixty-hour weeks for eight weeks that they would have gotten the *same* amount of work done had they just worked forty-hour weeks that whole time. At higher levels, the outputs equate much faster: When you get up to eighty-hour weeks, it takes just three weeks to match the output you would have produced averaging forty hours a week.

Although there is an amount of work that has a negative impact on output (errors, duplication, and the like), we refuse to accept it. Doing so goes against our national credo.

Everyone loves to talk about how people in the Nordic countries seem so darn happy all the time. They wear flowers in their hair and dance around maypoles and forage for weeds that they eat with lots of fish that make them live forever, etcetera, etcetera. They take like half a year's worth of vacation, get paid to spend some twenty months cuddling their newborns (even dads!), and have universal health care, free college, all that good stuff. (If it makes you feel better, they also have to deal with the world's smelliest food: a rotting fish called *surströmming* that won the stink factor award in a study of global cuisines. So I'll take my apple pie any day.)

Then everyone else likes to retort that we Americans shouldn't be so envious or unrealistic about trying to become more like those countries because they are scarily homogeneous and have tiny populations. They don't have problems like the ones we have here in the United States.

I get it. I buy it all. And living there is probably not the fairy tale it seems like from across the Atlantic.

But to shed some perspective on ourselves and our penchant for working ourselves into a tizzy, it's worth lifting up the hood on a less-overwrought dinner party conversation, and that is the Nordic concept of work itself.

I was on a hike with a Swedish friend, and she was talking about how stunned she is by the amount of time people work in the United States. On the positive side, she has noticed that many people here seem more passionate, creative, and entrepreneurial in their jobs compared with workers back home. Now, take this with a grain of salt since she lives in San Francisco and is surrounded by filmmakers and artists.

But she asked me a simple question about the sheer number of hours we work: *Why?*

She was absolutely dumbfounded when I explained: Putting in the time proves your value. She laughed at the idea and said, "In Sweden, if you're working more than the hours absolutely mandatory and expected of you, people's reaction is, 'What's wrong with you that you couldn't get your work done in time?'" In other words, it's an efficiency question—"You're working late tonight? Oh, you must be slow."

I stopped in my tracks. Mind blown.

This Swede had just taken something so elemental, so deeply engrained in my psyche, and turned it completely on its head.

While this perspective is profound, it's actually not true that we're all terribly inefficient in America. In fact, I'd say we're efficient to a fault. We're so outcomes oriented—furiously multitasking and optimizing our routines and our tasks to have as much to show for our time as possible—that we often miss out on the experience itself. Rarely do we allow ourselves to take the scenic route. The real problem is that we've married that efficiency orientation with our natural bent toward excess. After all, we're the super-sized nation, with the biggest portions, the biggest cars, the biggest home theaters. Consensus is, more-is-better also applies to hours of work.

Our industriousness is arguably our economic edge around the globe. And it stems from the very core of our national identity: the American Dream. In school and in children's books, we're taught from a young age that there's nothing more heroic than the self-made man. You can do anything if you put your mind to it. So the long hours aren't just for show. In the United States, they're for self-worth.

Given this landscape, what is the future of food because of work, and food at work?

What Is a Meal?

Market researchers and their clients are often shocked when they hear what people consider a meal, compared with how they actually eat. Michael Barry, a professor at the Stanford University School of Mechanical Engineering, is also founder of Quotient Design Research, an innovation consulting firm that conducts ethnographic research to understand consumer behavior. When Barry has asked consumers how they define a "meal," they describe a combination of foods, home-cooked and plated. This sounds about right to me too. But when he asks them the last time they had a meal like that, responses vary from "a couple of weeks ago" to "maybe Thanksgiving." One of the fundamental themes of eating behavior is that there is a difference between what people say they want and what they actually eat. It's often the difference between intention and action, between goals and reality.

But increasingly, the difference is due to the fact that, like TV dinners and delivery pizza before them, snacks have overhauled the definition of a meal in America. A major change in how we eat is that snacks have begun to dominate our main meals. Today, we are more likely to cobble together several prepackaged foods than, say, buy the necessary ingredients and assemble a sandwich. A packet of almonds, a bag of chips, a bar, a yogurt, and there you have it: lunch. Again let's hear from Harry Balzer: "Are you too lazy to make a sandwich to put in your kid's lunch bag, for God's sake?" He answers his question with a yes.

We're not only assembling snack foods to collectively equal "a meal," we're eating more snack foods altogether. As "grazing" has been taken to a new level, snacks have assumed a greater role in our lives than ever before. The experts at the Hartman Group—a consumer research firm in Bellevue, Washington, that specializes in advising food and beverage companies—refer to this phenomenon in American culture as "the dissolution of meals." Their research has found that a whopping half of all eating occasions are now snacks.

You can consider a snack "anything small, increasingly nutritional and portable that complements or replaces a meal." This definition, offered in *The Wall Street Journal*, succinctly covers all the bases.

Some people forgo the traditional three squares in favor of

more frequent, smaller amounts throughout the day. (It's all a little murky whether to designate these as "large snacks" or "mini meals.") This style of eating is driven by some nutritionists and health professionals who endorse it for boosting metabolism, keeping blood sugar steady, and avoiding the overcompensation that can happen after feeling very hungry. But the jury is out on the best approach, in part because it's not so easy to be so disciplined: For plenty of people, snacks more likely fall in the "complement" than the "replace" part of the definition.

One big result is: We eat more total food than before. Between 1978 and 1996, calories consumed from dinner decreased 37 percent, and increased 16 percent from breakfast, 21 percent from lunch, and 101 percent from snacks. You can do the math to see that this nets out in the positive. Between 1970 and 2010, the average daily calorie intake in the United States increased by 505 calories total, up to 2,544, according to the Department of Agriculture. That's a 25 percent increase. (To be fair, average daily calorie intake has decreased somewhat since 2003, but we've still got a long way to go.)

Part of the issue is that the grazing throughout the day idea hinges on these more frequent amounts actually being smaller than traditional meals.

For an example, let's turn to the burrito. Many Americans consider a burrito a "snack." When probed, the explanation might go something like this: Say you skipped breakfast, grabbing a Red Bull on your way out the door. Somewhere around 11:00 A.M. your stomach starts rumbling. But it's not quite lunchtime, so you buy a burrito. It seems relatively healthy, and it doesn't come with a salad or dessert.

The Hartman Group has a team of anthropologists and social scientists who have been conducting a quarter-century-long study of American food culture. Along with administering surveys, they actually go into people's homes and watch them eat. The results are fascinating and bizarre, full of quirks and contradictions. Their vice president of consumer insights, Melissa Abbott, told me that people explain to her that because the burrito was eaten on its own, it doesn't constitute a meal. Instead, it gets logged in their minds as a mere snack. It's pretty standard protocol to eat dessert after eating a meal, not before. So for many people, dessert's job is to mark the end of a meal. It turns out, though, that dessert may also be crucial for signaling a meal was had in the first place.

Because the definition of a meal has changed, so has the definition of a snack.

As discussed, a snack used to be infrequent, a special occasion. Now it happens throughout the day, every day.

A snack also used to be for kids, mostly. They've got a lot on their plates—what with all the growing and the freeze tag. Who can blame them for being hungry 24/7? So they've mostly been excused from having to wait until mealtime to eat with others around a table. But snacks are no longer just for kids. They're for adults of all ages. Unlike in the 1980s, the majority of Americans no longer feel the need to avoid snacking. The reason is that snacking is now a social norm. And that's because we can all relate to the underlying force: We're nearly all starved for time. As anyone who has recently tried to coordinate a group of people knows, we're an overscheduled bunch. So we empathize when you're running from one meeting to the next, from a teacher-parent conference to pick up the dry cleaning and go to spin class, and all you have time for is a bag of peanut butter pretzels and a string cheese.

Another reason, though, is that marketers have tapped into this desire and made an ever larger array of snacks and portable foods available to us. The flood of bars and nut packs and fruit leathers filling our food environment also shapes our sense that snacking all the time is normal.

We've been heeding shortcuts and taking it to go for a good long while now. Just think of the drive-thru or instant oatmeal, canned goods or automatic pot stirrers. No one *needed* cake mix. But when it came on the market, people thought, *Why not*?

We want everything to be more convenient this week than it was last week. And next week we want it more convenient than this week. Consider the banana slicer. That's what knives are for. Or the egg separator. That's what fingers are for. Some of this isn't driven by the collective "us" but by product engineers. Did we demand an apple corer, or did they invent an apple corer and so we started using it? You could ask the same of just about every gadget in your kitchen.

There is a tendency in the marketplace to create a new product or a new food and then convince consumers we need or want it. Case in point? The iPad.

Finally, a snack used to be a treat, an indulgence. A few cookies or a handful of chips. Snacks were higher in sugar and less "nutrient dense" than most of the snacks we're looking for now. Today, consumers want low sugar, they want less processed, and they want healthy. Plain old fruit has become a more common snack, for one, but that's just the start. Walk into any grocery store and the outpouring of new kinds of snacks is astounding. Many are marketed as superior in nutritional value, and some actually are: from chips, crisps, and crackers made with oats and black beans and flax seeds and seaweed, to an astounding number of ways that fruits and vegetables have been freeze-dried and dehydrated and pureed and molded into portable forms. No washing, peeling, or slicing required.

So did the idea that eating throughout the day create more healthy snack options, or did more people start eating throughout the day because more healthy snack options became available? One thing is for sure: Inextricably tied to snacking in

America is a national obsession with protein. It's the thing we look for most in a snack.

To see this trio of factors—snacks as daily habits, consumption across all ages, and the protein craze—in action, take Oscar Meyer's Lunchables, the ready-to-eat meal kits for kids. They've been rebranded for adults. The core contents are the same, plus some nuts and minus the Capri Sun, except now the Lunchable is called P3, which stands for Portable Protein Pack. You can read all about it on the official website, ProteinProteinProtein.com. And no, I'm not making this stuff up. The best part of writing about the food industry is that you don't have to.

Protein Can Do No Wrong

As a country, we bought $16 billion worth of food containing protein claims in 2014. That represents a bump of over 5 percent compared with the previous year.

Nearly 60 percent of Americans are actively trying to increase their protein intake. That's according to the Hartman Group, who call protein "the new low-fat" or "the new low-carb," even "the new everything when it comes to diet and energy."

"Soccer moms feel they can't be anywhere without protein," says Abbott. It's like a crutch. In her research, she always seems to be finding beef jerky in gym bags and purses, protein bars in laptop bags and consoles.

Snacks now account for 14 percent of all restaurant traffic. Keep in mind that "restaurant" in this context means foodservice outlets, not necessarily places where you *dine* per se. Brands like Starbucks and Dunkin' Donuts that have been traditionally breakfast oriented have added afternoon snacks like high-protein sandwiches.

The power of portable protein means yogurt and nuts are also stars in the snack show. Andrew Cuomo, the governor of New York, signed legislation crowning yogurt as that state's official snack. Yes, yogurt is a fan favorite, but this might also have something to do with the fact that Chobani and Fage have major production facilities upstate. Both of these brands are Greek yogurts, which has, of course, especially taken off, probably because, for about the same number of calories as regular yogurt, you get about half the sugar, assuming you pick plain, and about twice the protein (roughly equivalent to eating a few ounces of lean meat). When considering Greek yogurt versus other high-protein snacks, customers also go for Greek yogurt's probiotics, which are said to promote digestive health. Until cottage cheese makes its resurgence, it's hard to find a more dietitian-approved dairy item than Greek yogurt.

Americans like nuts of all kinds, but almonds especially. Almonds alone are packaged and sold in a stunning *forty* different forms, everything from trail mix and portion-controlled packs to clusters and chips.

But far and away, bars are the game changer in the snacks-as-meals phenomenon—you've got nut bars, granola bars, dried fruit bars, and countless bars made with patented protein blends of ingredients like soy protein isolate and pea and whey protein. You've got savory bars that are marketed to men, bars that are good for the heart, good for pregnant women, good for kids, good for Grandma. And so on. Cheap, individual-size instant hits of calories, and in many cases, protein.

Over the last thirty years, snack bars have been among the twenty fastest-growing food items in the American diet. Whenever we think we can't possibly imagine yet another kind of bar, out come new product lines with new niches. There are now 2,000 different bars on the market. Two *thousand* different combinations of fruit, nuts, grains, protein powders, and whatever else they put in there (glue?).

And get this: Six of the top ten fastest sellers are from the Kind brand. Put another way, of the ten bars we're most likely to buy on a given grocery run, only four would *not* be Kind bars. Kind emphasizes what have become known as "clean labels," a short list of recognizable ingredients. And you see them everywhere—the Starbucks counter, the grocery checkout aisle, even Amtrak trains, hockey arenas, and Bed Bath & Beyond. It's all but the Kind Bar Occupation. It is estimated that their sales surged from $15 million in 2008 to $120 million in 2012, and more than tripled in the years following. Talk about a swift invasion!

Bars are also taking the place of meals for many people, and the one most often replaced is breakfast. It's what Rabobank, a Dutch bank that does research and analysis for the food and agribusiness industries, calls "snackfast": a sequence of morning-oriented products spread throughout the first half of the day—a Kind bar on our way out the door, a yogurt around 9:30, and maybe a handful of nuts or a banana to get us across the finish line till lunch.

So what's the protein bonanza all about? And what are snacks replacing?

In a way, the decline of breakfast is a response to that most iconic of foods: cereal.

In the 1800s, the purpose of breakfast was for a person to load up on a huge storage of calories to draw from throughout the busy day. It's not that this was considered an optimal way of eating, but the circumstances didn't leave much other choice: For most Americans who worked, the long hours were spent on a job that was physical—farming or manufacturing. Eggs and meat were relatively cheap in the United States compared to other parts of the world, allowing this combo to become established as the classic American-style breakfast.

Then, along came two enterprising Midwesterners named John Harvey Kellogg and C. W. Post. They recognized a growing middle class of office workers who didn't move around much and weren't performing demanding manual labor. These entrepreneurs turned breakfast into an opportunity to gain not a massive fuel supply but a calculated start toward racking up one's daily nutrients.

With all that sausage and bacon had come a nationwide affliction of what was termed "dyspepsia," or as one called it, "Americanitis." It basically meant feeling bloated and gassy all the time. In the late 1800s, eager to cure the gas, John Harvey Kellogg started a now-infamous health resort in Michigan called Battle Creek Sanitarium, or "the San," where health fanatics were subjected to unusual treatments like lying in bed with sandbags on their stomachs. It was a huge hit.

One day, while traveling, John Harvey met another entrepreneur and liked his idea of a shredded wheat breakfast cereal. He started serving it to his guests, and his younger brother, Will Keith (W.K.), got hold of the concept, baking flakes in a barn out back. These eventually debuted as the brothers' joint product: Sanitas Toasted Corn Flakes.

Then, in 1906, W.K. did something crazy: He added sugar to the corn flake mix. And so began the Dessertification of Breakfast in America.

But ask any kid in the grocery aisle, and she'll tell you at least one name is missing from the story. The name is Post. A former guest of the sanitarium, C. W. Post had in 1892 started a rival health spa nearby. He too wanted in on the cereal game, and he did so by launching Grape-Nuts, a wheat-barley cereal, and Post Toasties, another sweetened corn flake cereal. General

Mills soon entered the picture, rounding out what are called "the Big Three," and by 1911, there were 108 brands of cereal coming out of Battle Creek.

The sugar ante was upped in several major, stunning ways. In 1949, Post introduced Sugar Crisp, which became immensely popular, and General Mills and Kellogg's answered with, among others, Sugar Corn Pops, Sugar Frosted Flakes, and Sugar Smacks. Cereal sales only grew from midcentury until 1975, when, as Michael Moss writes in his book *Salt Sugar Fat*, "sugar—the keystone of the cereal makers' fortunes—suddenly became a matter of vivid distress to consumers." Mostly this was caused by dentists who worried about cavities, though there were a few early doctors sounding alarm bells about diabetes. Cereal companies came under fire and suddenly removed "sugar" from the names of many popular brands. Frosted Flakes, for example, were once called Sugar Frosted Flakes.

Some of the names might have changed, but for several decades, cereal kept tasting more and more like dessert. Along the way, we saw the birth of products like Cocoa Puffs, Oreo O's, and Smorz. And marshmallows somehow made their way into cereal bowls as reasonable things to eat at 7:00 A.M.

Many of these cereals are still available on grocery shelves today. The absolute worst on the list of high-sugar varieties is Kellogg's Honey Smacks, at nearly 56 percent sugar by weight. That's according to a review of eighty-four popular brands of children's breakfast cereal by the Environmental Working Group. Its report found that one cup of the cereal has more sugar than a Hostess Twinkie. One cup of any of forty-four other cereals, including Honey Nut Cheerios surprisingly, delivers more sugar than three Chips Ahoy! cookies.

The cereals that vaguely have something to do with fruit are also often among the worst culprits. Apple Jacks is 42.9

percent sugar by weight, Cap'n Crunch's Crunch Berries is 42.3 percent—with the OOPS! All Berries iteration weighing in at 46.9 percent—and Froot Loops, which touts itself as a "good source of fiber" and "made with whole grain," is 41.4 percent.

But there's a reason we let this happen. It's not like we wrote letters to General Mills and said, "Hey, why haven't you put cake in my cereal bowl yet?" Cereal companies know the struggle parents face in trying to find no-fuss foods for their children. So they made these products available, and kids responded because of the sweet taste and the appealing cartoons and the games on the boxes. Parents responded because it was often the only thing they could get their kids to eat for breakfast.

Not to mention the debut of breakfast pastries that dance dangerously close to the dessert line: Frosted Chocolate Fudge Pop-Tarts and Quaker Oatmeal Chocolate Chip Breakfast Cookies, to name just a few.

The United States is far from the only country eating dessert for breakfast. In fact, other countries are arguably far more indulgent: the many European countries eating chocolate- or Nutella-filled croissants each morning, or the Dutch, who every day consume 750,000 slices of buttered bread topped with chocolate sprinkles called *hagelslag*. That is, bread, butter, and sugary sprinkles of varying types.

But in America today, sugar is nearing tobacco status in the public-health world. Excessive sugar intake has been tied to obesity and its related medical conditions, as well as a lack of other nutrients because of what sugary foods and beverages replace. And consumers have started to change their ways.

The lineup of brands that makes up the nutritional scum of children's cereals is, interestingly, the category of cereals in greatest decline: sales of children's cereals dropped 10.7 percent between 2003 and 2013, according to Euromonitor, a market research firm that analyzes trends in dozens of countries including the United States. In a piece in *The Atlantic*, James Hamblin—my all-time favorite health writer—cut to the chase: "Sugar puffs are not 'part of a complete breakfast' any more than Skittles or toenails."

The mid-1990s were cereal's heyday, and although it still remains the leading breakfast-food category—$10 billion in sales in 2013, with 90 percent of all U.S. households purchasing cereal—sales have declined significantly since 2000.

"To turn the tide, we suggest a renewed focus on innovation, a rebooting of the message to consumers, and, for children's cereal, an embrace of what you are, even if that means new positioning in a different grocery aisle," said Nicholas Fereday, executive director and senior analyst of food and consumer trends at Rabobank, in a press release for the firm's report, "The Cereal Killers: Five Trends Revolutionizing the American Breakfast."

Translation: Maybe it's time those Smorz and Oreo O's and chocolate Pop-Tarts just own up to being the desserts they truly are—and skip the whole cereal act altogether. At home in the cookie aisle, they might regain their footing.

"Snackfast," Fereday says, is one of the key explanations behind the decline in cereal consumption. Part of this is that convenience and portability have reached new heights in the breakfast world—with more and more people looking for breakfast to be *handheld*. Fereday says other factors at play include demographic shifts, our lower birth rate (cereal tends to be more of a kid food), and the observation that millennials just aren't that into cereal. A good number of us tend to be more health conscious, eager to avoid processed foods, and leery of marketing ploys that distract consumers from weird hidden ingredients. Basically, we don't trust Toucan Sam, Tony the Tiger, the Cap'n, or any of the other breakfast table companions of our youth.

———————

It's great that we're slowly moving away from dessert as breakfast and calling out cereal companies for masking the fact they have been *selling* us dessert as breakfast. If you think about it, cereal was already a shorthand version of the sit-down, multi-component breakfast of our forefathers. And the bar-as-breakfast is really an even shorter-hand version, with the appeal of delivering a higher dose of protein than cereal more efficiently. Which is why tossing in some protein is one tactic that seems to help many of the fumbling cereal companies manage to hang on. It's like when they just removed "sugar" from the names, except now their focus is protein, giving us names like Special K *Protein* and Cheerios *Protein*.

The crazy thing about all this is: We eat way more protein than we actually need. This, friends, is the Great Protein Myth.

Every human cell contains many proteins, and we need them to help our bodies repair cells and make new ones. Proteins are made up of amino acids, which are the building blocks of life. Some of these amino acids, called essential amino acids, must come from food because our bodies don't produce them. Nonessential are the ones our bodies make on their own.

Part of the protein myth is that it only comes from animal-based foods like fish, meat, and dairy. A second part of the myth is that plant proteins are missing some of the essential amino acids. Not true. All plant foods have protein, and the protein in plants has all twenty amino acids, including all of the essential amino acids. The difference lies in the proportions, where it's fair to say the proportions of the amino acids in animal foods are optimal compared to the proportions we need, while in protein from plant foods, the proportions of amino acids are still well matched, but lower than what is considered optimal. This all becomes moot, though, after considering the *quantity* of protein consumed in the average American diet. Which brings us to the final part of the myth, the part most responsible for the over-the-top consumption of protein bars and cereals and powders: that we aren't getting enough total protein.

In reality, many believe that their requirement is higher than it is and that their intake is lower than it is. Most American adults eat about one hundred grams of protein per day—or more. That's roughly double the Recommended Daily Allowance. Even on a vegan diet it isn't hard to get sixty to eighty grams of protein per day. And it adds up over the day (beans, legumes, nuts, broccoli, whole grains, and so on). Despite our penchant for asking vegetarians and vegans how on earth they get by, you may have noticed that their hearts do somehow continue to beat.

So while protein malnutrition is a problem for millions of people around the globe, for most of us eating here in the United States, it's hard *not* to get enough protein on a daily basis.

As a nation, protein-wise, we've gone off the deep end.

(Full disclosure: I'm as guilty as the next person. I ate a pack of almonds a few pages ago, and I'm thinking about grabbing a dark chocolate nuts and sea salt Kind bar from the cupboard. You know, for insurance.)

Even those Hartman researchers—who say consumers' "perceptions are our reality"—recognize that we're taking this protein thing a bit too far. Exhibit A of taking things too far is a brand called ips, which stands for intelligent protein snacks. Resembling *chicharrón* (fried pork skin), their product is a type of chip . . . made of egg whites.

So if regular foods provide protein, and hardly any of us fail to get enough protein, what's all the fuss about?

One factor in packing protein into our snacks seems to relate to how some people feel after eating foods high in protein versus sugar. There is a very specific mood with a very special name: "hangry"—a combination of hungry + angry. Consider it the adult equivalent of a small child's blood sugar meltdown: Some men turn sullen, some women turn snippy, and the only way to quell the stirring storm is to shove something in our stomachs—and fast. Hangriness is much more likely to set in not only after a long time without eating any food, but after eating a lot of processed crap. Eating a protein-rich food like nuts or yogurt instead of a food that is primarily refined carbohydrates, like cereal or a cookie, might be more helpful in fending off hangriness.

"We find that people are realizing this whole connection to sugar and simple carbohydrates now like never before," says Melissa Abbott of the Hartman Group. People notice the sugar crash they experience, and how it has a cascading effect. Maybe they won't get that load of laundry in or ever make it to the gym, or maybe they lack the energy to play with their kids. "Consumers from all different demographics all across the U.S. freak out if they didn't have protein for breakfast," she says, adding, "Really it's that we've been eating so many highly processed carbs for so long. Now it's like, you try nuts, or you try an egg again, or fat even, and you feel a sense of satiety—consumers never use this word—but they're feeling like they can get through the day."

If we all went to confession together, we'd reveal that the reason we fuel up on portable protein is our fear of crashing. It's like "bonking" in athlete lingo: As the intensity in schools and workplaces has risen, people have a lot of anxiety about their energy levels. It's about the need to perform, to be "on."

So we arm ourselves with snacks.

We accept as a given that our schedules will be jam-packed and carried out at warp speed. Mere passengers, we will be swept along the tracks, inevitably facing repeated derailment (buzzing texts!) and a siege of bombs (chiming e-mails!). Our sentences will be punctuated by how "insane" things are, how "slammed" we feel every minute, perennially "in the weeds," "in the trenches," "in the muck," or in whatever ecosystem we feel is most apt to portray ourselves as drowning. With no certainty that we'll surface in time to squeeze in lunch or make it out of the office before 7:00 P.M., it's only natural to think, *Snacks to the rescue or bust.*

Instant Gratification

A second driving force behind snacks as meals—and not just protein-based snacks, but all of them—is convenience taken to new extremes, and an increased need for immediate gratification. *Because* we feel so pressed for time, we will go so far as to purchase a four-minute microwaveable entrée over a five-minute microwaveable entrée.

And in the single-minded pursuit of efficiency, what's falling by the wayside?

We are no longer the home cooks we once were. Instead, "cooking" at home is often really mere *assembly*. (In surveys, people consider tasks like adding frozen peas to a premade soup to be "cooking.")

Americans spend less time cooking than people in any of the OECD nations. Just thirty minutes per day. In 2014, under 60 percent of the dinners we ate at home were actually *made* at home. In 1984, it was nearly 75 percent. Of all our eating occasions, 42 percent involve exclusively prepared foods; 77 percent involve at least some prepared foods.

When we do actually break out the pots and pans, Americans' favorite home-cooked dishes are baked goods—chocolate chip cookies, for one—dishes with only a few ingredients (i.e., baked garlic chicken), and simple comfort foods—mac and cheese, lasagna, chicken pot pie. Anything that can be made in a slow cooker tends to score well with us too. These are the findings of an analysis by *The Daily Meal* of the most-searched recipes on Allrecipes.com, the Food Network, and similar websites, along with social media data boasting of our accomplishments in the kitchen. As these results reveal, and as we'll explore throughout this book, we're far more daring when we dine out than when we eat in.

Though there are slight differences by income level, all socioeconomic groups of Americans are cooking less than they used to. Along with these changes, nearly all of us have become more willing to embrace alternative channels as legitimate ways to obtain food. Take, for instance, home delivery—not just community-supported agriculture, or CSA, boxes with farmers' produce, but subscription services like NatureBox, which provides deliveries of packaged snacks straight to your home or office. There are also delivery dinner kits like Blue Apron, Din, and Plated, where the planning and shopping and most of the chopping has already been done for you, but you have to follow the recipe and put it all together. These hybrid approaches to preparing meals at home give the sense of having cooked your own meal, but with the degree of convenience and in the amount of time you can accommodate given your busy lifestyle.

You might even find yourself eating sushi from Walgreens, or inserting your credit card into an ATM-like machine that dispenses Sprinkles cupcakes, or a Burritobox, the "world's first burrito kiosk." Picture a Redbox kiosk that spits out a warm, rumored-to-be-delicious burrito. You can even tack on a side of guac and sour cream with the press of a button. (And while you wait all of ninety seconds, the kiosk plays a video to keep you entertained.)

So why are we so determined to consume food immediately? Why do we need cupcake ATMs and burrito boxes? The same reason we need our protein to be portable: overwork.

I'm not suggesting we go back to washing clothes by hand or spending all day getting the stove hot, but it's worth thinking about how convenience changes the way we act—and the way we eat. It's not a straight one-for-one trade. Before automatic washing machines, people just washed their clothes and sheets less often; we lived with a little more dirt in our lives. Before vacuum cleaners, we just let the rugs go a little longer before smacking the dust out of them over a balcony. But the greater availability of convenient foods doesn't just save us time and get us back to work or on to whatever else we want to do—it leads us to eat more *because* the foods are there and they're easy.

If it's midafternoon and I'm only a tad bit hungry, I'm not likely to go into the kitchen, pull out some ingredients and prepare myself a nice sandwich. That seems like a whole ordeal, and I'm not *that* hungry. I can probably wait until dinner. But there's a bag of trail mix in my drawer, and all I have to do is pull it out and eat it. And I do.

When Is a Meal?

It's not just greater quantity per meal that explains America's overall increased eating, but greater frequency. More than half of Americans now snack two to three times daily. Consumer behavior expert Michael Barry is finding people eating a hundred calories or more every two hours.

With all the rules out the window, there are huge implications of not only *what* is a meal—increasingly an amalgam of snacks—but *when* is a meal.

It has become socially acceptable to eat anywhere, any time. In observing Americans' eating habits, Melissa Abbott says, "There's food at every gathering—boy scouts, soccer club, office meeting; there's food everywhere, whereas it was not like that before. There were times when we ate, and times when we didn't eat."

And with all of this eating around one another—at the hardware store and the vet's office and the study group—we can't help but be influenced by other people's food choices. A recent study found that participants were 13 percent more likely to make a healthy food choice when told that others before them had done so. When participants in the survey were told that others had made an unhealthy food choice, they became 15 percent less likely to make a healthy food choice. So as more people around us eat more snacks, we eat more snacks, and so on and so on.

"As Americans, we feel it's our right to snack," Abbott says. "If you try to take it away, like 'You can't eat here,' Americans will get angry, like, 'How dare you?'"

While snacking is unquestionably a global phenomenon— only 9 percent of consumers surveyed in sixty countries in 2014 did *not* snack at least once a day—Abbott sees the social taboo of snacking in other countries. In Brazil, India, China, and Russia, her research shows that you might be looked down on if you eat on the street. She once observed a woman in Brazil take a bag of chips and walk to her car to eat it. She clearly didn't want to be seen snacking.

We simply don't have that in the United States. I have heard of women bringing Tupperware containers to Nordstrom, and have personally seen a shopper stroll through the shoe store DSW with one hand submerged in a bag of Snapea crisps. No one seemed to notice. Or care.

When it comes to snacking, it may only be the beginning. "Driven by consumer demand, some trends might be fads, some might be a new paradigm," wrote the trade publication *Food Processing* in 2013. "But with sales that could hit half a trillion dollars in the next 15 years, snack makers will be facing continued challenges to come up with the right crunch, the right munch for a snack-addicted world."

So again, what's driving this constant munching is a combination of being efficiency oriented—I suppose we can use our hands to feed our mouths while we use our eyes to look at shoes—and our concerns about following the latest nutritional guidance, which, in some cases, has been the slow trickle approach to calorie intake.

For generations, we established the three-meals-a-day standard, and those rituals gave us clear social guidance about what times to eat and how much. "We're seeing people eating more often, and there isn't a lot of language about what they're doing," says Michael Barry. Today, he says, we've turned to convenience and technology for answers about how to feed ourselves without working out all the customs of the provisioning. Instead, "We're kind of reinventing this all along the way."

Each of us is rewriting our own rules as to what constitutes an "eating occasion." And we have more eating occasions now than ever before.

So whether we realize it or not, we are all participating in a revolutionary experiment.

CHAPTER 2

Food at Work

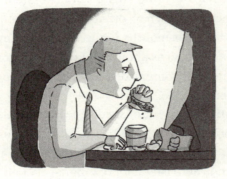

At San Francisco's historic Ferry Building, workplace well-ness execs, professors of design and nutrition, and some of the country's most distinguished leaders in food and health gathered to discuss American eating habits at a place less sexy than restaurants, less obvious than homes, but no less import-ant or intriguing: the American workplace.

This conference has stuck with me because of a startling re-alization I had there: Many of us all but *live* at work. And no one sees this changing any time soon.

All the extra time we're spending at work means we're eating more at work. At the Ferry Building, I paused for a moment to imagine how things used to be—workers bringing a sandwich in a pail or grabbing a quick bite at a bar around noon.

Those days are behind us, but what does eating on the job look like today, and why has it changed?

On one end of the corporate food spectrum is Sad Desk Lunch. Today, we are more willing than ever to keep our heads down and work through lunch. Just one in five workers in North America takes regular lunch breaks. The rest usually just power through until dinner (most likely snacking to get through the day).

I've certainly been there myself—hunched over a plastic container, semi-productive but mostly staring at the screen, spewing crumbs across the keyboard. Glancing over at a colleague, I might see him eating any of the thousands of types of microwaveable meals on the market, a food category that goes hand-in-hand with the widespread practice of solo dining. Not to mention a lack of concern for the aroma it might be piping through the office.

On the other end of the spectrum, we can look to companies like Google, which offers its employees free food. Employees are pampered with copious spreads, global flavors from high-end chefs, and the assurance that food is never more than 150 feet away. There's just one problem: Googlers have been gaining weight. Employees sometimes acknowledge the "Google fifteen," referring to the fifteen pounds some of them gain in their first year there. The cafeteria does try to nudge people toward healthier options by labeling some foods as "red" for ones to avoid, and "green" for the ones to load up on—but the ubiquity and variety of food are far more powerful. Many can't help but chow down.

By contrast, Apple employees have to—gasp!—pay for their own lunch there. "[At Apple,] you're not getting lunch from daddy—you buy your lunch like most grown-ups do," as Adam Lashinsky, author of *Inside Apple,* once explained to *Business Insider.*

More radical still is the increasing number of employees—particularly young engineers in Silicon Valley—who eat *all* their meals at work. (See Dave Eggers's *The Circle*.) As a result, we may be raising an entire generation of the workforce that never learns to cook for itself—an entire generation of food illiterates.

Work plays a hefty role in the American food psyche, and there is a distinct subgenre of American food culture unique to the workplace. It presents a particularly fascinating laboratory of American behavior because the rules are unlike those anywhere else. Again, I'm not talking about the actual rules—like a dress code prohibiting flip-flops or hats—I'm talking about the cultural rules. What is socially acceptable and even encouraged, what's *routine*. Daily life.

In a study done at the University of Illinois at Urbana–Champaign, researchers placed containers of thirty chocolates in varying arrangements on and around office workers' desks. Participants had been told merely that the study related to candy. When they received the candies, they were told they would later be asked about them. Each night, when the office workers had gone home for the day, the researcher elves crept into the office and recorded how many chocolates had been eaten. Then they replaced the containers with thirty fresh chocolates for the next day. They repeated this procedure every day for three weeks, then tallied the results.

They found that, when the candy container was left on the desk, the workers ate on average about nine chocolates per day. When the researchers put the candy in each participant's desk drawer, the number per day dropped to about six. And when the researchers moved the chocolates to a shelf six feet away from the desk—just far enough out of arm's reach that the participant would have to stand up and walk over to the container—the number dropped to three.

The takeaway from the study is supposed to be that convenience is a major factor in candy consumption, and so is visibility. Merely creating a psychological barrier with a drawer or lid can cut consumption. For certain employers, campus dining professionals, K-12 administrators, and anyone else feeding people in a cafeteria-like setting, this finding can help guide the design of eateries and the ways that foods are offered. Those strategies, in turn, may help lead diners toward healthier options and control how much they take. For example, if visibility and convenience lead people to eat more, then prominently displaying fruit bowls in central locations might lead them to eat more fruit. Placing soda cans on the bottom shelf of a refrigerated case, behind frosted glass, may lead people to drink less soda. As the thinking goes, it's not about taking away people's choices or forcing them to eat certain things, but making the healthier choices easier and the more indulgent ones less mindless.

But my takeaway revolves around the study's having been conducted *in an office*. It reveals a great deal about the eating mores of American office culture and the relationship between food and work.

For one, the workers in the study didn't think it was strange that giant containers of chocolates were out on people's desks and in drawers and on shelves because it's a regular occurrence in an office. But people rarely leave giant containers of candy scattered around their homes. Maybe some people do, but culturally we think of candy (and especially chocolate) as essential furniture of the work environment.

The office supply chain Staples has a candy section to rival that of most grocery stores. Candy has become as standard a business operating expense as paper clips or Post-Its. As a result, introducing the candies into the office was not strange, and the study was just a matter of where exactly in the office the candy was placed.

It's everywhere you turn. That little dish of lollipops is right next to the pen-on-a-cord at the bank, and assorted hard candies can be found in the eye doctor's waiting room. Andes mints adorn the dry cleaner's counter. Or my favorite: A former coworker referred to a section of her desk as the "emergency chocolate drawer." She had more visitors than anyone else in the office.

Candy at work is so widespread today that it's easy to imagine the American economy coming to a screeching halt if we ran out.

So what is it about the workplace that it might take nine chocolates to get us through a single day? That the woman with the emergency chocolate drawer would have the most popular cubicle in the office? What is it about *work,* and what is it about *us*?

Food at work comes in three major stripes: Food you bring yourself. Food you get from colleagues. Food your employer provides. Let's take a look.

Food You Bring Yourself

Lunch is the meal most likely to be eaten away from home. So we'll start with this not-at-all comprehensive quickie history of lunch in America.

For most of human history, people ate just one meal a day. What with all the finding of the food, the building of the fire, the grinding of the wheat into flour, it basically took all day to put together a meal. Agricultural societies mostly ate as families except during harvest time when a communal lunch was had with friends and neighbors. By medieval times, Europeans started eating two meals—"dinner" at midday and "supper" later on—a tradition they brought with them when they settled in North America. These meals were both typically consumed with the family, though with most settlers' lives revolving around farming of some kind, men commonly ate lunch in the fields together while colonial housewives ate at home in between chores.

In the early 1800s, gaslight came along. That allowed for less sleeping and more doing things. Factories could extend their hours and therefore their production. If smartphones marked the End of Having an Excuse Not to Work, surely gaslight marked the Beginning of the End. No longer could you use "It's too dark to see" as an excuse to call it a day at 4:00 P.M. in December.

With more awake time, and more work output, people needed more meals to keep themselves moving.

Whereas agriculture was the main industry from the time of colonial America until the early 1800s, and most people grew their own food, both people and jobs migrated to cities as part of the Industrial Revolution. Since then, workers have mostly eaten lunch at or near their jobs. By the mid- to late 1800s, streets were teeming with crowds of workers searching for a quick bite before returning to the factory line. Unless you were an executive, in which case you could lounge and feast in a men's club or pricy restaurant.

The significance of lunch *in public* cannot be overstated. We now had a new urban phenomenon of being surrounded by people who were not members of your family while you ate. To preserve some decency given this radical new development, men and women ate separately: men lured by saloons offering free chow with a purchase of a beer, women sitting on street curbs, eating items bought from nearby shops or leftovers brought in folded napkins. (Later, someone started using old coffee cans as lunch boxes, and they became all the rage.)

Then, in the first half of the twentieth century, we had

two world wars, and the men were sent overseas, and women worked and then didn't, and then worked again. During the 1920s, both we and the Canadians went completely nuts over grilled cheese sandwiches for lunch. Called "cheese dreams" in Canada and "toasties" here in the United States, they were served by most lunch counters and were the rare lunch item that was both cheap and warm. Surely a landmark step forward for mankind. One for which we have Kraft's sort-of-cheese squares and the invention of sliced bread to thank.

Along the way, there were luncheonettes (think: dining at a drug store) and automats (think: room-size vending machines, stocked in real time by real people). Then came post–World War II suburbanization, which meant even more people staying at the office and eating lunch there.

In that era, you had Mad Men–type urban office employees getting wasted at three-martini lunches in the name of the "creative process." But all this midday glee came to a standstill in the early 1970s when a recession hit and everyone had to start using "brown bag" as a verb. While some high rollers carried on during the austerity period with their fancy white-linen power lunches, many a boss had to join the office plebs and desk dine—that lunch reality that Megan Elias, author of *Lunch: A History,* sums up as "a brief pause in unremarkable surroundings to eat something from a container."

Next, the entire lunch-at-work paradigm was revolutionized by the invention of two magic-inducing boxes. First, the microwave oven. Second, the desktop computer. Together, they turned white-collar workers into keyboard-clogging victims of early onset hunchback.

While it couldn't have happened in the way it did without the personal computer, it was the microwave that really did a number on our workplace eating. The microwave transformed the kitchen, and offices often have kitchens.

Its origin is an all-too-American tale. An orphan with just a sixth-grade education who was a self-taught engineer, Percy Spencer invented the microwave oven—by accident—and it landed him in the Inventors Hall of Fame.

In the 1930s, before the Pearl Harbor attack drew the United States into World War II, some British scientists had begun experimenting with pulse radio waves, and they developed a tube called a magnetron that produced microwaves. These waves bounced off metal objects and returned a signal, which made it possible to locate enemy ships. But by 1940 Britain was already drained of resources from fighting the Germans, so they shared their scientific discoveries with the leading American electronics companies in the hopes that they could manufacture magnetrons at the scale needed for the war effort.

Percy Spencer was working for one such company called Raytheon when some British scientists presented the top-secret tube. Percy took it home over the weekend to see what he could do. On Monday he showed up with a plan to mass-produce the magnetron and was declared a war hero and a genius. Then we beat the Nazis. The end.

After the war, Percy continued to fiddle with the radar system. One day he noticed that a candy bar he kept in his shirt pocket (for emergencies, of course) had started to melt.

That made him even more curious, so he played around with some other foods. He discovered, for instance, that if popcorn kernels were placed beside the magnetron, the kernels popped. Doing the same with an egg sent a burst of cooked yolk across his face. Recognizing that this might be a handy device in the kitchen, he next built a metal box to hold food, then channeled waves into the box. The food cooked!

He spent two more years testing his oven before going to market with it as "The Radarange." It was not a success out of the gate. The $3,000 price tag probably didn't help. Second, the oven was six feet tall. Six *feet*. (The ovens were so massive they were used to roast coffee beans and to dry items like paper and potato chips.) Plus, you had to cool the magnetron using water, requiring plumbing and the whole nine yards.

Over time, the technology improved. First introduced to the domestic consumer market in 1955, the microwave took off in the 1970s, when cookware companies started introducing microwave-safe dishware and Pillsbury started marketing microwaveable products. You may recall the famous scene in the film *American Hustle*, set in the 1970s: The Rosalyn Rosenfeld character, played by Jennifer Lawrence, gripes about the alien "science oven" that has just arrived in her kitchen—and promptly sets it on fire.

By 1975, more people bought microwave ovens than gas ranges. The percentage of Americans who consider the microwave a "necessity" more than doubled between 1996 and 2006, up to 68 percent. The percentage has dropped since then, as have sales. But still, today, only one in ten American households does *not* have a microwave.

The merits of the microwave should not be overlooked. You could argue that it helped free many American women to work outside the home because family meals could be prepared more quickly. Plus, microwaveable meals are affordable and certainly more satisfying than a hodgepodge of cold snacks and bars. And they (usually) contain chunks of foods you can recognize.

By 1993, more than 75 percent of American workplaces had a microwave. Which brings me to Lean Cuisine, Stouffer's, and Amy's Kitchen: the sad poster children of Sad Desk Lunch.

Frozen entrées are one of the runaway success stories over the last generation. "It's kind of the golden age of quick meals," says Richard Wilk, a professor of anthropology at Indiana University, where he directs the Food Studies Program and codirects the university's Food Institute. He says, "My wife has in her lab a refrigerator and a microwave, and she just puts something in the microwave for lunch everyday." It used to be that if you did eat lunch at work, it was bound to be a sandwich, he says. But the sandwich has been replaced. Nowadays, the options are endless.

Wilk argues that the food industry has provided us with a greater variety of individual-size, premade lunch options than ever before. Lean Cuisine, for its part, offers 148 varieties, from "simple favorites" like mac and cheese to its veggie-forward "spa collection."

Interestingly, the market for frozen fare has been slipping in recent years—due to greater concern about the products' nutritional value, especially sodium content, and a more widespread priority on fresh food—but as a $44 billion industry, it's still sitting pretty. (For context, $2.7 billion of that is for handheld frozen foods; frozen fruit rakes in another $422 million annually, and frozen vegetables are just shy of $6 billion.)

Today we have more options than ever out in the real world, yet the appeal of the office kitchen—stocked with, at minimum, a toaster, microwave, fridge, and coffeemaker—is universal. Employers dig it because it keeps employees within the confines of the building and decreases the odds that, instead of obtaining food in the fastest manner possible, their employees are actually out napping in a massage chair at Brookstone. And employees like it for all kinds of reasons: convenience, freeness (when cabinets are stocked by employers), and the cultural permission to eat all day long at the office rather than just at lunch when ducking out to buy food.

Today, the microwave has helped transform the workplace . . . into a hotel. An extended-stay hotel, that is. With everything from high heels stored under the desk to deodorant in the back of the file cabinet, many employees today basically move into the joint, except instead of everyone having their own room, everyone has a personal pantry. People do entire grocery runs

Monday morning, filling the communal fridge or freezer with their week's worth of meals.

Once, I saw a beige mottled blob emerge from a vacuum-sealed plastic package. Kind of like a jellyfish, minus the tentacles. My colleague plopped the blob into a bowl, zapped* it in the microwave for a few minutes, and walked away as the timer counted down. I poured myself some coffee while rapidly running through ideas in my head of what the blob could be. Maybe she had brought her child to work that day and was heating up some kind of frozen applesauce. Maybe it was one of those weird meal-replacement packs you order from infomercials where you can only eat what they send you in the mail.

By the time she returned, I was still there, puzzled. So I had to ask.

"It's oatmeal, of course," she replied with a smile. That squat, cylindrical brick was a yet-to-be-stirred serving of steel-cut oats from Trader Joe's. (For the record, they are surprisingly tasty.)

What dawned on me then was a vision of the future: an orderly lineup of sparkling, stainless steel freezers in a warehouse-size office kitchen, each freezer engraved with an employee's name, and each paired with a matching stainless steel microwave on an adjacent counter. With a freezer all to oneself, each employee stocks an entire *career*'s supply of frozen meals and snacks. Lives made up of days spent like zombies, every day the same pattern: from the desk to the freezer to the microwave, from the desk to the freezer to the microwave, and on it goes.

––––––––––

* It is still unclear to me why people say "zap" when referring to heating things in the microwave. But they do, and I don't, usually, except I spent a whole month of my life writing about microwaves, so I couldn't resist.

Unlike what you choose to eat in the privacy of your own kitchen or couch or car, what you eat for lunch is on display.

And there are all kinds of unspoken rules and judgments that take place around it. Take gender, for instance. Salads boomed in the early 1980s and even rivaled the mighty lunch sandwich, a staple since the 1950s. This was in part because of the health craze at the time (never mind that often the salads were so buried in bacon bits and blue cheese dressing that those calorie-conscious diners would have been better off just enjoying a sandwich), but also in part because of the increase in the number of women in the workforce. Females—and yes, I'm generalizing here—tend to avoid being seen scarfing down a towering pastrami melt. A salad looks more kempt.

Or consider class, for another example. You know you've made it if part of your job involves *dining*. I'm talking about the business lunch, at a restaurant. Like with napkins. It's where deals and eye contact are made, and everyone orders iced tea. While the lavishness may have dropped a notch since the recession, the business lunch is alive and well. That's because, in the age of conference calls, webinars, and saga-length e-mail threads, in-person interaction may be more powerful than ever before.

One tier down, you're still doing mighty fine if you can afford to bring a $12 noodle bowl back to your desk every day.

And if you're brown bagging it, well, colleagues may make any number of judgments about you: "Whoa, smelly tuna sando sogging up the bag." Or "Is that a note I see in there? Do you . . . still live with your parents?" Not to mention what a range of leftovers might suggest: a gradually curling, whitening Domino's pizza slice stamping you "Bachelor"; a Pyrex container filled with an elaborate romanesco curry stamping you "Foodie"; and so on.

But whatever you're bringing, you're likely to take it back to your desk for another episode of Sad Desk Lunch. What might floor you is that this practice is so common, so deeply entrenched in American culture, that it even influences the *design* of food products themselves.

"We work more hours than any other culture, and we eat at our desks more than any other culture," says Melissa Abbott of the Hartman Group. "Whether it's ramen, or things that won't stain your keyboard, it's really gotten to that stage. Cupholder food and that kind of thing—so many manufacturers ask us about packaging innovation, and hand-to-mouth snacks that you can eat in your car or at your desks. Our clients are constantly requesting new products like this."

Companies are actually inventing foods—and ways of delivering foods to us—that take into account that we eat them while at our keyboards. Especially snack foods. They are doing this because they've figured out that we won't leave our computers just to eat. Ramen, you see, is a clear liquid. Or take popcorn. If you're eating it at home watching TV, you might be fine with a cheddar seasoning of some sort, but popcorn makers are looking for innovative flavors for work occasions that won't leave finger residue.

Now, to be fair, not everyone works in an office sitting at a computer all day. There are teachers, construction workers, restaurant workers, health-care professionals, members of the armed forces, and countless others whose days look a lot different. Then there are the 34 percent of American adults who aren't in the workforce at all; perhaps they are retired, disabled, in school, or taking care of children or elderly parents. So this portrait of an office worker may not resonate with everyone. But the point remains: Sad Desk Lunch—and the array of microwaveable, handheld, keyboard-safe foods that accompany it—is a full-blown cultural phenomenon of the American workplace.

————————

In general, lunch breaks are one way we might increase the number of minutes per workday that we focus on food. And they bring up heated debates. More and more people are catching on to the productivity–lunch break relationship. Consider the movement called Take Back Your Lunch, where participants pledged to take real lunch breaks. They asked, *Are we really going to be lying on our deathbeds wishing we'd eaten* more *of our meals at our desks?*

Others decide they get to leave earlier when they desk dine than if they take a real, leave-the-premises lunch break, meaning they'll have more time at the gym or with their family. Assuming they *like* spending time at the gym or with their family, this boosts well-being and so offsets the bummer of no break.

I'll personally opt for the advice of Kimberly D. Elsbach, associate dean and professor of Organizational Behavior at the University of California, Davis Graduate School of Management. She says to go ahead and take the brain rest. Tease out my mental floss knot. (If not at least for the restored blood flow for my mean case of keyboard elbow.) Some research shows that even just fifteen to twenty minutes away from my desk might sharpen my concentration, increase my shot at a jolt of creative genius, and grease the wheels on my decision-making machine.

Food You Get from Colleagues

Food makes people do weird things.

After a Florida woman's dining companion refused to buy her a McDonald's McFlurry, she set his car on fire.

A Massachusetts woman ordered a steak-and-cheese sandwich at Nathan's Famous Hot Dogs. When she received her order, she punched the guy behind the counter because the sandwich had "too many pickles."

In Washington State, a prowler came upon an unlocked SUV in the middle of the night and stole three boxes of Girl Scout Cookies the owner had left inside—nothing else.

But food *in the office* makes people do especially weird things, and we have some strange ways of viewing food in the office.

Example #1: Food You Get from Colleagues—That Your Colleagues Don't Want You to Have

Jeanne Hamilton has a website called Etiquette Hell, with over 6,000 tales of jerk moves in all kinds of social situations. Stunningly, far and away the top complaint about the workplace is fridge theft. That's right, stealing your colleagues' food from the office kitchen.

Such larceny is so rampant that employees nationwide have taken to all sorts of creative means to combat the issue: labeling their sack lunches as "poison curry," or leaving cat food sandwiches as traps.

I've even heard stories around offices about people writing letters like this:

Dear Heartless Sandwich Thief,
I find myself in a state of acute emotional distress at the loss of my Caribbean roast pork shoulder sandwich. With each minute that passes, I ask myself whether it is right to loathe you—or pity you. Perhaps you took this sandwich due to insufficient disposable income derived from generations of institutionalized inequities, in which case, this one-of-a-kind artisanal sandwich is the very least I can offer, and I hope that you thoroughly enjoy every last morsel.

If, however, you snatched this sandwich for no other reason than you took one look at its succulent figure and simply could not help yourself, that would suggest an act that one could only describe as repugnant and unforgivable. Do you understand, mister/miss/ma'am, that you have misappropriated not only my midday nourishment but a piece of my happiness? Have you no honor? No decency? With all due respect, how do you sleep at night? Given the reputation of this law office for distributing five-figure checks for mere holiday bonuses, all signs point to this as an unthinkable wrongdoing. And so, for the remainder of your sandwich-eating days on this earth, may you have nothing but cold cuts encased in slimy film, bread so stale it nicks the gums on your back molars, tomato slices the color of turnips and cheese slices still stuck to their paper separators, and ~~a disfavorably disproportionate amount of mayonnaise in your mustard-mayonnaise spread~~ a complete moratorium on selling you condiments of any kind, to ensure only hoagie experiences akin to slow-chewing one's way through the entire wad of cotton in an Advil container until jaw lock sets in.

Sincerely,
George, the Aggrieved

Example #2: Food You Get from Colleagues—That You Want but Pretend Not to Want and Didn't Ask for but Your Colleagues Want You to Have to Make It Okay for Them to Have Too

Let's turn to something that unleashes an especially high amount of weirdness: The Pink Box. You know the one. It's the one full of donuts.

In an office where I used to work, an e-mail would arrive on a scarily regular basis that more or less said:

то: All Staff

subject: Pink Box

body: . . . is on the counter. You know what to do.

Juuuust in case we didn't see the glistening rows of plump pastries, peeping their heads out from the cardboard box sitting right on the counter that we had to walk by to get to our desks. Or juuuust in case we *did* see the box and had already settled the conversation with ourselves about whether or not to take a donut from said box: *You're not going near that thing. You already ate oatmeal for breakfast!* And *you brushed your teeth. It won't even taste good. Plus, even if you only take half of one, that's like your entire workout in calories.* So *not worth it.*

But then that e-mail arrives, and you have the conversation with yourself all over again, slightly different this time: *You eat so healthy every day—you deserve to indulge from time to time! And that minty toothpaste residue? I bet it would pair nicely with chocolate frosting and sprinkles. Plus, you're working out later, you'll totally burn it off.*

It certainly used to brighten my morning to see the pink box. But there's something odd about office donuts. It seems that maybe people bring the box "for the office" so they have an excuse to eat donuts themselves. Or what about the economics of office donuts—productivity surely plummets with the sugar crash that inevitably follows. Funnier still are the etiquette and psychology associated with office donuts. Something I was guilty of myself was a phenomenon I've named Denial Dicing.*

---

* Some of the phenomena I name are real things with names given by experts; others are real things that, to the best of my knowledge, no one has yet named, so I named them; others are just observations of mine, that may not be universal or widespread but instead anecdotal, and which I have given names for ease of reference.

Let's call my colleague Jane. On office donut days, Jane would approach the pink box, poke her head around it from varying altitudes and vantage points, pick up the white plastic knife that lay in a pile of crumbs, pause, stare hard at the contents of the box, then make up her mind about which flavor she wanted, cut the donut in half, and put it on a napkin to take back to her desk.

This little dance went on throughout the day, with Jane finding reasons to "need" to walk to the other side of the office and pass by the box again. As the hours went by, colleagues sliced and poked and partitioned the donuts so that a minefield of slivers and nubs remained. By the afternoon, Jane might grab what looked to be someone else's half subsequently cut in half a second time, pop that into her mouth, and walk back to her desk.

All told, Jane would eventually eat $\frac{1}{2} + \frac{1}{4} + \frac{1}{3} = 1.0833$. As in, greater than 1. If you'd asked Jane whether she planned to come to work and eat an entire donut, she likely would have laughed and said, "Of course not!"

So is it just that we're bad at fractions? Well yes, in fact, we *are* bad at fractions: In the early 1980s, the A&W restaurant chain decided to take on the McDonald's Quarter Pounder by offering a burger made with a third of a pound of beef, for less money. But it didn't work because customers thought the 4 in $\frac{1}{4}$ made it larger, and that they were being overcharged for the $\frac{1}{3}$ pound.

Back to Denial Dicing, though. The moral of the story is that humans are funny creatures, and when it comes to food, we do not act rationally.

Surely most of us can relate to Jane's predicament. There is a lot of emotion that comes with food, and something like office donuts brings with it a cocktail of guilt, reward, comfort, and pleasure. When faced with an indulgence, we feel deprived if we choose to avoid it, but when we go for it, we do so in this Denial Dicing way that mostly involves torturing ourselves. Mind games and bargains like "Okay, but this is my *last* bite." In the end, we eat more, but enjoy it less.

Example #3: Food You Get from Colleagues—That You Don't Want and Didn't Ask for but End Up Eating Because Your Colleagues Want You to Eat What They No Longer Want

The free table. Often located in the office kitchen or an empty cubicle in the corner, the free table is that communal dumping ground where people bring things from home that they want to get rid of. Things like . . . a rubber Hertz magnet, or a partly chipped mug from their alma mater, or a 2012 "Ins*paw*ration" dog calendar they bring in right around September of 2012.

But more than anything else, people bring food. And what kind of food do they bring? Food they themselves don't want to eat.

Food people don't want to eat falls into three categories:

1. Food that people have allergic, religious, or ethical aversions to.
2. Food that is so flavorless or revolting that virtually no one would want to eat it.
3. Food that is so scrumptious that virtually anyone would want to eat it.

Most of what happens at the free table is a practice I call Artificial Altruism. These are "gifts" from our coworkers that are really gifts to themselves—saving them a trip to Goodwill, or the guilt of tossing unwanted foods in the garbage, or sparing them the torture of something so irresistible but bad for them that they can't bear to have it hanging around the house. They don't care if *you* get fat on Funfetti frosting, so long as *they* no longer have the temptation lurking in the cupboard.

At no time of year is this phenomenon more pronounced than the week after Halloween. The free table is inevitably overflowing with plastic jack-o-lanterns full of exclusively lame candy. Long gone are the full-size Reese's peanut butter cups (dubbed "the limousine of Halloween candy" on BuzzFeed's "definitive list" of the holiday's offerings). What's left are bound to be fun-size Mounds bars ("literally barf city," wrote BuzzFeed, rating it the absolute worst candy on its list) and Almond Joys ("slightly less bad than Mounds"). Let's face it, folks: the bottom of the barrel. Any fourth grader could tell it how it is.

So why is it that we'll go ahead and eat other people's Halloween candy when that very day we brought in a bag of our own rejects—plain Hershey's milk chocolates, Good & Plenty, Smarties, and those weird vanilla- and orange-flavored Tootsie Rolls—to deposit on the table?

One answer: sensory specific satiety. This is the thing where we want and eat a food less after eating that food, compared with the appeal and amount we'll eat of foods we haven't yet eaten. It's why you can be full on spaghetti but still have "room" for dessert. It's why small-plates and tapas restaurants are so popular. And it's considered the leading explanation for why we seek such astonishing variety in our diets. So I may be disgusted by *my* bottom-of-the-barrel Halloween candies but thrilled to scrape out the sewage lining the bottom of *your* barrel.

It's also because of a riveting revelation about how we view our own eating, and one that applies to more than just the free table: In our minds, food from a colleague doesn't really "count." During studies on eating behavior at the office, people will explain that they consider these calories "free." Not in the sense that the calories don't cost money, but they don't need to be included in one's daily log of foods consumed. As Melissa Abbott at the Hartman Group says, "Consumers will say, 'I ate it in the office kitchen—I didn't bring it, so it's almost like it didn't happen.'" *It's almost like it didn't happen.* "It becomes this desperate act of consumption, and it has so much to do with the fact that we are so wedded to our work."

Is it something about the office that causes people to act particularly funny about food there?

Or do people act funny about food at the office because people act funny about food *in general*? And it's just that when we're in the confined social environment of an office, we are exposed to habits normally hidden within the privacy of one's home?

Our affinity to grazing applies regardless of whether we're in the office or at home or at a party because we are a highly visual culture, and our judgments about portion are less precise when we don't see the total amount of food all at once (as we would on a plate). But there are at least three major factors unique to the workplace, and the American mores within the workplace.

One is unpredictability. You walk into the office kitchen for some tea and oh, what do we have here, a cheese pizza sitting on the table. You take a slice, walk back to your desk—popping a handful of M&Ms into your mouth on the way—and so the day goes on. Consumers will tell Abbott, "'I can't believe I just ate six Costco cookies over the course of the day'" or "'I don't know why I ate that.'" Her research shows that, as far as weight management and overall lifestyle quality, "Those who plan versus those who don't—it's like night and day." So some of our grazing-at-work can be attributed to the fact that it's not planned.

A second element that is specifically applicable to the workplace: social permission to indulge. With all the pressure Americans feel about constantly striving to be healthy and sticking to a regimen, Abbott says, "When something's put before us that's not regulated, we turn back into children, like there's no gatekeeping." Your colleague isn't going to shake her finger at you for eating that pizza or those M&M's because he or she is likely doing the same thing. And in that environment, there's an addiction quality, with habits formed almost subconsciously day after day: "I talk to a lot of consumers who say, 'I worked for X company and I got lots of cavities because there were candy bowls everywhere,' or 'I gained a bunch of weight,'" says Abbott.

Some of what is now called the national scourge of "mindless eating" is intertwined with a third major factor at play in the office, that trinity of subfactors of stress, fatigue, and boredom.

Seventy percent of American workers are either "not engaged" or "actively disengaged" at work. That's according to a Gallup report, "State of the American Workplace." This means they are "emotionally disconnected from their workplaces and less likely to be productive."

There is, of course, much discussion about unemployment and the quantity of jobs available, but this stat raises concerns about the *quality* of jobs available. Feeling this way at work affects how we eat at work, which is to say, with our minds elsewhere. It breeds a certain apathy. Bored by the tasks filling most of the time, a surprising treat might be the highlight of our day. Pressured by deadlines and tired from long hours, we can feel as if the walls of the building might contain us forever, and we might never see the outside world again. Probably without realizing it, we seem to feel we might as well eat whatever's put in front of us before our colleagues beat us to it.

One thing is for sure: We often eat at work for reasons that have little to do with hunger.

Food Employers Provide

Fact #1: People like praise.
Fact #2: People like drinking instead of working.
Fact #3: People like moving up in the world.
Fact #4: People like feeling important.
Fact #5: The thing people like *more* than praise, drinking instead of working, moving up in the world, and feeling important, is free food.
Fact #6: The only thing people like *more* then free food is money.

These rankings come from an Employee Appreciation Survey released by Glassdoor, a website with a large database of job openings, salary information, and company profiles. According to the survey, free food—which they termed "unexpected treats and rewards"—beat out all nonmonetary forms of appreciation an employer can provide. It outweighed personal recognition, social events like holiday parties on the employer's dime, opportunities for career growth, and being included in company decision-making.

In general, everyone appreciates being appreciated. It's the puppy in us all. A "way to go, Baxter!" goes a long way in both puppy and human behavior. In the Glassdoor survey, 81 percent of employees said that when their bosses show appreciation, they feel compelled to work harder. But *how* that appreciation is conveyed makes all the difference.

Free drinks work too. Hence the companies offering Friday happy hour. In the early 1800s, men would often show up at work having already stopped by the tavern, then grab another drink at 11:00 A.M. for the "elevenses." But it didn't last. The Industrial Revolution in midcentury brought a need for dexterity and alertness throughout long workdays using fast-operating machines. And for that, tea was the ticket. It sharpened the mind and improved concentration. Coffee too, of course, and both beverages have been the lifeblood of nearly every American workplace.

So today, on-the-job boozing is primarily reserved for the no-holds-barred event that is the company holiday party. It's a gesture made by about 90 percent of U.S. companies. And each year, a whole new set of social norms arrives. Hot toddies are had, hair is let down, lines are crossed. While the costs and gaffes can run high, it's all done in the name of morale.

Not only is food valuable currency to workers, but it is to employers as well. Food makes people feel happy and, interestingly enough, happiness makes people productive. A series of studies conducted at the University of Warwick in England found that happier workers are 12 percent more productive.

The studies involved measuring both productivity and happiness before and after certain interventions, including showing people a comedy clip or giving them chocolate, snacks, and bottled water, as might actually happen in some workplaces. Granted, these studies were done in laboratory settings, and the boosts were not measured over the long term but in short intervals, yet the point remains: Free chocolate bar → happiness hike → 30-plus minutes of significantly greater productivity. And because of the randomized controlled design, the researchers were able to conclude decisively that it was the extra happiness that caused the increased productivity.

Naturally, the appeal of free food works outside the office, too. Supermarkets reap reliable rewards from offering product samples. In the short term, free samples lead us to purchase items we might not have given a second look. Think of the free samples at Costco. Since when do I eat pigs in a blanket? *The Atlantic* reported data from a company called Interactions, which provides demonstrations of products in stores like Costco: Over the course of a year, offering samples increased beer sales by an average of 71 percent, wine sales by over 300 percent, and frozen pizza sales by 600 percent. Those are some serious boosts.

The reason samples prompt such an eager response from our wallets is the powerful human instinct of reciprocity, explained Dan Ariely, professor of behavioral economics at Duke University's Fuqua School of Business, in the *Atlantic* piece. Once we have received something from someone, we feel we owe something in return. In the long term, offering free samples makes a store feel like a fun place to hang out, increasing our loyalty to that company, and the likelihood of our returning time after time.

Coding and culinary have officially gotten hitched. Today you can hardly say "tech company" without "free food" in the same sentence—and people want specifics.

What snacks are stocked in the office kitchens? What global cuisines are represented in the cafés? What special social events are sponsored? Recognition banquets and team-building off-sites like white-water rafting would be nice, or for goodness' sake, do they at the very least do bagel Wednesday?

Catered lunch at start-ups is now all but expected. And while we may think of food at work as *lunch* at work, increasingly it's breakfast and dinner too—along with all manner of snacks and treats in between. You'll find just-baked cookies and boba tea at Dropbox, and frostings dyed with watermelon radishes and herbs plucked from the rooftop garden at Zynga. Zillow's candy wall is legendary. At a company called BandPage, they hold a *Game of Thrones*–themed feast featuring sixteenth-century recipes, the show's soundtrack playing in the background, and crowns for all.

So why has tech turned to food?

Clearly companies like Google and Facebook have the funds to provide food in the first place. But the logic diagram has a bit more to it: In the modern American economy, engineers are like kings and queens. I think of them as the Lewises and Clarks of our day—willing to venture into the (digital) unknown, capable of charting the future. Whether the tool they create is a new operating system or a smarter car or an e-mail interface we're all glued to all day, we'll likely spend years of our lives, and much of our disposable income, on it. As a result, tech companies offer free, good food as an incentive to get the best people to work there.

Google recognized early on that providing its employees with food was not only an incentive for people to take the jobs, but also led to productivity, loyalty, and happiness. Food is part of its, ahem, secret sauce.

The fifty-sixth employee hired at Google was not a programmer or a project manager, a user experience designer or a sales strategist. He was a chef. And that chef was Charlie Ayers.

Charlie, who had previously cooked for the Grateful Dead, among other clients, was first approached by Google in 1998, when the company was less than a year old. It had a mere dozen employees in a crowded office in downtown Palo Alto, yet Sergey Brin had determined that what would set Google apart from other companies was good food for its staff—all of it free.

(Sergey wasn't the first to see the power of food as a tool for recruitment and talent retention. Family farms had been using this tactic long before tech and the battle for gifted engineers. To lure the best seasonal farmworkers, wives of neighboring farms would duke it out to offer the most sumptuous spreads: platters of pork roast, breads, jams, and homemade pies.)

Google was scrappy and couldn't pay much, and Charlie took one look at the operation and passed.

But eight months went by. Which, in Silicon Valley time, is like . . . a decade. By that point, Google had grown to forty-five employees and proclaimed itself one of the valley's "hottest and fastest growing Internet companies." The chef position was offered with stock options no less. In its ad calling for chef try-outs, Google called itself "a group of people with well traveled refined palates with a craving for epicurial delights." At the time, that group's nearby options ranged from McDonald's to Krispy Kreme, which simply would not do.

This time Charlie had to audition. The judges were the employees—who had already turned down twenty-five chefs. Charlie was hired and came aboard in November 1999, helping to carry out Sergey's vision of getting the best out of people by keeping productivity high, keeping employees on campus, and keeping them guessing with new menu options to tickle their fancy. It was clear that people place a high value on good food—as long as they don't have to be the ones preparing it.

By the time Google moved into its headquarters in Mountain View about four years later, the tech giant was already widely known for its world-class free meals. When Charlie left Google in 2005, there were ten cafés across the Mountain View campus, with five sous chefs and 150 foodservice employees. And that culinary reputation has become an indelible factor in Google's ranking as the top company in the country to work for.

The food we choose to ferry from our houses—or the nearest take-out spot, or Whole Foods' Grab & Go, or a gas station on the way to work—says a lot about us. But the environment at our workplaces—the office kitchen, everyone eating at their desks—says a lot about America. Among other things, it says: Time is a priceless resource, and it is to be used productively, to accomplish goals and deliver deliverables. Food is the fuel to be shoveled, like coal into a steam engine, as quickly as possible into the worker's mouth so the worker can continue to produce. The Digital Revolution might have more in common with the Industrial Revolution than first appears, because the office hasn't come as far from the factory as we may think.

As our offices have become extensions of our homes, the reality for most of us is: We cohabit with our coworkers.

We're sharing space, and we're spending time. Time spent in a space eventually involves some food. And with cohabitation come all the quirks and conundrums and drama of living with roommates. But more broadly, with those social microclimates come social cues that we bring in from the outside world—our values as Americans—and also cues we collectively, invisibly shape within the workplace. Those, in turn, influence what food we eat at work and in what ways we eat that food.

I'm not picking on the Googlers with their "Google 15," or corporate America for its Sad Desk Lunch; consequences are all over the place. In nearly every industry, the ironies of overwork abound: Retail food and foodservice workers are paid so little they often must work multiple jobs and multiple shifts, leaving not enough money or time to eat decent meals. Medical students, interns, and residents—providing care to help others be healthy—are so sleep deprived and starved of basic needs like showers and laundry, living off cafeteria fast food, that they're often in need of care themselves. Public health professionals study how stress kills, yet are drowning in stress themselves under the workload that is the norm in their field. Management consultants work such long, grueling hours advising companies, on the road Monday through Friday, eating every meal out, they'd need to hire their own life consultants to get back on track. Employees at food start-ups and lifestyle organizations—inspiring others to improve their quality of life—work so much they don't have time to cook, garden, or exercise themselves.

And innovators are doing everything in their power to combat those consequences. They've launched solutions like delivery dinner kits, on-site farmers' markets, and cooking classes, even vending machines selling salads in jars—stocked fresh that day, no less.

What's a little scary, though, is that most of the innovations promising healthier food-at-work habits are solutions only to a very white-collar problem, not the daily realities of the working class or the working poor. Take transportation workers, for instance, who suffer by far the worst health outcomes of any job sector. For them, eating "at work" means eating on the road *by definition,* not by laziness or preference. Just imagine the opportunities that might surface should we apply the disruptive spirit of Silicon Valley not only to corporate lunchrooms but to the work sites of construction crews, truck drivers, custodians, and the 20 million Americans working along the food chain itself.

These solutions also take as a given that we will only continue to work ever longer hours—inevitably eating *more* food at work.

They don't begin to imagine an America that heeds the calls of groups around the globe: Work . . . *less.* (!)

One three-day work week proposal argues that with people living so much longer, we shouldn't be retiring at age sixty anyway. Instead, workers could enjoy higher quality of life but work longer throughout our lifetimes, retiring at, say, seventy or seventy-five instead. The New Economics Foundation, based in the UK, calls for a twenty-one-hour work week, arguing that there is nothing "natural or inevitable" about what we consider a "normal" work week today.

The New Economics Foundation isn't against people working more or less than twenty-one hours a week, but just resetting our social and economic norms. They say:

the logic of industrial time is out of step with today's conditions, where instant communications and mobile technologies bring new risks and pressures, as well as opportunities. The challenge is to break the power of the old industrial clock without adding new pressures, and to free up time to live sustainable lives.

Sustainability means different things to different people, but basically the idea is that lots of people with jobs don't have time for anything but work, and lots of people don't have jobs. More people could have jobs if people who already have jobs worked less.

That would also leave everyone with a lot more time on their hands. More time for sewing, growing vegetables, building things. More chewing before swallowing. More sleep. More thinking and processing. Thinking before speaking. Thinking before e-mailing.

Radical? Absolutely. Tempting? Clearly.

A good idea?

In theory, but first you'd have to pay people more. Wages have been stagnant in the United States, and 40 percent of people can't cover their basic expenses. A huge number of Americans have fallen out of the middle class. You can't just say "enough with all the overwork." People have to be able to *afford* to work less.

But there is one thing I can promise you: Working less would sure as hell affect how we eat.

CHAPTER 3

Having It Our Way

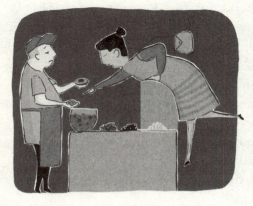

Decaf Double Tall Nonfat Capp, for Bruce."
"You got it, buddy." [Response]
"Yeah, that's a wonderful choice, Bruce."
"Thank you, Sam."
"Yeah, it certainly is."

"One Caramel Macchiato. It's very hot."

"Good morning. Vanilla Grande No-Foam Latte—that's a wonderful choice."
"Thanks, Sam."

The opening scene of the film *I Am Sam*, and the validation of each person's four-adjective-long Starbucks order, speaks to a most American element of the American food psyche: customization.

Among the first to recognize this consumer desire was Burger King, with its now-famous slogan, "Have It Your Way." While the slogan hints at individualizing each diner's eating experience, Burger King's menu is a far cry from the truly customizable experiences consumers actually want most—and the customizable experiences they're able to have now, thanks to the rise of the fast-casual restaurant sector, online ordering and other new technologies, and a cultural shift that has made personalization the expectation in nearly every part of our lives.

Did you know there are eighty-seven *thousand* different drink combinations at Starbucks? The company has bragged about this at public appearances, on its website, and in full-page ads in *The Wall Street Journal* and *The New York Times*. It's as if they're saying: No two individuals are the same, so neither are their frappuccinos. Just like . . . snowflakes. (Sigh.)

Nowadays, there's a Starbucks on every corner, a Chipotle in every strip mall. Each diner designs her own burrito or bowl or tacos exactly to her liking. From 500 flavors of individual-size Keurig cups of coffee and tea to the countless assembly-line style restaurant chains, we are living in the Era of Infinite Choice. Americans are hardwired to personalize and individualize our eating experiences. Customization, it seems, is our birthright.

Having It Our Way, *At a Restaurant*

In 1974, Burger King's "Have It Your Way" commercial debuted on TV: It's a bright, clear day, and a blond, cereal-box-model-looking family of four spills out of a blue and brown station wagon, racing toward the door of Burger King as if late for a Bee Gees concert. After reaching the counter, the father—whose head, like his wife's, floats above a shelf of pointy, patterned triangular collars—places the following order: Two Whoppers, Two Whopper Juniors, and four Coca-Colas. He then tilts his head coyly like Bambi would and leans slightly toward the cashier, who looks like a supermodel. With a gee-whiz kind of deference, he asks, "And, would I have to wait long if you made one Whopper with *no* pickle and *no* lettuce?"

"No sir," she replies, with heaps of pep. Wearing an orange and red pontoon hat, she then grabs the intercom microphone and belts out their famous jingle. It encourages customers to make special orders like not having pickles or lettuce, ending with "All we ask is that you let us . . . serve it your way!"

The mother, emboldened, says, "Oh, well, in that case, could I have the other Whopper with extra ketchup?"

"Sure!" the cashier replies.

The mother's face lights up as if she's just won *The Price Is Right* showcase. The second Broadway solo follows, describing how you can have any toppings you want: "Any way you think is proper, have it your wayyy!"

The family collects their Whoppers, and the father turns to them to say, "Now *that*'s the way to do things—*our* way."*

---

* Stunningly, this ad with the family and the singing cashier is among the least bizarre in Burger King's history of bizarre commercials, especially a string of ads from 2008 to 2009. There was the one in 2008 where they portrayed "Whopper virgins"—rural villagers in places like Romania and Greenland— taking their first bite, with lines like, "If you want a real opinion about a burger, ask someone who doesn't even have a word for burger." Then there was the one in 2009 that showed a woman showering in a bikini made of hamburger buns, as part of a campaign to "win a date with our shower babe," and another showing a woman with bright red lipstick, mouth agape, as a "BK super seven incher" moved toward her mouth. The tagline read, "It'll blow your mind away." Chief global marketing officer at Burger King at the time, Russ Klein, told *USA Today* in 2005 that given their core customer is age eigh-

As a *New York Post* article said, "Anybody who started getting serious about clogging his or her arteries with animal fat during the '70s knows that jingle."

The slogan stuck around until 2014, when Burger King changed it to "Be Your Way." Just barely not the same as "Have It Your Way." Aside from the new slogan's grammatical issues, it is unclear what on earth it means. Burger King's press release stated that Be Your Way "reminds people that no matter who they are, they can order how they want to in BURGER KING® restaurants and that they can and should *live* how they want anytime. It's okay to not be perfect. Self-expression is most important, and it's our differences that make us individuals instead of robots."

To paraphrase: *What's the most compelling reason to come eat at Burger King? Is it our delectable semi-food? Our romantic mood lighting? No, no. It's because here at BK, you can order whatever you feel like, you nonperfect, nonrobot!*

The release goes on to remind us that Burger King has always been "a place where you come as you are, eat what you want, how you want, with whom you want." It urges us all to "step out of this world of standardization" and be different enough to "bring on the eyeballs."

Values shape what's considered normal and expected in a culture. And what's normal and expected in a culture shapes our daily behavior.

Psychologists Heejung Kim, at the University of California, Santa Barbara, and Hazel Rose Markus, at Stanford University, have conducted a range of studies looking at how cultural

---

teen to thirty-four, " 'We understand it's more important to be provocative than pleasant with this group.' "

And to think, all this before the bacon sundae stunt! (See chapter 8.)

values shape a person's preferences, from the relative appeal of certain visual images to magazine ads. Kim and Markus have found that, across the board, Americans prefer to think of themselves as unique. Consider the following scenario.

You're in the San Francisco airport, traveling alone, and you're wandering around the terminal, waiting to board. A stranger with a clipboard approaches you and asks you to complete a short questionnaire. You've got some time to kill, but what you really want to do is read a magazine and buy a neck pillow. Then they mention: To thank you for your time, you'll get a free pen.

Sold!

You fill out the questionnaire, and the research assistant reaches into a bag and fans out five pens. They all look the same except four are orange and one is green.

Which pen do you choose?

American citizens of European descent (classified as "Americans" in the study) picked the green pen 77 percent of the time. By contrast, citizens of China or Korea (classified as "East Asians") chose the unique colored pen only 31 percent of the time.

You see, the study wasn't about the questionnaire; it was about which pen each person chose and how that matches their cultural background.

The study showed that the pen people chose was determined by whether or not it stood out from the group.

When informally chatting with researchers, participants stated their choices were based on color preferences. *I picked it cuz . . . I just like green!* But the results showed the choices held regardless of which color was the more common among the five pens. This finding matches earlier research establishing that people are often unaware of what leads them to make a certain decision.

Granted, this study took place at an airport, so you might be thinking the sample could be biased, that the participants share some specific traits of people who travel by plane. They must have enough money to buy an airplane ticket and find themselves milling around the terminal in the first place. And in fact, another study did find that social class affects how strong this tendency is: Middle-class Americans are more likely than working-class Americans to pick the pen that stands out. Yet this tendency is shared across all socioeconomic groups.

In addition, there are all sorts of problems raised by considering "American" to mean "American of European descent," and that opens a can of worms beyond the scope of this book, but it's safe to say Americans come from an enormous variety of backgrounds, and those backgrounds are tied to certain values that affect our actions. For instance, if your cultural background considers extended family to be very important, that may affect whether you prioritize the wants and needs of your parents, siblings, cousins, or grandparents over your own—skipping, say, a movie you're dying to see with friends to attend a weekly family potluck. It's also safe to say that Americans of European descent have contributed significantly, and perhaps disproportionately, to the values system at the base of our nation's founding.

And that values system means that in the United States, being average has always been something of an insult. Few of us want to be pegged as merely "normal"—we want to be extraordinary!

Still not convinced? Here are two more examples to chew on: Ninety-four percent of professors in one study rated their IQ above average compared to their colleagues'. Of course, that's statistically impossible because everybody can't be above average. Thirty-two percent of employees at a software company rated their performance higher than 95 percent of their colleagues'. That too is clearly impossible.

This phenomenon, called the "Superiority Illusion" in psychology, is defined by *Scientific American* as "the belief that you are better than average in any particular metric." Ask people in East Asia the same types of questions, and you get the opposite pattern.

The desirability of uniqueness is part of the broader American cultural context in which we all live. It is so second nature to value individualism that we don't even realize that it affects how we think and act—especially about food.

Ohhh, but it does. Every time you step up to that restaurant counter, you are committing an act of intentionally and joyously deviating from a prescribed box.

"If a person orders a decaffeinated cappuccino with nonfat milk in a café in San Francisco, he or she can feel good about having a preference that is not exactly regular," write Kim and Markus in the *Journal of Personality and Social Psychology*. "The best taste is one's individualized taste," they say, yet in a café in Seoul, a person "may feel strange about being the only person who is getting this specialized beverage."

They go on: "Ordering a cup of coffee is a social act saturated with culture-specific meanings. Liking and ordering a cup of decaffeinated cappuccino with nonfat milk is a result of being in a cultural context where individuality is valued and the communication of one's individuality is required."

Think about what all those different Starbucks orders might say about who you are.

Venti Caramel Cocoa Cluster Frappuccino, soy, half-caff, extra whip. This says, *What I really wanted was an ice cream sundae, but I'm out running errands, and what if I run into that guy I've been eying at the gym?* This satisfies a craving you have but looks more dainty when sipped from a straw.

Short, nonfat, no-foam latte, quad, 120 degrees. You're a purist. A very amped-up purist. Ordering four shots of espresso, in a cup so small it's not even on the menu, below the normal temperature says, *I have to give an important presentation in an hour, and I don't have time to mess around. All I need is a splash of milk to wash this down so I'll be on my game.*

So while you may think nothing of your order, think again. In the United States, conformity is unpatriotic.

Having It Our Way, *At a Restaurant 2.0*: Fast Casual

Food marketers have taken our desire to reduce the effort and time spent on meal preparation and consumption to such extreme levels that the hassle of sorting through all the options has gotten "out of control," says University of Pennsylvania food psychologist Paul Rozin. Now, Rozin laments, you can't even find the fish sandwich, or the shake, that was the reason you went to a given fast-food joint in the first place.

At last check, McDonald's—once a destination for four simple choices: French fries, hamburgers, milkshakes, and soft drinks—had 107 items on the menu. There you stand, beneath panels and panels of menu items in tiny print, eyes scanning up, down, side-to-side, unable to make up your mind, until you're ready to just throw a dart at the thing.

This speaks to the now-famous "Paradox of Choice," the situation explained by Swarthmore College psychology professor Barry Schwartz that having more choices can actually make us feel *less* satisfied. Paralyzed even. Many consumers simultaneously say they are satisfied by having personalized choices when eating out, *and* that there is an excessive amount of choice at many places.

"I think there's going to be a response to these menus that take fifteen minutes to read," Rozin told me in the spring of 2014.

He turned out to be right. Recent figures from Datassential Menu Trends show that, basically, Americans don't like to read. Er, when it comes to the menu-as-textbook, they're over it. And in the last several years, restaurants have been responding. New restaurants classified as "fast casual" have been offering fewer items to start with, on average about forty items fewer. Instead, they emphasize quality: both in the food (often made in-house that day, with seasonal and/or local ingredients), and in the experience (often more upscale décor, with more gentle lighting). Existing chains—including McDonald's but also others like Olive Garden and IHOP—have been paring down the number of items on their menus.

Some places, such as The Cheese Board Collective and Sliver in Berkeley, California, have just one option on the menu each day. If, on Wednesday, December 10, you don't like pizza with citrus zest, garlic olive oil, Emmentaler, baby chard, and roasted kabocha squash, you will be dining elsewhere. Come back and see what they have the next day.

For decades, many restaurants gave us customization in the sense of providing an ever larger number of permutations of mood × price × dietary restriction × taste preference. For example: feeling guilty about this morning's bear claw × no restraints on cost × lactose intolerant × picky eater might lead to the Grilled Chicken Sandwich at Chick-fil-A, which is a marinated, boneless chicken breast on a toasted multigrain bun that's only 320 calories. It comes with lettuce and tomato but no cheese, and you skip the Honey Roasted BBQ Sauce, but make it a meal by adding a large fruit cup and a large diet lemonade. This classic system meant greater odds that during a given visit, every customer would fall into one of the buckets generated by those permutations. But now, we want to build our own damn bucket.

According to food industry research experts, customized dining options are now more available to us than ever before. A major driver is the growth in fast-casual restaurants. Your Paneras and your Baja Freshes, your Shake Shacks and your Noodles & Companys. And don't you dare call them fast food. The number of diners visiting fast-casual restaurants grew at ten times the rate of traffic to fast-food restaurants from 1999 through 2014. Double-digit growth is expected to continue through 2022, compared to an increase of just half a percentage point for the rest of the restaurant industry. Sales at numerous fast-food chains have been dropping.

Fast casual is all around us, yet a mere 5 percent of consumers are familiar with the term. So let me take a stab.

Think of fast casual as the Goldilocks of restaurant-going.

Wendy's, Burger King, KFC, Pizza Hut—those places sell ungodly quantities of low-quality food from a menu of scripture-length choices that are highly processed, prepared far away, in bulk. The food is made using standardized, mechanized cooking methods to ensure transportability and uniformity, sold at rock-bottom prices, served within so little time you can keep your engine running. On the other end, fine dining sells teensy quantities of the best-quality food from a menu of single-digit choices that are prepared on the premises, by humans trained in culinary excellence. The food is prepared from scratch to ensure optimal flavor and presentation, sold at sticker-shock prices, served within so much time it's worth having a pimply teenager valet park your car in a lot somewhere.

Fast casual, however, sells reasonable quantities of reasonable quality food from a menu listing a reasonable number of choices. The food is prepared partly far away and partly on-site, to ensure adequate freshness and temperature, sold at decent prices, served within enough time to gather your napkins and beverage and secure a booth.

In other words, for many, fast casual is *juuuust* right.

Plus, fast-casual restaurants tend to appeal to environmental and social responsibility concerns you might have, or at least feel you're supposed to have—from their locally sourced ingredients and compostable cutlery to the reclaimed wood beams that line the booths.

Part of why fast-casual menus feel approachable and infinite at the same time is that many follow the create-your-own-meal concept. For example, at Blaze Pizza, Custom Fuel Pizza, and that one with the funny name, &Pizza, you can pick your dough and cheese, point to your favorite toppings, and have your personal pizza baked in just minutes. At the DC-based Mediterranean spot Cava Mezze Grill—which Zagat calls a "Greek spin on the Chipotle model"—you start with a base of anything from salad to mini pitas to a rice bowl, choose up to three dips or spreads, from harissa to "crazy feta," throw in a "hearty protein" and some toppings, and finish it off with a dressing. Everyone from the vegetarian yogi to the carnivorous football player is happy.

At the Encinitas Fish Shop in Southern California, you pick your type of fish, your marinade, whether to have it grilled or fried, and whether to have it as a sandwich, taco, salad, or plate with sides. The Counter gives diners a clipboard with an order sheet to "Build Your Own Burger." The chain, which boasts 312,120 possible burger concoctions, urges customers on its website to "Create something special. Show us what you've got."

Whether it's salads or rice bowls, wraps or noodle bowls, at Sweetgreen or Asian Box or Tava Indian Kitchen, you're given a set of starting blocks, and you construct your masterpiece. At all of these places, you can add a little flair, take up the heat, or go wild and combine sauces.

And because you work your way through different menu choices one batch at a time, the decision as a whole doesn't feel as daunting.

Not only do these restaurants not reprimand you for making special requests, they *require* that you be a participant in the process. That's a long way from don't you dare hold the pickle!

It's not only Chipotlified restaurants that are successful, though. To make sure we don't lose sight of this fact amid the landscape of next-generation have-it-your-way concepts, consider these two stats:

1.   80 percent of Americans live within twenty miles of a Starbucks. (For fun: Over 70 percent of married Americans live within thirty miles of their mother or mother-in-law. Awww.)
2.   About one in seven Americans received a Starbucks gift card during the 2014 holiday season. That's 46 million people.

Clearly, the harbinger of the customized consumption craze is still wildly popular.

Consumer insights researcher Michael Barry calls directing your order—adding tomato, subtracting onion, doubling the pepper jack—"cheffing." A professor of mechanical engineering at Stanford, he is also a founder of Point Forward, a boutique firm of innovation consultants who uncover hidden insights about how people behave. For example, in the late 1990s, the major aluminum manufacturer Alcoa came to Barry and his team with a concern about competition from plastic bottles. Point Forward consultants went into people's homes and discovered they had trouble finding room in their refrigerators for multipacks of aluminum cans, so they'd leave them in the garage, often forgetting about them altogether. Point Forward connected Alcoa to a major paperboard producer and developed a prototype for what became the almighty Fridge Pack. The long, narrow box of cans now fits neatly on a shelf, and strategic perforation makes it easy to grab one cold can out at a time. It was a huge leap forward in the history of beverage packaging, and it was just one of many times Barry and his colleagues at Point Forward, as well as his new firm, Quotient Design Research, have helped clients translate detailed ethnographic research into innovative products and services.

Barry says that cheffing has been happening at places like Subway and Baskin-Robbins for years, and it's so widespread we don't think twice about it.

By contrast, psychologist Rozin says, "The French, for example, have a very strong national cuisine that they love, so you don't fuck around with it." You would never walk into a French restaurant and start adding your own ketchup or salt and pepper to your entrée, he points out.

In the United States, though, cheffing is expected. And it's about more than nailing your favorite combination of sandwich toppings. It's about not feeling like a "cog in a machine," Barry says. "When you go to McDonald's, and see it with fresh eyes, it's pretty terrifying . . . There are data displays, chutes that stuff flies down, things are beeping and buzzing. So it's this idea of, 'I won't be processed.'"

Removing and adding and dictating even the smallest specification goes a tremendous distance in our minds. You could order a chicken sandwich that's been lying around for weeks in who knows what dank corner of the walk-in freezer, but then a deli counter worker heats it up, tops it with a lettuce leaf and the pesto aioli you sub for standard mayo, and your perception is that it's been transformed. According to Barry, when a fast-food worker merely looks at customers while preparing their meals, they report their food actually *tastes fresher.*

He explains: "The standard at this point for fast food is so incredibly low that to have someone make eye contact, give you a little more guacamole, it's like 'Wow, that was truly done for me. That was having it my way.'"

Cheffing, he says, is in many ways about regaining some amount of control; it's about seeing who is making your food and what kind of treatment it receives before arriving in your belly.

Barry continues: "Anything that allows this to feel in some way more like an actual meal . . . ways to reduce the guilt of like, 'I am a good mom, but I'm holding down two jobs and I'm commuting fifty miles to pull all this together, so at least I'm giving [my kids] hot food. God, I wish it were just a little healthier. I wish it weren't made by a machine.'"

So cheffing is also about freshness, yet another trait we value in our food. One that is at odds with other values. Depending on our individual situations, most of us don't have time/make time/feel like spending time preparing our own food. Yet the machinery designed for mass production is not built for delivering food that is either fresh *or* individualized. The processing and preparation happen far away from the site of consumption, and the result will be nearly identical for every customer. Adding that lettuce or tomato is about denying this reality.

Having It Our Way, *Thanks to Technology*

Today's technology has revolutionized the importance of customization in American culture. You can customize the photo on your credit card, create your perfect bike from the pedals up, select from more than a hundred color combinations of Jambox speakers, and design an Indochino suit to match your every dimension. There's a company called YouBar that combines Americans' passion for protein, convenience, and customization all in one by letting you create your own energy bar.

For a limited time, it was possible to get Pepperidge Farm Goldfish crackers "your way," so I decided to order a box for my Goldfish-loving friend. I visited www.GoldfishMyWay.com, picked an occasion and two colors for the fish, wrote a message, and uploaded a photo of us together. What a rush!

She was giddy at the sight of our faces on the box, which was a relief because my own expression must have revealed how creepy I thought the red fish turned out in the, uh, flesh. But still: It made her day. The Goldfish people gave me an opportunity to create a personalized, meaningful gift for someone.

I'm not alone in my gratitude: According to research firm Datamonitor, the strongest factor in consumers' assessment of good value for their money is feeling that the product meets their personal needs. Customizing our eating is a way of "resisting the standardization and homogeneity of modern life," writes leading food scholar Warren Belasco, professor emeritus of American Studies at University of Maryland, Baltimore County, in his book *Food: The Key Concepts*. A Bain survey of shoppers shows that having the opportunity to customize a product inspires brand loyalty. This was the first time I had ever considered that Goldfish crackers *had* a website, much less made a point of visiting it. But apparently, I'm now more likely to engage with Pepperidge Farm, visit their site more often, and linger longer on a given page.

Customization isn't a new concept. But it's now more possible for the customer to experience exactly what he or she wants. The Internet and its many pathways to technological innovations have brought this on more than anything else. As a culture, we have shifted from customization as a nice-to-have experience, or a luxury even, to a must-have, an expectation.

Today, we have so many choices we may not even realize how unprecedented it is to have them all. We have the food scientist and industry consultant Howard Moskowitz to thank in part. In 1986 he proposed a radical *three* iterations of a similar product, Maxwell House coffee: weak, medium, and strong, turning coffee from a one-size-fits-all to a segmented grocery product. As Michael Moss writes in *Salt Sugar Fat,* "This was a novel concept at the time. The American consumer was viewed as a singular target, uncomplicated by variation, and every food company making every grocery product was focused on finding the one perfect formulation."

To see why all this is a big deal, let's pause to remember how it used to be. When shopping for a blender, you had your choice of maybe three brands at your local department store, and they came in maybe beige, mustard, and pistachio. It wasn't just foods and home goods, though; limited options were pretty standard in most aspects of life. When shopping for boyfriends, for instance, you had your choice of your dad's colleague's son, your parents' neighbor who became sorta cute after college, your aunt's personal trainer, or maybe your fling from back in high school.

In today's dating world, you can step up to the counter and tailor the life partner you'd like to, ahem, order: "Uh yes, hi, I'd like one athletic, twenty-eight-year-old working professional, available for pick-up, today, in the 206 area code. Let's add a college degree, a slack-key guitar, a Jewish mother, and . . . a knack for craft brewing. Extra curly hair on top, but skip the back fur. And no cats. Oh, and if it's not too much trouble, can we make that a double tall? I like to wear heels."

Bringing the topic back to food, *Time* magazine's Belinda Luscombe said it best: "In terms of choice, that's like going from eating whatever Mom is serving for dinner to carrying a plate around an all-you-can-eat buffet stocked by every restaurant in the world while people dump food onto it."

With the meal-tailoring floodgates flung wide open, we're doing a lot more me-centric eating. Today, over half of our eating and drinking occasions are alone.

According to the U.S. Census Bureau, the percentage of households with married couples and kids was down 50 percent in 2012 compared with 1970. Twenty-seven percent of U.S. households in 2012 were single-person households, compared with just 17 percent in 1970. Compared with 1950, ten times as many Americans age eighteen to thirty-four lived alone in 2012. And the change is especially noticeable among men living alone, for whom the percentage doubled from 6 to 12 percent between 1970 and 2012.

These stats affect who is out buying food, and therefore *whose* way is being had.

Today, only two in ten "primary shoppers"—the person who does the majority of grocery shopping in a household—are mothers with kids under eighteen. And stunningly, nearly half of the primary shoppers are male. So the old model of Mom out buying groceries for the whole family is, well, an old model.

The Internet and iPhones and other new technologies have led to two major cultural shifts related to individualized eating. The first is a new shade of customization beyond individual tastes: We now customize our eating throughout the day to fit our *moods,* our specific biological needs and urges.

"We can actually decide almost hour by hour, meal by meal," says Melissa Abbott of the Hartman Group. "It's not the idea of, 'I'm gonna thaw out this chicken breast for dinner.' That doesn't work. Everyone decides half an hour or so before what they want for dinner, because it's like, 'Oh shoot, I had a chicken Caesar for lunch, I actually don't want that anymore.'"

It's no longer worth expending the energy to decide in advance what to eat, because not only will you likely change your mind by the time dinner rolls around, you have all the tools to meet those changed needs. You can evaluate and re-evaluate on an hourly basis. Did you get enough sleep, how's your energy level, did you have a stressful meeting, was there a birthday celebration at lunch, or did you end up grabbing burgers at Five Guys with coworkers last night?

Convenience is no longer compromised quality—McDonald's drive-thru, say—but paying a small premium to meet your exact desires at a given moment.

To see how, let's go back to grocery shopping for a moment. It used to be that you'd map out your meals for the week, take stock of what you already had, and make a list of what you needed. You'd likely make one major grocery run a week. And it would typically be to the same supermarket each week. But this way of obtaining food is becoming less and less common.

Instead, grocery trips are more frequent and less planned, with lists made right before the trip as opposed to a week in advance. And the experience is more fragmented, buying different items from different places at different times. Consumers might make a trip to Costco or Safeway twice a month for staples, but fill in throughout the week with one-off trips to the closest drug store or a neighborhood grocer. Better yet, they might realize on the bus home from work that they just *have* to bake snickerdoodle cookies that night. They can pull up any number of recipe apps and grocery delivery apps, and have baking soda, cream of tartar, and butter delivered to their door by dessert time.

Minute-by-minute customized eating is also linked to the "quantified self" movement. Maybe you wear a Fitbit or one of countless other activity trackers that monitor things like heart rate, sleep, and how many steps you take and how many calories you burn in a given day. Around 6:00 P.M. you see that, aw shucks, you didn't get in as many steps today as you'd hoped. Better go for the salad for dinner. So you pull up one of any number of a third category of food apps—prepared foods from stores and restaurants in your city—and they'll deliver it to wherever you are.

The reasons for these habits are clear: Eighty-two percent of smartphone users feel technology has improved how well they eat, according to Abbott.

Millennials—and the stream of technologies we adopt early and fervently—are the drivers of this change. According to *The Washington Post,* market research suggests that "this more spontaneous approach to meal-planning reflects broader changes in food culture that are likely to remain endemic to this generation."

On top of all this is a change in the ordering and payment platforms now available, from kiosks to mobile apps. These enable diners to customize a meal, whether making it a combo, adding avocado, or picking light, medium, or heavy on the aioli. It's cheffing by touch screen. Even better, these systems save your purchase history so the next time you don't have to enter all your personal specs. The digital age has given us what we've all dreamed of: That local eatery where they greet you by name and ask if you'll be having "the usual." A couple of taps is all it takes to get whatever you want, however you want it.

The second major cultural shift brought on by the Internet and iPhones and other new technologies is best captured by the poet Kelly Clarkson: "Doesn't mean I'm lonely when I'm alone."

Surveys show that 43 percent of Americans *enjoy* eating alone as a way to catch up on other activities like social media, TV, and reading. An increased number of single-person households plays a part in more eating alone, but so does the way we as a society look at eating alone.

When the occasion presents itself, chances are you're an eat-with-one-hand-scroll-with-the-other kind of diner. You might get off work and dive into a microwaved chicken tikka masala from Trader Joe's while sifting through scores on your Yahoo Sports app, checking whose birthday is coming up on Facebook, and reading Yelp reviews for this weekend's brunch outing.

Technology has enabled more alone eating than ever before just by making us *feel* less alone. You arrive at the fast-casual restaurant Qdoba Mexican Grill, by yourself, "check in" on social media, take a photo of your burrito, post it, and before you know it a chorus of people you vaguely know are telling you what they think of your burrito, what they think of Qdoba, what they too are having for lunch, and what they would have ordered if they were you. It's like you *do* have dining companions after all! They just can't, you know, smell, or hear, or taste what you can.

Having It Our Way, *At Home*

Dinner has become a litmus test for family values in America. According to recent data from Gallup, 53 percent of American adults with children under age eighteen say their family eats dinner together at home six or seven nights a week. On average, families share 5.1 dinners together, down only slightly from 5.4 in 1997. And there aren't strong differences across political or religious lines.

So more than half of American families actually gather at the same time most nights and eat dinner together. I'll admit, this figure is higher than I would have given us credit for. In the words of Stephen Colbert: "Nation, this makes me proud to be an American."

But if you dig deeper into the family meal, it gets more interesting. See, when you happen to know a consumer behavior expert like Melissa Abbott, you learn the stories behind the numbers. My favorite kind of stories.

It turns out that a good number of families eating dinner "together" aren't eating the same thing. Family meals are following more of an à la carte model. "Consumer households are becoming more democratic when it comes to decisions regarding food," says Abbott. More than half of families cook multiple meals or dishes to cater to each family member.

Let's try to picture what this might look like.

Richards Family Dinner Version 1

It's 6:37 P.M. on a Monday in May, and the Richards family of four sits down for dinner. They hear about Jackie's spelling bee at school, and Luke's classmate's birthday party coming up on Saturday. Mom spills raspberry dressing on her sweater, and they all laugh. Dad takes a sip of his beer and pats Luke on the head.

Richards Family Dinner Version 2

It's 6:37 P.M. on a Monday in May, and the Richards family of four sits down for dinner. Jackie does her homework at the table while she waits for her tofu stir fry that Mom is sautéing. Standing at the stove stirring with one hand, Mom tries to dress for herself a salad kit with the other hand. She spills. Meanwhile, Luke finishes his baby carrots and plate of Dino nuggets, one foot on the ground, sitting on his other leg, folded at the knee. Dad glances over at the TV in the other room as he bites into the grilled chicken breast he picked up at the grocery store deli counter.

So even families who sit down together are increasingly eating meals tailored to different preferences and sensitivities. That's all well and good when the food is prepared by restaurants and retailers. But try being the home cook with all those special orders. Family dinner à la carte means outsourcing most of the meal making.

Why does this happen? Why do we care about customization in the first place? And why is it socially acceptable and normal to eat alone?

Personalized eating seems to stem from America's fundamental premium on personal freedom. Food psychologist Rozin ties it back to our country's Protestant roots, based on individualistic values that include, for instance, notions that you alone are responsible for your health, religion is about you and your relationship with God, and so on.

In a 2014 Pew Research Center survey of people in forty-four countries, one of the factors that made Americans stand out most was our individualism. Even our country's founding national documents set out to create a positive cultural emphasis on being distinct from others.

Culture can be thought of as a fuzzy set of attitudes, beliefs, and behavioral norms shared by a group of people. Culture affects not only our own behavior, but *how we interpret the meaning of other people's behavior.*

It means that everyday actions that seem on the surface to be mundane or meaningless are actually expressions of specific cultural values and basic assumptions. As explained in psychology, these are like water to fish or air to humans. Always there, hard to see, yet difficult to imagine life any other way.

As an American, I select the unique pen, and I chef at Blaze Pizza, and I use a Keurig capsule to brew myself a caramel vanilla mocha, and I eat by myself, and I observe my parents and friends selecting the unique pen, and cheffing at Blaze Pizza, and using a Keurig capsule to brew themselves a decaf gingerbread latte, and eating by themselves, and I interpret all this as a natural expression of our most basic right as humans.

But in reality, it all comes from a very American view of what it means to be an individual. We see ourselves as separate wholes, not, as Markus and Schwartz write in the *Journal of Consumer Research*, "a part made whole in relationship with others and their actions." *Inter*dependence, as opposed to *in*dependence. These psychologists see subcultures within the United States that share this interdependent value, the feeling of being inextricably linked to others, adhering to a strict hierarchy, and feeling certain social obligations to a group. But the prevailing national norm is still independence.

"The most treasured U.S. ideals—freedom, equality, self-governance, and the pursuit of happiness—are based on the idea of the 'free' individual who has the right to govern himself or herself and to pursue the achievement of his or her full potential," write Markus and Schwartz.

For an illustration of how this psyche affects our behavior, let's look at a study on puzzles. Children ages seven to nine were brought to a lab and given six minutes to solve word puzzles—anagrams specifically, written on index cards, in categories like animals or food. They were assigned to one of three test groups. The first group was told to work on puzzles the researchers had picked for them. The second group was asked to choose which puzzles they wanted to solve. The final group was told to solve puzzles their moms had supposedly picked for them ahead of time.

All the children were native English speakers and were growing up in the United States, so they were surrounded by the independence-centric cultural context. Children whose parents were born in the United States and were of European descent, called "Anglo Americans" in the study, solved the most puzzles when they were in the second group—when they could pick the puzzles themselves. The rest of the children had parents who were born in East Asia, called "Asian Americans" in the study, so they were also surrounded by an interdependence-centric cultural context in their homes. Those children solved the most puzzles when they were working on puzzles they believed had been chosen by their moms. That group solved more total puzzles than Anglo Americans in any group.

Here's the stunning thing: Anglo American children solved the *fewest* puzzles when working on the ones they thought their moms had picked for them. Fewer than when solving puzzles assigned to them by a researcher they'd never met. These kids were like, *No chance I'm gonna do zoo animal anagrams when I'm a trucks anagrams kind of guy!* Or, for some analysis by actual psych experts: Anglo American kids "balked at the very suggestion that their moms would know what kind of puzzle they should do or would like to do," write Markus and Schwartz about the study, which was conducted by psychologists Sheena S. Iyengar of Columbia Business School and Mark R. Lepper of Stanford. All four are experts on decision science.

Culturally, in independence-oriented America, we don't berate Jackie for asserting herself as a vegan or Luke for insisting he only eats foods that are orange on Mondays or foods that start with D for dinner. We say, "Whatever you need, Jackie," and, "Wow, Luke, you're so creative! Such an independent thinker." And we don't trash Dad for testing out yet another diet. We say, "Good job, Dad, you're giving the whole weight-loss thing another go, trying to be your own best self."

(It also turns out that family dinner may not even do the wonders people think: A new study shows it won't help much for kids who have a weak relationship with their parents, whereas it can benefit kids who already have close bonds with their family members. Meaning that the credit we've been giving family dinner may actually be owed to the family itself. It's likely they make time in other ways for interactions as a family, with or without food, that produce the positive results.)

You know how there is a "Got milk?" slogan for everything from car insurance to concert tickets to faith in the transforming love of Jesus Christ? And a "Keep Calm and [Do Something]" for everything from eating cupcakes to running a marathon?

There is also a widespread marketing template for "Not your mom's [insert name of object]." The slogan originated from a 1988 Oldsmobile ad campaign, announcing the new model was "not your father's." Having made the jump to moms, today it's become a general way of saying: *The times? Yeah, they've changed. Go ahead and do your thing.*

Type in "Not your mom's" in the Google search bar and you get "Not your mom's jeans/beach waves/meatloaf recipes." To name a few. There are books like *Not Your Mother's Make-Ahead and Freeze Cookbook* and *Not Your Mother's Slow Cooker Recipes for Two;* even *Not Your Mother's Divorce.* For another, Not Your Mother's hair products say: "Don't follow others, make your own statement" and "Stand out, be different, and embrace your style."

All of this speaks to that broader American outlook. All around us, guidebooks and consumer products, advertisements and recipe titles are telling us to embrace our Americanness, to break free, be our own person.

"Family dynamics have mirrored the cultural shift from clear social roles and rules to valuing an egalitarianism in which rules and roles are transient," says Abbott.

At least when it comes to eating (beyond Gerber), the flow of influence is not fixed as Mom imparts stuff to kid, kid does stuff. We don't have a Mom-knows-best kind of eating culture. Not only is it our birthright to carve out our own niche, it's our right to shed whatever rules our parents followed and create our own.

Food industry expert Balzer says that in addition to Chipotle wannabes and innumerable food apps, the greater availability of personalized eating options extends to packaged goods. There's a whole subset of popular food products—the multitude of yogurt and Keurig coffee varieties—we may not even think of as customized. But our food culture thrives on "mass customization," which sounds like an oxymoron but means taking existing processed foods and delivering them in individual-size portions that meet a wide range of specific demands.

A cup of coffee made with a Keurig capsule costs about three times more than one made with supermarket grounds and a drip machine. That Keurig habit can add up to spending $400 more on coffee in a given year. Apparently the exact flavor we get from Keurig, made fresh at the precise moment we want it, is worth *that* much.

In the United States, it's not only socially acceptable to dine alone, it's the norm and it's even encouraged. So we consume frappuccinos in our cars, energy bars on the walk to the subway, and individual-size entrées with one hand while scrolling through Twitter with the other. But over the course of our daily rhythms, we don't focus on food. We don't go out of our way to make eating an activity in itself, or to eat with other people. When we dine with others, it tends to be the exception not the rule: the Wednesday team lunch or the Saturday dinner party.

We not only spend the least time preparing food of any of the OECD countries—we also spend less time *eating*: just one hour and fourteen minutes per day. That's twenty-seven minutes less than the average across those countries.

So is individualism in our eating so bad? Do smartphones at the table signal the end of community and harmony and civility as we know them? We'll probably need a few decades to see if we all get carpal tunnel in our scrolling hand, but maybe solitary dining is an opportunity to eat our food in peace. No watching your friend get crumbs in his beard, or listening to your sister chomp-slosh her way through a noodle bowl.

Maybe it's all just a different way of experiencing food.

But one concern about eating alone is that we end up eating in ways we might not eat when dining with others. Having it our way often means eating faster, which can mean eating more; it means eating while no one is watching, which can lead to any number of things (read: single-handedly downing that carton of Ben & Jerry's or share-size bag of Skittles).

"It's why there's rampant overweight, because we're eating by ourselves too much," Abbott says.

How much you eat when you're with a dining companion really depends on who your friends and family are, their weight and how they eat, but there's some truth to Abbott's statement to be sure.

Another concern is the loss of sharing tastes with each other. "We like the idea that we're going to get exactly what fits [our] personal hedonic profile," says Rozin. "It's a much less communal idea than we're going to eat what has always been eaten, and is tested by time."

Going communal usually requires dining at restaurants

serving cuisines from around the world, where the collective sharing of flavors is built into the experience: from Spanish tapas and shared Ethiopian *injera,* to Chinese meals eaten family style, served from dishes on a spinning lazy Susan at the center of a round table.

Most of the time, though, our focus is on what I want to eat, where I want to eat it, how much time I want to spend, and with or not with whomever I want. I expect to break the mold, be my own snowflake, and yes, have a burger that meets all my peculiar effing needs.

The irony in all the cheffing and individual-size products is that there is a much simpler way you can, actually, have it your way: cooking a meal from scratch. You can pick the ingredients at the store or farmers' market or online and prepare them however and whenever you want.

Unfortunately, many people don't feel they have the skills. Myself included. But maybe we can take all that passion for personalization, that constant quest for customization, and channel it toward reclaiming confidence in the kitchen. Because *that* is the ultimate control over what we eat.

CHAPTER 4

Selling Absence

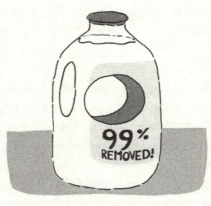

How many calories are in a hamburger? That's a question two marketing professors at Northwestern University's Kellogg School of Management asked participants in a study published in 2010. They also asked the number of calories in that same burger when it came with a salad. Stunningly, study participants guessed that the combination of the burger and salad contained *fewer* calories than the burger alone.

What the chuck? How could this be?

It can't have been lack of knowledge about calorie content, because all participants were shown a "reference" hamburger and told it was 500 calories. Instead, the professors explain that the flawed calorie estimation is actually due to something called "averaging bias." The averaging happens because of how we place foods into good or bad buckets, and the professors attribute this bias to the human tendency to process information qualitatively. People make value judgments about foods by balancing opposing goals of health and indulgence, virtue and vice. When eating a healthy food and an indulgent food together, we end up averaging the two in our minds.

Countless studies show how tragically, laughably misguided we are when it comes to assessing the healthfulness of a food, but this example speaks volumes. This study's views of our distorted sense of food virtues and vices helps explain a far more prevalent, and equally puzzling, practice: Selling Absence. That is, how marketers convince us to buy foods such as fat-free milk, low-sodium pretzel sticks, and 100-calorie packs of cookies. What we are doing is purchasing a food not for the crazy reason that it contains worthwhile ingredients—but because of what an item lacks.

Emily Green, a writer for the *Los Angeles Times,* has dubbed this genre of foods "nonundelows," because their labels begin with "non-," "un-," "de-" and "low-."

"This started with fat-free," as Marion Nestle, professor of nutrition, food studies, and public health at New York University, and author of numerous books on food including *Food Politics,* explained to me in an e-mail. "People are interested in their own health, and it's easiest to reduce health to the absence of one nutrient or food." A physiologist named Ancel Keys set off nationwide alarm bells in the early 1960s about fat causing heart disease. By the 1980s, this association was set in stone, and the dietary directives were clear. As a result, reduced-, low-, and nonfat foods became mainstays of the American diet, hitting their peak in the 1990s.

And since 2002, the percentage of new food products making claims of any kind about health and nutritional attributes has been on the rise.

Today, with the proliferation of air-popped snacks and ones

without artificial flavors or colors, gluten-free and GMO-free products, and the like, the "nonundelow" genre now has even more subcategories.

As mentioned, there are 42,214 items in the average American supermarket, according to the Food Marketing Institute. Even the small neighborhood grocers offer an overwhelming number of choices. How on earth do you manage to make it out of the store with just one basket's worth?

You walk by special display cases of new Tostitos Fajita Scoops, promos for limited-edition holiday Post Sugar Cookie Pebbles, and offers to save 10 cents on Nabisco Brown Rice Wasabi & Soy Sauce Triscuit Thin Crisps, but only if you buy twelve boxes. And—quick! Eat this sample! Your watch is ticking, you turn down each aisle and stand there, paralyzed, gazing up at rows and rows of salad dressings, dozens and dozens of sliced breads, towers and towers of canned soups.

What causes you to put Newman's Own Sun Dried Tomato Lite Vinaigrette in your basket instead of Hidden Valley Farmhouse Originals Homestyle Italian Dressing? Or Annie's Homegrown Bunny Pasta with Yummy Cheese instead of Kraft Scooby-Doo! Macaroni & Cheese?

The fruits and vegetables in the produce section call to you in ways that are different from foods in other parts of the grocery store: There is, say, color. Waxy perfection. Lack of blemishes. Little orbs shining like Christmas ornaments. There's also touch—maybe you feel up some avocados to test their ripeness. Or maybe you even smell the cantaloupe.

But almost everything else in the store is not foods so much as what author Michael Pollan calls "edible foodlike substances." These highly processed products rely on their signage to speak to us as consumers. Impulse buys account for as many as eight of ten items we might purchase at the supermarket, according to retail studies. Price plays a key role in these decisions, of course, but so does packaging. Think of organic food products with their scenes of a farmhouse surrounded by rolling hills of wheat and soft, brown paper-y feeling bags, or children's food products with their large, kid-friendly lettering, bright colors, and popular cartoon characters.

And then there are the words on the package. So forget about *Words with Friends*. Let's play Words with Foods.

What words are powerful enough to flip the switch from scanning thousands of products on a shelf to actually taking one home to live in your house, and ultimately to be put into your body? What causes you to shift from eating a little of this "edible foodlike substance" to downing the whole bag?

"Low-Fat"

For two days in 2006, nearly 400 incoming university students and their families attended an open house. Exhibits on food science and nutrition were on display, and guests received plastic bowls and sanitary gloves. Then everyone was invited to help themselves from one of two gallon-size bowls of M&M's.

The bowls were in different areas, hidden from one another. Both were filled with uncommon colors of M&M's (gold, teal, purple, and white), but one had a label that read, "New Colors of Regular M&M's," while the other read, "New 'Low-Fat' M&M's." Keep in mind that a standard bag of M&M's contains 30 percent of the U.S. Food and Drug Administration (FDA) daily allowance for saturated fat, and 14 percent of the allowance for total fat.

The researchers found that people eating from the "low-fat" bowl ate 28 percent *more* M&M's than those who ate from the regular bowl. Among overweight participants, the increase was far greater: They consumed 47 percent more, or ninety calories more than participants eating from the regular bowl.

Of course, the M&M's were all the same. No such low-fat product was actually available. But the *perception* that the M&M's were low fat led people to eat more of them.

Other research has found people pouring themselves 28 percent more than the recommended serving size of milk when it was labeled skim versus whole, and serving themselves 71 percent more than the recommended serving size of coleslaw when it was labeled reduced fat.

We attribute all kinds of health benefits to foods labeled "low-fat," in a phenomenon called "health halos." For decades, we've had linked in our minds the ideas of fat and disease, eating fat and *being* fat. For these reasons, among others, we associate fat with "bad" and assume that removing it makes the food "good." For people who read nutrition labels, fat content is the first thing we look for, as Michael Moss reports in his book *Salt Sugar Fat*. We believe that foods labeled as reduced fat are lower in calories, higher in quality, and more natural. (In reality, foods labeled low fat, on average, contain about the same number of calories per serving as foods without that label.)

The reasons we do all of this are not that we are crazy or ignorant, but that we listen to the science. Our cultural faith in progress and innovation, and by extension, our reliance on new products and their labels to tell us what to eat, happens alongside those qualitative value judgments—pegging foods as positive or negative, resulting in situations like the averaging bias. These judgments are just part of human nature.

Nutrition science has tremendous ripple effects throughout society, not least of which is shaping policies that affect millions of Americans, such as school lunch programs.

But the science is constantly evolving. There is much that's not yet understood, and it takes time to earn funding, design studies, analyze results, and publish papers. And researchers often disagree.

Then there's the problem that new study findings make catchy news headlines. These bold statements often make it appear as if the nutrition field as a whole has swung the opposite direction from the day before, when the reality is far more nuanced. And as soon as the pendulum of food wisdom appears to have swung, new products emerge on supermarket shelves, from low sodium and no sugar added to 0 grams trans fat and gluten-free. We do our best to navigate the complexity of it all—fat is bad, fat is good, carbs are bad, carbs are good—with information coming at us from so many different people and places. And with such an enormous number of choices, it's no surprise we're all left scratching our heads in the super-market.

In its 2015 review of all the evidence on fat, the Dietary Guidelines Advisory Committee concluded that no longer should there be a focus on limiting the amount of fat in a person's diet. It's the *type* of fat that matters most.

The committee—a group of experts from around the country charged with making evidence-based recommendations to the U.S. Department of Health and Human Services and the U.S. Department of Agriculture (USDA), which jointly publish the Dietary Guidelines for Americans every five years—still advised limiting saturated fat, considered the second-worst "bad" fat after trans fat, as it may increase risk of heart disease.

Gallup surveyed Americans about a month after the committee's report was released, and—lo and behold—the percentage of Americans avoiding fat dropped 9 percent compared with the previous year.

Monounsaturated and polyunsaturated fats, found in plant oils, nuts, avocados, and fish, are considered "good" fats. We *want* these fats in our diets, to make our hair glossy and help us live long and stuff, like the Greeks. The Mediterranean diet has plenty of fat, but not the artery-clogging kind.

So while a shift has begun away from reducing the total amount of fat in our dietary pattern, for now the total absence of fat is still one of our strongest drivers of how healthy we perceive a food to be. Lack of sodium is up there as well. How we make sense of the meaning of health drives which demons we ask the food industry to first *remove* from the foods we desire. Once we see that this something has been taken out, we'll put our grocery dollars toward it.

But when looking so carefully at the removed fat, we overlook what *replaces* it. When fat is taken out, sugar and salt are added to make up for the product now tasting like garbage. Or, at best, tasting like nothing at all. In addition, a product might get packed with extra carbs and weird thickeners and additives. All of these replacement ingredients are often worse for us than the apparent offender.

There are a couple of problems with replacing fat with carbs and additives. A benefit of eating foods that contain fat is that they make you feel full, and you stop eating. But when we eat foods with added refined starches and sugars, we burn through them quickly, without time for them to travel through our digestive tract and trigger the *pause* button. Fat has more than twice the calories of carbs, but those low-fat labels on carb-heavy food products give our brains the green light to eat more of the product than we would if these labels weren't there. The equation doesn't balance in carbs' favor.

In addition, a "low-fat" product has less fat, but it's not all gone. Not only are you consuming more sugar, salt, and additives when you eat a low-/non-/reduced-fat product—you're likely not eating as little fat as you think.

The FDA has some strange rules when it comes to the language on nutrition labels. How many grams of trans fat do you think a product with a "zero trans fat" label contains? This is not a trick question. However, you should know that "zero," in this case, means an amount that is actually greater than zero. Products can have up to 0.5 gram of trans fat per serving and still be called "zero" trans fat. So if you eat just two servings, you'll have eaten up to a gram of trans fat. (We are primarily exposed to it in processed foods as the ingredient "partially hydrogenated oils," so the way around this is to check the ingredient list for PHOs.)

The medical community has been in agreement for a while about the relationship between heart disease and trans fat. It is considered the most harmful fat in the food supply gram for gram. And in 2015, the final rejection of trans fats came when the FDA concluded that PHOs are no longer generally recognized as safe (GRAS). Food manufacturers have until 2018 to remove them from their products.

Plus, that "zero trans fat" label might just be distracting you from noticing that a product packs twenty grams of *saturated* fat per serving. The same game applies to "fat-free," which doesn't mean exactly no fat, because "fat-free" foods can contain up to half a gram per serving.

Given our inclination to eat far more of something *because* of a "low-fat" label, we may end up eating the same amount of fat—or more—but just at a lower concentration. This will often result in more calories consumed.

According to the FDA, reduced fat is defined as at least 25 percent less fat than the regular version. So if an original ice cream started with 4 grams of fat per serving, and you ate two servings, you'd be at 8 grams of fat. The "reduced-fat" version, at 25 percent less, would have 3 grams of fat per serving. So if you ate just one more serving of the reduced fat than you would have of the regular version, you'd be at 9 grams. Meaning you would have eaten *more* fat. You also would have consumed more calories.

The serving sizes listed are often grossly out of touch with how people actually eat. So this scenario is all the more likely because of the fact that I chose ice cream for my example, a food notorious for having a serving size set artificially low: It's a measly ½ cup. You might have a bone to pick with Ben or Jerry, because a pint has *four* half-cup servings.

More fun with numbers: Do you ever find yourself standing in the milk cooler at the grocery store, agonizing between skim, 1 percent, and 2 percent? Seems like 2 percent would mean 98 percent fat-free, right? Wrong. That percentage refers to the percent of the milk's total weight that is fat. Whole milk is only 3.25 percent fat.

Alongside our many decades of avoiding saturated fat in milk—the average American drank twenty-five gallons a year of milk in 1970, and today drinks only six—has been an increase in the amount of cheese we eat. In 1970, the average American ate eleven pounds of cheese—then eighteen pounds in 1980, twenty-five in 1990, thirty in 2000, and thirty-three in 2007 when the recession dropped the rate temporarily until it continued rising. So although we have pulled back on fat consumption by skimping on milk, we've shown a *gain* of 200 grams of saturated fat per person per year.

What were we thinking!? Well, we were responding to the countless new ways cheese has been used as an ingredient in new food products. Food manufacturers started selling products like soups with processed cheddar and four-cheese artichoke dip; Paula Deen helped Kraft get women to use more cream cheese in home recipes; and companies like Nestlé tossed some cheddar onto frozen entrées like Stouffer's Grilled Mesquite-Style Chicken.

———

How did we get to this point? Large volumes are dedicated to answering just that question, so I'll give you the short version:

As an American, it used to be that you were going to die from the flu, pneumonia, or tuberculosis. There's a saying that the public health field is at its best when it's invisible: the water so clean you don't think twice about drinking it, the cigarette smoke you no longer breathe at a restaurant. But since about 1930, the leading cause of death in the United States has been heart disease. (Though cancer is a close second.)

The rate of death from heart disease peaked throughout the 1960s, and though it has decreased, by the mid-1980s nearly a million Americans a year were still dying of heart disease—that was 1 in every 238 people. Naturally, the U.S. government was concerned, and that led to a series of dietary proclamations in the late 1970s and early 1980s that fat is evil. The message was that unless you like the idea of collapsing on the sidewalk, gripping your chest in agony, you need to eat less fat. Oh, and less cholesterol too.

But recently many leading physicians, nutrition scientists, and epidemiologists have concluded that the war on fat was misguided. The idea that cutting back on fat would help Americans lose weight and prevent heart disease turned out to have the opposite result.

The thinking had been that if people were told to eat less saturated fat, they'd all start eating spinach and berries by the bushel.

By now most people know the story. And spinach and berries aren't the star characters.

The food industry reacted to these warnings about fat by providing consumers with lots and lots of new, highly processed *products*.

We got the message and stopped eating eggs and pot roast, but we started eating breakfast cereal and SnackWell's cookies by the cupboard load, all downed by glasses of skim milk, of course. And we all got . . . fatter. And sicker. Type 2 diabetes and other obesity-related chronic medical conditions have all increased since 1980. (This is not just in the United States; one of our most influential exports, fast food, has us playing a role in the global epidemic.)

New York Times columnist Mark Bittman has called the substitution of fat with carbs and sugars and additives "probably the single most important factor in our overweight/obesity problem."

As a country, we haven't eaten any less since jumping on the low- and reduced-fat bandwagon. We have eaten *even more*. Average calorie intake increased from 2,039 per person per day in 1970 to 2,544 calories in 2010, according to the USDA. The percentage of our total calories from fat went down, but that's just because we ate so much more of everything *else*! Mostly carbs, and plenty of foods branded "nonfat." We've eased back a bit since around 2003, but we're still eating at least 400 more calories a day, on average, than we did forty years ago.

For a period, public health professionals made some headway in getting people to understand that it's the type of fat that matters more than the quantity of fat.

Then, in March 2014 a meta-analysis published in the *Annals of Internal Medicine*—conducted by an international group of epidemiologists and led by one from Cambridge University—rejected the idea that saturated fat is the Voldemort of our foodscape.

The study reignited decades of debate.

One of the foods highest in saturated fat, of course, is butter—about a third of the daily allowance per tablespoon. Bittman wrote a column in the *Times* entitled "Butter Is Back," and about three months later, *Time* magazine proclaimed on its cover, "Eat Butter."

Bittman said, however, "This doesn't mean you abandon

fruit for beef and cheese; you just abandon fake food for real food, and in that category of real food, you can include good meat and dairy." (By "good meat" he means *not* meat from animals pumped with corn, antibiotics, and scary chemicals, and stuffed into concentrated animal feeding operations [CAFOs] to endure short, miserable lives inhaling their own poop gas.)

There was a lot of controversy about how the authors of the *Annals* paper had analyzed their data, but they continued to stick by their takeaway, which is that more research needs to be done on saturated fat. It wasn't a thumbs-up to eat donuts every day, but a suggestion that less is known than we have been admitting or acting on.

For the time being, the conversation is changing, and low fat has been turned into a myth. So after all the fuss, it's just one big national oopsie.

The point is not so much who is right about saturated fat or unsaturated fat, or what future studies will tell us about these fats. But why are we arguing about saturated fat or unsaturated fat in the first place? We don't eat isolated globules of fat. We eat *food*.

"Natural"

Market research has shown that, in consumers' minds, when it comes to nutrition, negatives are easier to understand than positives. Warren Belasco, in his book *Appetite for Change,* says the most clear-cut negative in the United States has been the fear of too much of a bad thing. The bad thing in question has evolved over the decades, from additives and pesticides to saccharin and nitrates, to calories, fat, cholesterol, and sodium, and now on to sugar and gluten and antibiotics.

And the way to escape these bad things is to buy products that assure you they're nowhere to be found.

On the other hand, we have a harder time grasping the idea that a food has too little of a good thing, like vitamins. Belasco says we react this way because the solutions are less clear: You can take dietary supplements, of course, but otherwise you'd have to, what, eat more vegetables? Eating vegetables raises all these confusing questions, like fresh versus frozen, raw versus cooked, and whether or not adding bacon to Brussels sprouts cancels out their healthiness.

In a process Belasco calls "nutrification," manufacturers of food products first remove the good stuff, say, the germ and bran from wheat kernels, then add back in fiber and vitamins and minerals that would have been in the whole grain to start with, slap a label on the box of the refined grain product touting these attributes, and charge a bit more. Yet this ingredient-plus approach—adding fiber or what not—doesn't have as powerful an effect on us as ingredient-free.

Food psychologist Paul Rozin and his colleagues have studied the reason behind this in depth, and they've used the term "additivity dominance" to describe our tendency to perceive a food as less natural if something is added to it than if something is removed from it. Perhaps because so few of us ever really see food being processed, we have to imagine what actually goes on. Apparently, we associate processing with adding, not subtracting.

"Natural" is the leading claim on new food product labels in the United States, carried by 13 percent of those debuted each year.

According to a recent survey of Americans by *Consumer Reports* magazine, here's how we perceive the "natural" label:

▸ 64 percent or more think it means no artificial ingredients or colors, toxic pesticides, or genetically modified ingredients.

▸ 85 percent or more think it *should* mean no artificial ingredients or colors, toxic pesticides, or genetically modified ingredients.

▸ 68 percent think it means no artificial growth hormones (when the label is on meat or poultry products).

▸ 60 percent think it means it keeps out antibiotics or other drugs (again, when the label is on meat or poultry products).

All of these connotations we have are negatives, conveying the absence of certain ingredients or processes in our minds. That's why companies put "natural," or even better, "all-natural" on their labels.

But it doesn't mean *any* of these things. According to the FDA, a food manufacturer can use the word "natural" to describe their product if nothing fake was added "that would not normally be expected to be in the food."

"Under federal labeling rules, the word natural means absolutely nothing," wrote *USA Today* in 2014.

The problem with the FDA's guidelines is that what is normally expected to be in a food is open to interpretation. PepsiCo, for example, eventually had to remove the "Natural" label from its Naked Juice because of added synthetic "vitamins."

Interpreting the word "natural" prompts a philosophical debate best conducted in a high-ceilinged, wall-papered Parisian salon, surrounded by antique leather-bound books. With no federally regulated definition, you can take your pick among any number of philosophies.

Is nature any resource that emerges from planet Earth, including chemicals, meaning that everything from Ziploc bags to nail polish is natural in a sense? Or to be "natural," must something be free from human transformation, meaning eating as close to the original source along the food chain as possible? Some Americans argued in the 1970s that "natural" also meant homemade, so basically anything that takes a long time and a lot of labor and sweat, like making your own bread from yeast and air.

If you want to purchase "natural" grocery items, Belasco proposes two rules: "Don't eat anything you can't pronounce (i.e., no propylene glycol alginate, a stabilizer used in bottled salad dressing) and if worms, yeast, and bacteria grew on it, then it must be natural, for no self-respecting bug would eat plastic." Seek out decay and microbes, meaning the yogurts and tempehs of the aisles.

But ultimately, the way we view "natural" relies on a food product being, as Belasco says, "defined by what it was not."

In one survey in Europe and the United States, participants were asked to define the word "natural." The most common responses included no chemicals, no alterations, no additives, and no human intervention. Most people today think that processed products like cheese or meat can still be natural, so long as hormones and antibiotics are kept far, far away. Participants in all the countries were opposed to genetic engineering in their food, perceiving it to be the opposite of "natural," a term widely considered to be positive. People also associate "natural" with plants much more than they do with animals; this matches with green being the color most commonly associated with "natural."

We also prefer natural more in food than in medicine, and we often explain our preference for natural by saying it's healthier. But even when told that a natural medicine and an artificial medicine are equally effective for health, and chemically identical, most of the people who prefer natural stick with their preference. "This suggests that a substantial part of the motivation for preferring natural is ideational (moral or aesthetic), as opposed to instrumental (healthiness/effectiveness or superior sensory properties)," write Rozin and colleagues at the University of Pennsylvania Department of Psychology and the Rand Corporation in the journal *Appetite*.

People reported believing that adding additives is far more destructive to the natural state of a food than physical transformations like freezing or grinding. Finally, even a small amount of additives can reduce how natural a food is perceived to be.

Hold the phone; stop the tape. Do you realize what all this means? It means that we want natural foods and consider tampering and intervening to be forms of making something less natural. Yet, because we have such a positive association with the "natural" claim on packages, and rely on labels to provide assurance of a food's naturalness, we are turning to food products, which means, ironically, that the foods we are consuming in the hunt for natural are the ones that have been *most* tampered with and intervened upon.

"Gluten-Free"

"Gluten" is the term for a protein found in wheat, barley, rye, and a fun grain called triticale that's a cross between wheat and rye. Gluten is what gives dough its volume and elasticity. Blaming gluten for a host of hazards to our health, books like *Wheat Belly,* by a cardiologist named William Davis, and *Grain Brain,* by a neurologist named David Perlmutter, have helped set off an entire market for gluten-free products.

Already worth $10.5 billion, the gluten-free industry is expected to rise to nearly $24 billion by 2020.

Let's review a few more numbers:

▸ About 1 percent of Americans have celiac disease.

▸ About 6 percent of Americans have nonceliac gluten
sensitivity.

▸ About 33 percent of Americans are currently avoiding, or
trying to avoid, gluten.

Proclaiming himself as highly "pro-pizza," comedian Jimmy
Kimmel lamented that it bothers him how many people are "anti-
gluten." He wondered how many of us even know what gluten
is. After conducting man-on-the-street interviews, he found
that basically people are clueless; they just assume gluten is bad.
Kimmel said, "Here in L.A., it's comparable to Satanism."

People think eating gluten-free foods will help them lose
weight and feel awesome and energized. They see them as a
cure-all. And some become quite angry when you question
them about why. As the *Telegraph* writes, "Unfortunately, the
gluten-free community has even less tolerance for jokes than
for pasta."

So why begrudge people for giving gluten-free eating a try?
One risk of being gluten-free is the loss of whole grains in a
person's diet. As part of a healthy diet, whole grains have been
associated with reduced risk of heart disease, type 2 diabetes,
some cancers, hypertension, stroke, and even overweight and
obesity. In addition to missing out on healthy whole wheat,
barley, and rye, some people are also avoiding oats and other
whole grains that don't even have gluten.

Another problem with the growth of gluten-free products
is similar to one with fat-free products: Once the gluten is removed, it usually needs to be replaced with something. And
the junk fillers for gluten are usually flour replacements such
as tapioca starch, potato starch, rice starch, and so on. They're
also refined carbs, which give the bloodstream a jolt of sugar.

Glutino, the self-proclaimed gluten-free category leader (in industry speak) sells strawberry toaster pastries, among other products. Their strawberry toaster pastries say on the packaging that "you are our most important gluten free ingredient." You! And your trust is the glue of their operation, what keeps their "products pristinely gluten free"—pristinely!

In reality, the glue in Glutino products is some combination of gluey ingredients in its excruciatingly long ingredient list: "STRAWBERRY FILLING (SUGAR, APPLE POWDER (APPLES, CALCIUM STEARATE), GLYCERIN, STRAWBERRIES, WHITE GRAPE JUICE CONCENTRATE, WATER, MODIFIED TAPIOCA STARCH, PECTIN, CITRIC ACID, MALIC ACID, NATURAL FLAVOR, TRICALCIUM PHOSPHATE, BLACK CARROT JUICE (FOR COLOR), SODIUM CITRATE), WATER, WHITE RICE FLOUR, PALM OIL, MODIFIED POTATO STARCH, RESISTANT CORN STARCH, MODIFIED TAPIOCA STARCH, EGGS, TAPIOCA SYRUP, SUGAR, SUGAR BEET FIBER, INULIN, SALT, BAKING POWDER (SODIUM ACID PYROPHOSPHATE, SODIUM BICARBONATE, CORN STARCH, MONOCALCIUM PHOSPHATE), XANTHAN GUM, MODIFIED CELLULOSE, NATURAL FLAVOR."

Just as a fat-free SnackWell's cookie in 1992 was still a cookie, today a gluten-free toaster pastry is still a toaster pastry. Both give the impression of having removed the bad things, yet have arguably morphed into worse things. Both give the impression of being healthier and lower in calories than the original versions, resulting in increased consumption of the new versions, yet both are equally if not more unhealthy, and the same calorie-wise.

If "going gluten-free" means eating less refined carbs like crackers and cookies and cereal, drinking less beer, and eating more salad and tofu, then yes, odds are you're feeling like a million bucks right now. But that's not how most people are going gluten-free. Most are looking for labels to signal their favorite products have been reformulated, or new products have been created, and it's safe to plow ahead.

Ironically, as the Hartman Group points out, the gluten-free trend "or fad, depending on your definitions," was started about a decade ago by people who wanted to eat *less* processed foods. Then gluten went mainstream, books like *Wheat Belly* deemed it a toxin, and the shelves of grocery stores started making more and more room for new gluten-free products. Along the way, gluten-free has gotten credit for curing nearly all our woes: skin discoloration and obesity, depression and schizophrenia, arthritis and beyond.

100-Calorie Pack

In 2004, a new form of Selling Absence arrived on the market: 100-calorie packs. A few years earlier, Cornell University eating behavior expert Brian Wansink had told food industry leaders that customers wanted portion-controlled "mini-packs" of snacks. This shocked the snack company execs, and even made them laugh. You mean we can ask people to pay *more* . . . to eat . . . *less?* they asked.

Eventually a few companies took a stab, starting with Nabisco's Oreo Thin Crisps, Wheat Thin Minis, and Mixed Berry Fruit Snacks. They were an instant hit, and Kellogg's and General Mills soon followed.

Sales soared through 2008, with nearly 300 items labeled 100-calorie. But then, during the recession in 2009, the popularity of 100-calorie packs waned. Bang-for-buck overpowered pang-for-control. With results varying from person to person, it remains a point of debate whether the packs actually curb overeating.

Today, you see 100-calorie portions on supermarket shelves from all the major snack companies, from almonds to guacamole, crackers to cookies, chips to ice-cream bars. Clearly some of us feel it's worth paying a premium for at least the feeling that someone else is in charge of our restraint.

Air-Popped

From fortified cereals to chips made of every root vegetable imaginable, the number of new food products introduced each year has increased over the last decade. Each year, about 20,000 new products show up in grocery stores.

Sales for snacks are on the rise, and could reach a half trillion dollars in the next ten-plus years. The proliferation of new snack products is not only stunning for the sheer number, but for what they contain or do not contain. Chips have gone way beyond potatoes and corn, and are now made with everything from black beans and kale to quinoa and lentils, and there's been a serious surge in the number of "air-popped" products.

Take Popchips, for example. On its website, the potato snack introduces itself: "Thanks to the magic of popping, we found a way to pop all the flavor in, while keeping fake stuff and at least half the fat of regular flavored chips out." So what's its strongest selling point? Its expulsion of fat and "fake stuff."

Health magazines have praised Popchips, and celebrity investors include David Ortiz, Sean Combs (the rapper P. Diddy), and Ashton Kutcher (anointed "President of Pop Culture"). The website remains vague about what "the magic of popping" entails but assures you it's not frying or baking.

But when you shift from thinking about what you're keeping *out* of a bag of air-popped snacks, and ponder what you're actually getting *in* there, the picture changes. Mostly—you guessed it!—air. Occupying no more than a third of the bag's volume are some wispy potato slivers, which have essentially been shot out of an air gun in the company of a Top Ramen spice packet. For the record, I eat Popchips myself. But I recognize that I do so almost entirely because I get to eat 20 chips for just 120 calories. That's a terrible reason to eat something! It's an especially terribly reason when the texture is weird, the taste is off, and there's no real substance involved.

Sharing shelf space with Popchips are products from a company called Lesser Evil. They offer products like Chia Pops, similar to popcorn, and Chia Crisps, black beans and chia seeds that are also not fried or baked, but *puffed*.

Lesser Evil fills about 91 percent of the surface area on a given product's packaging with words. Consider one called Super 4 Snacks. Its package contains labels about what they keep out: no refined sugars; gluten-, yeast-, wheat-, and corn-free; all natural; and non-GMO. And it has labels about what they kept in: white beans, quinoa, lentils, chia, kale, and roasted garlic; "heavenly perfect crunchy baked bean bites"; "made better to taste better"; 3 grams of fiber and protein per serving; 110 calories per serving; "energy for the journey home"; and "made with only the finest ingredients."

Done reading yet? For more, they also say, "Go ahead! Flip me over," touting the transparency of their ingredients.

Super 4 Snacks gets to the heart of the good/bad confusion. With all this badness kept out of the package, goodness apparently ground up and smooshed together and molded into little noodle bites, and a bunch of neutral stuff—air—puffed in there, your brain is going to tell you to go hog wild. Yet there are 550 calories in the entire bag, which is five ounces. You also won't feel full or satisfied, though. It's a snack, not a meal, so you'll simply *add* this to what you already plan to eat that day.

Kale, quinoa, lentils—all things that are good for you, but there are so many labels on the package, you are distracted from noticing that the items inside are completely unrecognizable from kale, quinoa, and lentils.

More and more, we look to new food *products* to provide nutrients in inventive ways. And they couldn't be further from the taste and satisfaction that can be experienced by the real foods themselves.

Nutrition science has taken food and broken it down into building blocks of recommended daily intakes of this and that vitamin or macronutrient. Though it has been helpful in informing the public about what attributes foods contain, it has also given the inventors of new food products platforms on which they can take advantage of a titanic trio: our trust in the science, our fear of getting fat and sick, and our uncertainty about what to make of many of the real foods—from eggs and cheese to bread and apples—that have been eaten for centuries.

Food scientists will toss some fiber on flavorless, highly processed cereal flakes, and douse them in sugar, or mask the barely strawberryness of the berries used in a pie by cranking up the high-fructose corn syrup and Red 40 food coloring.

"Some nutritionists even boasted of their indifference to the aesthetics of food; taste, color, and appearance were relevant only to the extent that they fooled the mouth into ingesting the daily dose of nutrients," writes Warren Belasco in *Appetite for Change*.

Is that all food is? A vehicle for tallies and counts? Should you be, as Belasco says, "holistically minded," this approach might strike you as offensive. You might stand on a milk crate in a subway station and cry out for the loss of all that is good in this world, like a warm, chin-drip-juicy peach, gushing with flavor on a summer day.

Empty Promises
(and Often Empty Calories)

In January 2014, General Mills added the label "Not made with genetically modified ingredients" to Cheerios. Tom Forsythe, communications rep for General Mills—whose name, funnily enough, when shortened, is GM—explained the change and admitted on the company's blog that they didn't alter anything significant about the product itself. They switched to non-GM sources for the teensy bits of cornstarch and sugar used in cooking and flavoring, respectively. You see, regular Cheerios are mostly oats. And guess what? There is no such thing as genetically modified oats!*

"We did it because we think consumers may embrace it," Forsythe wrote.

Clearly it's a PR move, because most other cereals, and even *other* types of Cheerios, like Honey Nut Cheerios, contain so much corn or sugar or both that it would cost far too much or be operationally onerous to make the change and don the label. (Part of the reason for this is that 80 percent of U.S. corn is genetically modified.) So General Mills made the announcement because people will likely not know what Cheerios are actually made of. The name originally debuted in 1941 as Cheerioats, but since then customers have likely had to use their imagination to guess what the soggy little rings in their cereal bowls are made of.

---

* Why aren't there genetically modified oats? The demand for oats is too low, so it doesn't justify the hugely expensive research to develop the genetically modified seeds. The number of oat farmers to support such research is also very low. Compared with soybeans or corn, far and away the two leading crops in the United States, oats earn farmers far less for every acre they grow.

The strategy seems to have banked on our health halo-induced good will toward Cheerios and General Mills carrying over to their other products as well.

Our reactions to certain labels selling the absence of something we fear has led to a whole subset of new labels that take advantage of our lack of understanding of the food system. These can be blamed on the lack of transparency in the food supply, some might say. Hence GM-free Cheerios when the dominant ingredient, oats, couldn't be genetically modified in the first place.

Another example of a label that sells us on a product's absence of something, yet is also essentially meaningless, is "No Hormones" on egg cartons. You've probably heard the horror stories about cows being pumped full of hormones to make them grow faster or produce more milk ("recombinant bovine growth hormone," or rBGH). You don't want them in your cows, or the milk they produce, so it seems reasonable enough to think you wouldn't want them in your poultry and the eggs they produce, either.

The catch is that industrial chicken farms in the United States don't even feed hormones to their chickens *because it is illegal.* As NPR said, "It's like putting a label on a cereal box that says, 'No toxic waste.'"

The second empty claim (of many) on egg cartons is "No Antibiotics." Same idea as the images of cows being injected with hormones, except this one is slightly more reasonable to include on the label because chickens raised in the poultry industry do often receive antibiotics. The catch here is that antibiotics are used very rarely in the *egg* industry.

Not only do food companies display these labels to impart sunny feelings about their products so we'll consume more of them, but they also use them to distract us from the bad things they haven't removed, or have even added more of, to compensate for having removed some original bad thing.

Most of the salt Americans eat can be found in processed foods, including low-fat and low-sugar versions of leading brands' products. In processing, dialing one ingredient back inevitably means dialing another up. It's a classic technique, emphasizing the merits of one "good" ingredient in hopes you'll fail to notice the rest of the equation.

Take Wish-Bone Light Thousand Island dressing, for one. It boasts "$\frac{1}{3}$ Fewer Calories & $\frac{1}{2}$ the Fat" plus "Oils like those in Wish-Bone help better absorb vitamins A & E from salad." Yet, just 2 tablespoons pack 330 milligrams of sodium. That's over one-fifth of the total daily recommended limit for sodium among people in high-risk groups.

Trying to be healthy by eating products like these unleashes further ironies: We actually feel *hungrier* from foods we view as healthy, and we enjoy them less. (Perhaps this is also why people add salt to foods labeled reduced sodium, negating the whole exercise.)

So yes, we act strangely in the presence of ingredient-free or ingredient-low foods.

But it is because of what is done *to* us, and to the foods available at grocery stores.

We've seen a variety of these tactics, but one that is especially powerful is craveability, the ways manufacturers make their products taste better and lead us to buy and eat more of them. Now, that's their business, of course, to make foods we want to buy and eat. And they're very good at it. Many of the foods that are most craveable—pizza, French fries, potato chips—owe their success to salt.

But those of us who are not in the salt business, who have been warned by doctors about our blood pressure—or who just don't like the idea of being snookered when trying to be healthy by eating a granola bar, and getting blindsided by the

pile of salt we're accidentally pouring down the hatch with it—
are apt to look for assurance that foods are reduced-harm, low-
damage, heart-attack-free.

For food companies, as Moss explains in *Salt Sugar Fat,* salt
is magic. He notes that cornflakes taste metallic without salt,
crackers can be bitter and soggy, and ham can become overly
"rubbery." In other words, a food scientist can start with medi-
ocre to bad raw ingredients on the front end, knowing salt will
take care of flavor and texture on the back end.

And it's not just salt and sugar. As food processing really
came into its own, chemicals and dyes began cropping up in
newfangled food products more and more throughout the 1940s
and 1950s.

Moss writes that, in the mid-1940s, "The family-owned
American grocery store was fast evolving into the supermarket, and food manufacturers were scrambling to fill the shelves
with time-saving innovations that fed directly into the country's frenzy to modernize." General Foods was at the helm of
the movement, delivering new products called "convenience
foods" that would transform the industry and the very idea of
food in the American psyche.

In 1955, time-savers of every imaginable form appeared on
the market: two-step cake mixes, biscuits in a tube, dishwash-
ing detergent, and more. With its products like instant pud-
ding and dessert-for-breakfast cereals, General Foods helped
lead American consumers to an entirely new way of eating.
Now, every time people went to the grocery store, new products lined the shelves.

In the shift to convenience products, a host of additives were
thrown in to thicken, coagulate, rise, color, or do whatever it is
that would have normally taken, I don't know . . . time.

———

I'm a huge fan of nut butters. Crunchy and creamy alike, whether Jif or Justin's or freshly ground at the health foods store. So when something called PB2 came on the market, I had to try it. Powdered peanut butter! The label says 85 percent less fat calories, which they accomplish by removing the oil and fat inherently found in peanuts. The only ingredients are roasted peanuts, sugar, and salt.

Why do we go for products like this? In America, we apply our predilection for progress, our devotion to innovation, to food. Just as you can take, say, the idea of the telephone and continually improve it—from a clunky device with separate mouthpiece and receiver, to a clunky device with joint mouthpiece and receiver but a cord that always gets stuck in a knot, to a wireless land line, to a mobile phone, to a smartphone—why shouldn't you be able to take the idea of a peanut and improve upon that as well? Surely we can boil peanut butter down to the traits we wish to keep—spreadable protein—without being bothered by all those pesky calories and grams of fat.

As I measured 2 tablespoons of the beige powder and mixed it with 1 tablespoon of water, brow furrowed as if engaged in some lab experiment of my own, I watched in awe as it came together into a paste, forming a little dough ball. Looooks like peanut butter. Taaastes like peanut butter. But, wait. If you could simply reconstitute peanut butter in this way, it raised an existential question for me: What *is* a peanut?

We've seen our inclination to demonize and apotheosize different foods, and the strange things we do—and that are done *to us* by food companies—in our quest to make sense of nutrition.

There's at least one major problem with our reliance on studies to tell us what to eat: They study only one nutrient at a time.

And on that front, a shift is under way.

Many public health researchers are calling for a new wave of research, away from single-nutrient studies, toward *food* studies. As in, whole foods, in the context of how people actually eat.

There is also a call for greater inherent flavor to begin with, in something called "farming for flavor." In an educational material on sodium, the Harvard T. H. Chan School of Public Health, together with The Culinary Institute of America (full disclosure: my employer) call for a shift from an over-reliance on sugar and salt to add flavor in food served away from home, during home cooking, and in food manufacturing. Instead, they write, "we need to refocus our attention on enhancing natural flavors. As a practical matter, this means growing more flavorful tomatoes at the same time we try to reduce the sodium in tomato soup."

Some consumers are also catching on. The consumers most ahead of the curve in terms of health are already shifting away from an obsession with calorie counts and fat tallies to calorie *quality,* and looking at intrinsic value. They're seeking out foods not for what they exclude but what they inherently provide. This would be a much more holistic view of health.

These are examples of what you might call aspirational change for us as Americans. And I'm staying tuned.

Because for now, that's far from where we are. There always seem to be new influences keeping the ingredient-free, absence-oriented outlook central to our food culture. Our cultural mind-set is still nutrient-centric to a fault. Constantly pushing the new frontier, and our deference to science—unfortunately, these values compromise our eating. The ever-growing number of new food products distance us further and further from "real food."

I am also referring to an American belief in innovation so deeply engrained that we believe pretty much anything a person in a white lab coat tells us about what and how to eat.

"Your faith in science may actually make you more likely to trust information that appears scientific but really doesn't tell you much," said the Cornell Food and Brand Lab in a release for a series of studies they conducted. Showing trivial scientific information to study participants made them think medications were more effective. Lead author Aner Tal writes, "The scientific halo of graphs, formulas, and other trivial elements that look scientific may lead to misplaced belief." Just as we fall for health halos, we fall for scientific halos. And the former seems to stem from the latter.

I'm an enormous fan of vaccines, and if I didn't have contact lenses, I'd be utterly lost in the world. There's not a time I get off an airplane that I don't marvel at the fact that an aluminum capsule can zing me around the globe and deposit me safely from the sky. So I definitely don't challenge science on the whole. *Far* from it. Given factors like climate change and a growing population, the importance of food safety, and much more, there is, *of course*, a role for technology and innovation to play in our food system. I just think we have a tendency to exalt everything that comes from science without really questioning it, and without questioning whether it's the right guiding force for what we eat.

Because, what are we missing in the focus on ingredient-free foods? A guilt-free conscience, for one. Satiety and satisfaction as well. And taste! Pure deliciousness. In selecting the reduced-fat, air-popped chips, for example, we make a false calculation. We will eat more calories worth of the chips, enjoy them less, find they taste worse, and feel less full afterward. Just like the bag of air those powder-coated potato slivers came in, buying absence leaves us feeling empty.

CHAPTER 5

Secular Church

On more than one Sunday morning in 2011, my alarm would go off at 8:50 A.M., and I'd put on my glasses, throw on some sweats, and tiptoe out of my sand-kissed, drafty beach house in San Francisco's Outer Sunset neighborhood. Moving like molasses, I walked as briskly as I could up the two blocks to Outerlands, a restaurant just steps from the Pacific Ocean. The atmosphere is like the dining room of a ship, and their brunch is almost as legendary as their wait list. The list is placed out front at 9:00 A.M., even though they don't actually open until 10:00 A.M. After I put my name down, I'd go back to bed for another forty-five minutes.

Why did I have to bother with this nonsense? Because one time, as a weekend brunch naïf, I arrived promptly at 10:00 A.M.

and was told something horrifying like "Right now, it's looking like eighty to ninety." As in, minutes!

So the throngs who do not use my crafty approach—and I'm clearly not the only person who has developed one—and yet wish to enjoy one of Outerlands' acclaimed open-face breakfast sandwiches, will spend the better part of their Saturday or Sunday loitering on the street corner. Which—amazingly—many people seem positively *thrilled* to do.

San Franciscans aren't the only ones crazy enough to make this a weekly habit. From San Diego to Savannah, Chicago to DC, Denver to Portland (and there's a *Portlandia* episode to this effect), countless Americans are perfectly happy waiting in long lines for brunch.

The reason this ritual sticks out is that we usually seem determined to do whatever it takes to minimize the time spent obtaining, preparing, and cleaning up after a meal. Why doesn't that apply to weekend brunch? Part of the appeal of going out for brunch is you still don't have to prepare or clean up after the meal, but the obtaining can take half the day. What could compel us to spend hours simmering on a sidewalk for eggs, pancakes, and breakfast potatoes?

Clearly, weekdays are for deprivation, and the weekend is for indulgence. People tend to weigh the most on Sundays, decline steadily throughout the week, and weigh the least on Fridays. That's according to research conducted by Brian Wansink—a widely cited consumer behavior professor at Cornell University, where he is director of the Food and Brand Lab—and researchers from the VTT Technical Research Centre of Finland and Tampere University of Technology, also in Finland. They asked participants to weigh themselves each day immediately after waking up, before eating anything. Across three groups where people were either losing, gaining, or maintaining weight, this weekly pattern emerged.

Perhaps those waffles for brunch are the weekend's last hurrah.

Brunch is in America's roots, but its cultural status has been elevated lately.

If we are willing to admit that our Google searches are a reflection of who we are, then today brunch is more popular than ever. Evidence of brunching on Saturdays in addition to Sundays has been visible among many Americans since the 1990s, and interest in brunch has grown consistently since 2004.

With our working more hours than ever, and with that bringing about changes in what and how we eat, the weekend brunch ritual is also as much about *not* eating yogurt or a protein bar (alone, and on the go) as it is about the brunch itself.

The Meaning of Brunch

Ever since British journalist Guy Beringer first coined the term in 1895, "brunch" has carried deeper meaning than merely a cross between breakfast and lunch. It speaks to our weekly rhythms and signifies a slowing down, a pause.

The spirit of brunch is to make the meal drag on, even to be a focal point of your day. If you're eating brunch out, that might include all the things you do while *in line* for a table. Beringer writes, "By eliminating the need to get up early on Sunday, brunch would make life brighter for Saturday-night carousers." For many, it's about recounting foggy memories from the night before, commiserating about the hourly manifestations of the hangover. Sure, we might play games on our phones, but we also talk to complete strangers and catch up with friends and family.

If you're making brunch at home, much of the fun is in the

thinking about brunch: flipping through favorite family recipes or refining your search online—did you want orange or
vanilla icing on those cinnamon rolls? You undertake this research, of course, at the pace of a starfish. You shuffle around in
your PJs and your slippers, your bed head morphing into new
shapes as the hours tick by, and you slowly sip your coffee. You
read the news, or that magazine article that's been dog-eared
for weeks, collecting dust on your nightstand.

And brunch is not about fortification but reward. It's two
meals in one so you get twice the calories, right? In all likelihood, that no-carbs diet takes a break on Sundays, and you go
all in with your hubby on blueberry pancakes from scratch.
You know the ones. Or at least I hope you do. The ones so fluffy
the berries bounce right off. Unlike the usual toss of a Nature
Valley granola bar from your loved one on the way out the
door, brunch is about taking a moment to be together in the
morning for a change.

So the pace is different, the guilt is on hold, and often the
meal calls for company. That's true whether you're going to a
restaurant or cooking yourself. Beringer also said, "[Brunch]
would promote human happiness in other ways as well. Brunch
is cheerful, sociable, and inciting. It is talk-compelling. It . . .
sweeps away the worries and cobwebs of the week."

There's a lot more love in the kitchen making brunch at home
than in the car scarfing down a banana and a bagel. Maybe
you're crazy about your new girlfriend and the best way to
show her that is flipping an omelet like a pro. Or maybe it's a
roommate bonding activity, and you're each tackling a different part of the menu, from fruit salad to sausage links, mushroom frittata to French toast. Or maybe the kids are taking
over the kitchen and making smiley-face chocolate-chip pancakes for the whole family. Just the anticipation of homemade
brunch brings smiley faces to all. The oven heating up, the eggs

cracking in the bowl. The smell of baked goods, coffee, and bacon. Ohh, the bacon. Forget alarm clocks: With the rise of the "smart home," our vents should just start emitting the essence of bacon when it's time to wake up.

Brunch is one of the few elements of American culture that has remained relatively stable throughout our history. "Though an Englishman coined the word, brunch continues to take the form of high art in the United States," writes Heather Arndt Anderson in her book *Breakfast: A History*.

In 1896, the word "brunch" hit the United States and was instantly understood as something the wealthy did to pass the time. That was how it had first been conceived in Britain. A derivation of the hunter's breakfast of high society, it was usually held in late morning, featuring an extravagant assemblage of savory puddings and pies alongside the spoils of the hunt.

There is some debate about the first U.S. city to serve brunch, but it's either New Orleans or New York. New Orleans certainly had brunch by the late 1890s, with the title of the Mother of American Brunch going to the legendary Madame Begue. She is often credited not just with the idea of the meal, but with popularizing some of its most iconic dishes, including French toast and oysters Rockefeller. Brunch was also propelled among the New Orleans elite due to the era's stylish riverboats, where sumptuous brunch spreads were to be expected.

New York City claims to be the birthplace of eggs Benedict—an intellectual property it still takes very seriously a century-plus later—and the bearer was either Delmonico's Restaurant or the Waldorf Astoria hotel. Both are still serving brunch, and both credit themselves with the innovation. Brunch took off in the 1930s, thanks mostly to hotels. Restaurants were often closed on Sundays, and brunch was a niche that hotel restaurants could leverage.

In 1939, *The New York Times* declared Sunday a two-meal day. (Sometimes the paper calls trends before they happen. Other times they're late in catching on. Whatever the case may be, a declaration from the *Times* makes a trend official.) This announcement was an important signifier that brunch wasn't just for the wealthy but was firmly a part of middle-class American culture as well.

I have to pause on our trip down Brunch Origin Lane to tell you about an important history that intersects it: Cocktail Chronicle Boulevard. Prohibition became the law in 1919 and lasted thirteen aeonian years. Whether at private clubs or in people's homes, there were plenty of ways to keep the alcohol flowing, but the laws did make liquor less widely available. The stuff that could be had was less reliable in terms of flavor and quality. Mixing the hooch with another liquid helped mask these circumstances.

By the late 1920s, day drinking had come into vogue among the upper class, and mixed drinks and cocktails were served at brunch. These A.M. drinks usually combined vodka or champagne with something gentle and citrusy, pulling in the Parisian innovations of mimosas and Bloody Marys, but also Bellinis and Greyhounds. (The wisdom about the hair of the dog that bit you as the best way to cure a hangover was already well established.) That said, middle-class women were warned about how it might look to be hitting the bottle before noon. As opposed to, say, tequila on the rocks during the wee hours, mixed drinks cleared the path for day drinking as a socially acceptable activity for all tiers of society. And so, since at least the 1970s, moms nationwide have been getting tipsy on Mother's Day bubbly.

Brunch first appeared in cookbooks by the 1930s, and soon

after, it there were books devoted expressly to the meal. Though some items have certainly fallen out of fashion (you don't see as much creamed chipped beef or boiled grapefruit), the foods we commonly associate with brunch—the melons and berries, the pastries, the coffee and fruit juices, and the egg-, meat-, and bread-based dishes—have mostly stayed the same.

Early on, brunch was framed as the ideal eating occasion for professionals, who were too harried during the week to get together with friends for dinner, and definitely too harried to host them for one. Yet Sunday brunch was an opportunity to invite people over and enjoy a leisurely social meal for a change. Brunch was casual, no frills. It might be a potluck at someone's house, sandwiches, or even fondue during the 1970s.

As technology advanced and chores took up less of our time, we theoretically had more leisure time. Except then the work week grew more demanding than ever. So the weekends became even more sacred as a brief respite.

Our Omelets, Ourselves

In 2014, *Time* magazine declared San Francisco the brunch capital of America. (In case you're curious, *Time* also declared Denver the capital of beer, by a large margin, and Washington, DC, amusingly, the capital of Francophilia. Let's chock the latter up to either a lot of diplomats roaming the city, or the transferability of red-white-and-blue Jell-O shots.)

Yelp also knows a lot about what we eat. In one of the more interesting uses of big and scary big data, Yelp recently figured out which cuisine types are most common in each state by mining its monolithic directory of restaurant listings. What made their little study interesting is that they assessed each cuisine type as a percentage of the total restaurants in that state, and compared these percentages to national averages. In a map labeled "The Most Disproportionately Popular Cuisines In Each State," which the Huffington Post produced on Yelp's behalf, some of the results can only be described as predictable and underwhelming: Hawaiian cuisine is disproportionately popular in . . . Hawaii; Tex-Mex is disproportionately popular in . . . Texas. Steak blankets the plains. The award for most all-American food goes to: Minnesota. Dontcha know. And yes, Southern food is disproportionately popular in seven of the eleven states that formed the Confederacy.

But other results are unexpected: Colorado, for one, is the most gluten-free state in the land. What distinguishes Ohio is its love of soup—57 percent more than the national average.

So it's fun to see the pockets of different food trends around the country. But where does brunch fall into all of this? Google and *The Washington Post* collaborated in a project similar to the Yelp endeavor, but theirs focused specifically on brunch. They looked at Google searches of the word "brunch" as a percentage of all searches in a given state. They found that brunch's popularity was highest in Massachusetts, DC, New York, and Maryland. Though some suggest brunch is more popular in coastal states—Wyoming may as well be paved in ribeye, but good luck finding a veggie omelet—Illinois and Pennsylvania also made the top ten.

The reason behind these states' standing out is likely the finding that brunch is more popular in densely populated areas. So the growing popularity of brunch in general seems tied to the increased urbanization of the American population as a whole. More people are living in cities than before, and more people are living alone. This is particularly true among millennials. These trends are evident in census statistics as well as construction data from across the country, which shows a "'surge in urban apartment building,'" as David Crowe of the National Association of Homebuilders told *Time* in 2014. Add these shifts to the frenetic pace of the work week, and you get lots of young urbanites hungry for a Sunday-morning dining companion.

In her book *Brunch: A History*, Le Moyne College sociology professor Farha Ternikar writes that brunch is more than a niche or a fad. Since the 1970s it has firmly become "a permanent American meal." So although you might say that brunch is to the Northeast what barbecue is to the South, and although it appears *especially* popular in urban areas, brunch is widely embraced.

Sunday Service

Generally speaking, the wealthier a country is, the less likely its citizens are to be highly religious. In Senegal and Pakistan, for instance, nearly 100 percent of respondents to the Pew Global Attitudes Survey said religion plays a very important role in their lives. Compare that to about 10 percent of Japan and just over 20 percent in Australia, Canada, and Germany. The United States, however, is an outlier. We are the wealthiest of all thirty-nine countries in the survey, and yet 54 percent of Americans consider religion quite important.

But Americans are becoming less religious over time.

In its Religious Landscape Study released in May 2015, Pew Research Center found that 22.8 percent of U.S. adults say they do not have a religious affiliation of any kind. That's up from 16.1 percent in 2007. Meet the "nones." The unaffiliated now outnumber both Catholics and mainline Protestants, at 20.8 and 14.7 percent, respectively.

Interestingly, though, it's not as if this nearly quarter of the American population is a bunch of atheists. Only 3.1 percent of Americans are, with another 4 percent agnostic. Instead, the bulk of this group, 15.8 percent, is "nothing in particular."

These declines in Christian faith and rising nonreligious views are seen in most demographic groups, but the one that affects brunch is that younger adults are more likely to be "nones" than older adults. As a generation, millennials are much less attached to organized religion—over a third are religiously unaffiliated, compared with the general population, of which about 23 percent are unaffiliated.

Surprisingly, the nones are distributed fairly evenly among income categories, with the most notable difference being that 33 percent of the nones earn $30,000 or less, and 21 percent earn $100,000 or more.

The increase in the "nones" is related to the 18 percent of all U.S. adults who were raised as members of a religion such as Christianity but no longer claim any religious affiliation. For every American adult who has joined a religion after having been raised unaffiliated, more than four have become religiously unaffiliated after having been raised in a certain religion.

This study is the most definitive portrayal of religion in America because the U.S. government doesn't track such things, and individual religious groups who do track them aren't able to paint such a comprehensive picture. So these results have huge implications. In particular, that 1:4 ratio about the religiously unaffiliated tells a powerful piece of the brunch story.

Somebody who has been called upon by journalists and academics and many others to make many good points about many important things is Walter Willett, chair of the Department of

Nutrition at the Harvard T. H. Chan School of Public Health. And he's persistent about the importance of always considering what a food replaces. So instead of just asking how eating chickpeas affects your health, you have to ask how eating chickpeas *instead of* bacon affects your health. So when it comes to brunch, one way to think about its popularity is to ask what activity it is replacing. If people are sipping mimosas at a café with friends, what are they *not* doing on Sunday mornings?

The answer: Brunch is secular church. Sunday service for the socially starved. *Something* for the nothings. Specifically, something soulful and restorative.

I wish I had come up with the term "secular church," but it comes from Alana Conner, a cultural scientist at Stanford University who directs a center there called Social Psychological Answers to Real-World Questions, or SPARQ. Conner explains that, in parts of the United States where people aren't as religious, the brunch gathering is the closest substitute for the experience of church: getting out of the house, marking the turn of the calendar, breaking bread together. Perhaps most important, Conner argues, it involves spending time with friends or family.

"It's very peculiar in American culture how much eating we do by ourselves," she says. "We have biologized eating, and made it about getting nutrients, getting or not getting calories. We've really turned it into this *transaction*."

But Conner says it used to be that "if you're eating alone, you're doing something wrong." She goes on: "Brunch is definitely an institution that is trying to maintain, or resurrect even, the social practice of eating in a culture where we have been pulled further and further from the table."

Secular church is about affirming community, standing around on the curb with people—like at a block party—and then sitting down together to eat elbow-to-elbow for a change.

Or sitting around the table in your pajamas together as a family. Recharging our social batteries drained by a week of dining solo.

Not everyone is happy about the rise of brunch, and again religion plays a role in the tension. There was a so-called war on brunch in Brooklyn a few years back because of an outdated law preventing restaurants from seating customers at outdoor tables before noon on Sundays. The reason was to preserve the piety of the Christian day of rest. Loads of cafés violated the law, some knowingly and others unknowingly, and they got away with it in part because enforcement was lax. Customers would show up well before noon expecting to get their brunch on. And few people ever made an issue out of it. As you can imagine, the police have a few other things to worry about than what time of day the scrambled egg platters arrive on sunny sidewalk tables.

As more hipsters and professionals bought condos and settled into the historically Polish and devout Brooklyn community of Greenpoint, complaints were filed. The charge? Café patrons were blocking the path for people walking to a nearby church. (The law in Brooklyn has since been overturned, though it's still illegal to serve alcohol before noon on Sunday. Clashes over the larger issue, gentrification, are surfacing not just through brunch but a variety of other cultural symbols, such as bike lanes.)

I don't mean to celebrate or bemoan America's declining attachment to organized religion. Instead I am pointing out that it coincides with the nation's exhaustion epidemic. At the same time that we are overworked and busier than ever, causing us to skip lunch breaks and eat a collection of snacks instead of real food, we are more *available* on Sunday mornings than we've ever been.

———

Just as brunch is far from a Brooklyn-only trend, so is the controversy. Many of the issues around brunch have to do with alcohol and the sanctity of Sunday. Most of the Sunday blue laws—which date to colonial New England and banned everything from hair-cutting to traveling—had faded after the American Revolution, except those protecting Sunday as a day of rest, without alcohol. But many Americans want to go to church *and* drink alcohol. In fact, it was common in brunch's early decades for it to be served after church, around noon. After all, there was no reason you should only be able to do one or the other.

Prohibition ended more than eighty years ago, but many of its laws have lingered in some places. They're holdovers from deals with Christian temperance groups that put alcohol under state control under the guise of ensuring public safety. A dozen states don't allow liquor of any kind to be sold in stores on Sunday. Heather Long, in the British newspaper the *Guardian*, marveled at this incongruity: "That's right, in a country that promotes NFL Sunday Night Football and the partying that goes with it like a religion, you have to make sure to get your alcohol long before kickoff in some states."

In Pennsylvania, for example, the only place where you can purchase wine and liquor on any day is from government-run outlets. And they don't sell beer. For that you can go to a bar, where you point to your two six-pack maximum from a refrigerator. (The alternative is to buy from a licensed beer distributor, where you are required to buy a twelve-pack *minimum*. Until 2015, you had to buy by the case, meaning twenty-four bottles or cans.) Long adds, "America is often called a patchwork of different cultures, but [its] varying alcohol policies are akin to a crazy quilt."

In March 2015, the Georgia House of Representatives passed something known as the Georgia Brunch Bill. It would shift the time that alcohol can be served on Sundays from 12:30 P.M. to

10:30 A.M. The earlier time was selected because that's what is already in place for state-owned outlets like the Georgia World Congress Center. It's worth noting that Georgia was the last state to repeal Prohibition in 1937. So allowing boozing before noon—on a *Sunday,* as some brunch-goers like to do—indicates a seismic cultural shift. It's not just a matter of pleasing pancake lovers in the Peach State, though. Liquor has always been a big money-maker for the foodservice industry. It's estimated that this change would result in $100 million in taxable sales for the 4,000 Georgia restaurants that would participate. Sales in those two hours alone work out to an average of $480.77 for just one restaurant. That's about a $25,000 bump per year.

This brings us to the relationship between brunch and hangovers. That is, if you've got one from the Friday or Saturday night before, you're looking to brunch—and, in some cases, brunch cocktails—to feel better. And this, of course, is another reason for the brunch haters to scream in disgust. In an article in *The New York Times,* David Shaftel declared in his headline: "Brunch Is for Jerks," announcing he's had it with brunch. "The meal has spread like a virus from Sunday to Saturday and has jumped the midafternoon boundary," he writes. "It's now common to see brunchers lingering at their table until nearly dinnertime."

He argues that brunch is a reflection of a neighborhood pricing out the middle class, becoming more homogeneous, and that it's not just about bucking the standard schedule but immaturity, elitism, and a celebration of carefree carousing. For the countless young people in America who increasingly live in urban areas and often bounce around the country depending on internships or jobs or educational opportunities, their families are far away. In their adopted cities, friends become their family. Brunch, then, Shaftel says, has become the family gathering. His bemoaning crescendos to: "The friends aren't the problem, of course. Brunch is."

He's tired of the "brunch-industrial complex" and all its baggage: the "proudly bedraggled" crowds, the "rote menus," and the "well-off young professionals who are unencumbered by children" and "can fritter away Saturday, Sunday or both over a boozy brunch."

I'm with him (and the other critics) about pricing out the middle class. This issue is top of mind for all of us here in San Francisco. I've been shell-shocked by the price points on not just a simple ham and cheese scramble but everything from rent to parking tickets. And I hear Shaftel on feeling some bitterness about the unencumbered, given that he had recently become a parent. But it's the frittering I take issue with. We shouldn't shun a ritual that helps us feel more comfortable enjoying leisure time.

Time

When the weekend arrives, it's time to face up to our weekly realities, our relationship to time and who really owns ours. Whether we are in school or logging long hours at a salaried job or working multiple hourly jobs, this might be the first moment all week that we've not been watching a clock or optimizing our activities for efficiency—the first moment all week to relax.

Whether we are making a mess in the kitchen or waiting in line somewhere, spending half a weekend day in pursuit of *a meal* seems to be our way of affirming control (or at least the feeling of control) over our time.

It's like when people take a weekly "digital Sabbath" or "tech fast" to unplug from phones and computers and tablets and TV, affirming control (or at least the feeling of control) over our devices' presence in our lives. And it too is about consciously carving out time to slow down and connect with people.

With brunch, it's as if to say, *See, I have work-life balance—I've got all day to stand in this line, out of my sheer enthusiasm for eggs Benedict!*

Alana Conner, the Stanford cultural scientist, agrees: "Luxuriating on the sidewalk is like defying the man." Half-joking, half-serious, she adds: "When you finally succumb to working seven days a week, that's when you're really an American." She believes the propensity to wait in long lines for brunch is a way of creating an identity separate from your work self.

Of course, some might argue the opposite about its signaling control: Instead of getting caught up in the hype about certain brunch experiences, there are likely a dozen other restaurants you could go to instead where you'd be seated immediately. Either way, though, embracing the brunch ritual at the very least conveys that you have other dimensions. It suggests you care about down time and relationships, good food and letting a meal unfold at a casual pace.

An important element of our national psyche is "exhaustion as a status symbol and productivity as self-worth." That's how Brené Brown, professor at the University of Houston Graduate College of Social Work, described our collective thinking during an interview with *The Washington Post* a few years back. She has spent more than a decade studying a variety of the features of being human, such as courage, shame, and especially vulnerability—the subject of a TED Talk that over 20 million people have now watched.

"'Crazy-busy' is a great armor," she told *The Washington Post*. "It's a great way for numbing. What a lot of us do is that we stay so busy, and so out in front of our life, that the truth of how we're feeling and what we really need can't catch up with us." How people are really feeling, she says, is not just exhausted but "disconnected" from their families. But they can't confront those feelings head-on. In her research, people describe how, even if they go on vacation, they take their laptops to the beach and can't stop checking e-mails. She says their fear is: "If I really stopped and let myself relax, I would crater." So instead, it's like being on one of those moving walkways at the airport. But she warns: "A lot of our lives are getting away from us while we're on that walkway."

This is the stuff of Epicurus. Her insights are truly a mirror of modern American life.

Compared with the regimented, technology-addicted sides of ourselves that we most often exercise, the sense of community—and humanity!—brunch offers, can be, well, awkward. When we finally do slow down, we don't know what to do with ourselves. Some of us drink heavily at brunch because we're out of practice with social dining, uncomfortable with time moving slowly enough that we feel something.

As opposed to the numbing effect of "crazy-busy," at brunch we relish storytelling and reflecting over the past week, the passing of time, the changing of seasons, the milestones of life. Because our unhealthy relationship with time is not *only* about the cult of overwork, but also about the frenetic pace we have collectively ratcheted society up to—by increasingly overscheduling our time.

"The single biggest narrative underlying grocery shoppers' evolving behavior is their belief that their lives are 'more chaotic and hectic than ever before.'" This is the conclusion reached by the Hartman Group, one of the firms that studies eating behavior, in a report titled "Food Shopping in America." As a result, people don't want to spend time grocery shopping and preparing food. They are structuring and allocating the hours in their days to minimize that time.

The chaotic and hectic pace starts when we're teenagers,

with countless extracurriculars and mountains of homework. But with all this being our normal, it's hard to know any other way.

So we have to learn how to play more, rest more.

We have to *do* less.

The Meaning of Breakfast

To understand the importance of brunch in America, you have to understand breakfast.

A lot of our passion for brunch-going is that it's one of the only times many people actually eat foods from the breakfast category. I was stunned to learn from the Technomic Breakfast Consumer Trend Report, as reported in *Food Business News*, that just 26 percent of us eat breakfast every day. Eighty percent eat it sometimes. (But at least 63 percent of us feel that skipping breakfast is unhealthy.)

Nearly 40 percent of Americans say they skip breakfast because of lack of time. So when we do eat breakfast, speed and ease are the meal's enablers. Convenience is the one common thread among all demographics, who otherwise have a wide range of criteria for their breakfast. Yogurt is the single fastest-growing food item in the American diet over the last generation, and more than two-thirds of Americans eat a portable breakfast.

Breakfast is about fortifying you for the day ahead, and doing it as quickly as possible to get your butt out the door on time.

There are two great ironies of cereal: It was invented to be the healthy breakfast, and now it's demonized as dessert. It was invented to be the convenient breakfast, and now it's knocked as a chore. With cereal, you have to open the cupboard, pull out the box. Shake out some flakes into a bowl, put the box back in the cupboard. Then you have to open the fridge and take out the milk. Squeeze open the carton, pour the milk all around. Then you have to put the milk *back* in the fridge, and scoop out the cold, soggy bits one painstaking slurp at a time. Ugh. Who has time for that rigmarole on just another manic Monday?

Young people are so fed up with how long it takes to eat cereal that they hardly eat breakfast: About a quarter of millennials and Generation Z (those born between the mid-1990s and the early 2000s) skip breakfast, according to the USDA's analysis of data from the National Health and Nutrition Examination Survey. The rate of breakfast forgoers is even higher—30 percent—among males in their twenties.

There have been tremendous cultural shifts around weekday breakfast. "For many consumers, the cereal bowl has become redundant technology," writes food and consumer trends analyst Nicholas Fereday in the Rabobank report entitled "The Cereal Killers." This is because, with the increased insistence on speed in the morning, in order to get many people to even *consider* eating breakfast, it's got to be portable. Better yet, one-handable. Preferably hot and ready in a flash. What little nonpareil satisfies all three of those needs? The breakfast sandwich.

Much as it might *seem* easy enough to just toast an English muffin, microwave an egg and a slice of cheese, and run out the door—that's just too much work for people. Like the milk and cereal. But having someone else make one for you is a different story. Maybe they'll throw in some bacon (greasy mess in the kitchen, no good when you've got that early-morning meeting and you're wearing an ivory blouse), some tomato (which involves washing and slicing . . . you'd have to use a knife), or even some type of spread or sauce (no chance you're making that yourself). The satisfying yet simple flavors present near universal appeal.

The sandwich and salad chain Panera Bread has *ten* different breakfast sandwiches on its menu. The play-it-safers among us will go for the Egg & Cheese on Ciabatta, the dieters the Avocado, Egg White & Spinach Breakfast Power Sandwich on a sprouted grain bagel flat, and the manly men the Steak & Egg on Everything Bagel. A close contender in the breakfast sandwich game is Starbucks, with nine different options.

I wanted to try these two chains' spinach-related breakfast sandwiches, partly because eating eggs on weekends makes me feel like I'm having a real weekend, and partly because eating veggies for breakfast makes me feel self-righteous. By 12:15 P.M. on a Saturday, Starbucks had already run out of the spinach-feta egg wrap. 12:15 P.M.! At Panera on a Sunday, the cashier kindly told me they were "no longer serving breakfast." I checked my watch in disbelief: It was 11:54 A.M.! They informed me of their 11:30 A.M. cut-off. No exceptions. This goes against everything I know of weekend habits, which is that the eating is just getting *started* at noon. But my curiosity had gotten the best of me. Because what I really knew from the start is that neither of these chains is for brunch seekers. They cater to the on-the-go crowd.

Breakfast sandwiches are the number one breakfast item at fast-food restaurants, which have succeeded in positioning themselves as integral to many Americans' weekday morning routines.

In recent years, our tendencies have only moved to greater extremes on both ends of the spectrum, both of weekday time stressing and weekend time savoring. The weekdays are now even more about convenience than ever before.

On that note: Whoever invents the Go-Gurt equivalent of oatmeal is going to make bank. It should come in the usual dessert flavors of cinnamon apple and maple syrup and all that. Extra points if I can drive by, stick out my arm, and catch the oatmeal tube like one of those rope-toss toys for dogs, while my Apple Pay beacons my payment from my seat so I don't have to interact with anyone. While you're at it, adjacent to this contraption, please also invent a car wash for human bodies. Hear me out here: Instead of water and suds, you'd walk through a chamber that first sprays you down with coffee, seeping in through every pore, then tidies you up with one of those airplane-engine-sounding vacuum dryers. Sixty seconds tops and you're fully caffeinated by the time you exit.

The Psychology of Line Waiting

When I hear the phrase "waiting in line," I instinctively think "post office!" Giving it a few more seconds, "Disneyland" comes to mind as well. But I'm hard pressed to think of another element of American culture that stakes a better claim on third place than "brunch."

Americans spend about 37 billion hours a year waiting in line. That's a figure reported by Alex Stone, author of the book *Fooling Houdini* on how the mind works, and it works out to an average of 118 hours per person. It doesn't even count all the time stuck in traffic, a uniquely hellish "line" all its own. That's another thirty-eight hours a year per person, or more than sixty if you live in San Francisco, Los Angeles, or DC.

The first memory I have of this cultural quirk of being cheerful while waiting a long time was at a restaurant called Stacks in Menlo Park, California. My now husband's father was in town, and he's a big fan of pancakes. He's among the 72 percent of consumers who, according to the National Restaurant

Association, wish restaurants served breakfast foods all day long. (Some people probably just love the food enough to eat it for multiple meals, but others are contributing to the rise in "snackfast" during the week, so weekend afternoons are their only chance at waffles.) I was a sophomore in college, eating dorm food, which meant food was available . . . all the time, whenever you felt like it, however much you wanted. So I was stunned to learn that, when you go out to brunch, part of the experience is *expecting* to put your name in and immediately start sitting on the stoop.

That didn't seem so bad at first. But then, after about thirty minutes, we had already done all the catching up I figured we'd do during the meal itself. More important, I had come straight from a tough swim workout, and my stomach had begun to eat itself. I was dehydrated, sitting out in the sun, and my head was throbbing. This, of course, seems a tad extreme to me now, but when you're a college student accustomed to instant gratification, this was how it felt. I suppose embracing the brunch line is a rite of passage into adulthood.

When you look at the literature on lines, the brunch phenomenon is all the more intriguing. It naturally checks all the boxes to qualify for Exemption from Line-Waiting Freakout. "Psychology of Waiting Lines," a paper published in 1985 by David Maister, is the most cited material I've seen on the subject of waiting in line, or "queueing" as the Brits call it. It may be a thirty-year-old text, but boy does it hold up. Maister presents a Windexed reflection of some of our behaviors. He brings into focus the notion of time, how we perceive it, and how we wish to spend it.

Maister, now retired, was a Harvard Business School professor with a doctorate in Logistics and Transportation. From among his insights, what follows are the most fascinating in the context of brunch.

Interesting Maister Insight #1:
Unoccupied time feels longer than occupied time.

Like Disneyland, airports know a few things about lines. Passengers at one airport used to regularly complain about the long wait times at baggage claim. We've all been there, shuffling and strategizing our positioning, staring at the empty chute and the overlapping conveyer panels. The airport's execs were concerned about customer dissatisfaction, so they added more personnel to handle all the bags. The average wait dropped to just eight minutes. That's pretty reasonable by airline industry standards, and it seems hard to beat. But people still complained.

They were standing at the carousel for seven of the eight minutes. Just . . . standing there. The problem, it turned out, wasn't getting bags off the plane too slowly; it was getting passengers off the plane too quickly. The airport just needed to occupy more of the passengers' time between arrival and baggage claim. So they moved the arrival gates farther from the main terminal and sent the bags to the carousel farthest away. Passengers had to walk six times as long, meaning that now, all but two minutes were occupied. Stunningly, the complaining disappeared.

Elevator operators soon after World War II made a similar fix with similar results to a similar problem: They quelled complaints about long elevator rides in skyscrapers by adding mirrors to distract passengers.

In general, waiting at places like the grocery store checkout is so agonizing because you have this itching feeling that your life is passing you by. You think of all the things you'd rather be doing. But what sets brunch apart is: You're doing exactly what you want to be doing. Which is very little. And it doesn't hurt that many restaurants turn the waiting area into a morning cocktail party.

Interesting Maister Insight #2:
Waiting an unknown amount of time feels longer than waiting a known amount of time.

I'm convinced that part of why we don't mind the brunch wait is that the host tells you up-front that you're going to be waiting some obscenely large amount of time, instead of giving you regular updates as gate agents do about flight delays. Restaurants make a quick calculation, deliver the shocking news, and while you initially bristle and shiver in disbelief, you relax as you move on to the phase of acceptance.

Interesting Maister Insight #3:
The more valuable the thing you're waiting for, the longer you're willing to wait for it.

Think of the grocery store checkout again. The person with the cart overflowing with forty-three items has far more tolerance for a line than the person just grabbing toilet paper. Exceptions might be the single bottle of whiskey, or the single carton of ice cream, depending on other factors in your life at the time, but you get the idea.

A hot, luscious stack of pancakes is worth waiting far longer for than, say, a bowl of granola and yogurt. You probably had that on Wednesday. If you even ate breakfast, of course. Somewhere known or deemed to be exceptionally good tasting or trendy is also worth waiting far longer for than the just so-so café with the just so-so coffee and the forgettable scones.

The Meaning of Brunch, Continued

Sure, some call the brunch affair "conspicuous consumption." The pancakes are far too towering, the bacon far too dripping, the mimosas far too bottomless. But it's a form of consumption in such stark contrast to the rest of our week's consumption that it's not something to be embarrassed about but held on to for dear life.

Are we really so starved for indulgence? Not exactly. In a survey conducted by the Food Network, three-quarters of all American households have at least one carton of ice cream in the freezer at all times. One in sixteen homes has at least four. And 60 percent of Americans admit to eating ice cream right out of the carton. So we do decadence.

But our food is a reflection of who we are, and in the United States it reveals that we carry around a lot of guilt. The Skinny Cow "dreamy clusters" of chocolate and caramel, the reduced-guilt potato chips, the "CalSmart" Breyers vanilla fudge twirl ice cream, the extra twenty minutes on the elliptical to atone for the two pieces of bread at dinner the night before. Just as we feel guilt about indulgence and pleasure in our food, we feel guilt about leisure. When we aren't eating healthy, we feel guilty. When we aren't being productive, we feel guilty. We've got to clear out these plagues on our conscience. Because the problem isn't that we never treat ourselves—it's how we *feel* about it when we do.

"We're not really interested in *cuisine*," says Clifford A. Wright, author of *A Mediterranean Feast* and an expert on Mediterranean food and culture, noting that this is a trait unique to American life. "We're interested in nutrition, dietetics, and health. . . . Vegan, gluten-free, low-carb—it's all denial based, Puritan almost." This provocative statement is at the heart of our collective food psyche.

New research published in the *Journal of Health Psychology*
concludes that most of us value specific nutrients more than we
value the whole foods in which they reside. We've been trained
to eat bananas for potassium, oranges for vitamin C, fish for
omega-3s, milk for calcium, and so on. Not for flavor or texture
or the full package of a whole food that makes it good. This
approach misses the forest for the trees, nutritionally speaking. So explains the author of the study, an assistant communications professor at Cornell University named Jonathon P.
Schuldt. It's why the supplement industry does so unreason-
ably well for itself at the same time that fruits, vegetables, and
whole grains are greatly underconsumed.

It's also why we aggressively latch on to specific foods with
dizzying caprice, nominating a new trendy veggie each year
or suddenly putting *açaí* in everything, hoping to extract and
concentrate a healthy food's most death-defying components.
Wright adds that this way of perceiving food underlies the fe-
tishizing of certain healthy foods, like kale. "The superfoods we
seek, you would never hear anyone in a truly gastronomic culture talk about 'superfoods.' That's not about joy; that's about
dietetics."

Brunch, though, brunch is different. It's not about deprivation. The food at brunch is about feeling good. Brunch menus
are often romance novel-esque in their seductive descriptions,
rendering a diner defenseless, almost orgasmic, just conjuring
the image of the menu item in their minds. Upon sitting down
and casting their eyes on the menu, diners instinctively start to
read aloud, as one tantalizing item after the next calls to them:

*"Brioche French toast with Chantilly cream and brown sugar–
cayenne bacon!? Are you kidding me—how can I not go for it?"*

*"Banana chocolate chip pancakes with maple-pecan butter!?
Take me now!"*

"Short rib hash with fried duck egg, biscuits, and gravy!? Hea-VEN!"

Chicken and waffles. Omelets spilling over the plate. Pyramids of breakfast potatoes.

Sure, it's often over the top. But at least it's real. At brunch, there are no nutrition claims or luring labels to battle. No ingredient lists to decipher, no packaging to dispose of. There is just food on the table.

Other cultures have had brunch-like traditions long before us: dim sum in China, *le grand petit déjeuner* in France, the Sunday lunch saga in Italy, and the rancher's breakfast of huevos rancheros in Mexico. And brunch may not have originated in America, or even be exclusively an American tradition—it has also gained traction in countries around the world over the last few decades, and with that has taken on distinct variations— but an American tradition it unquestionably is. One that's been around longer than most food traditions to our name. And yet, it's constantly being reinvented. Because, in the United States, it can be.

What's interesting to think about is how the rise in brunch has dovetailed with the rise in mobile payment systems, food delivery apps, and grocery delivery services. These let you skip the line altogether, and with the latter two, you don't even set foot in a restaurant or store. Does this further reduction in human interaction during all the other parts of our dining and food-obtaining lives only heighten our need for tableside communing?

As we've seen throughout this journey so far, this book is about our national food psyche: our social mores, our collective mind and soul when it comes to eating. So in some ways, brunch is about the food. The omelet over the granola bar. But it's more about the *act* of brunch, the spirit of brunch, that's a boon to American life. As the *Chicago Tribune* said in 1980: "You do not eat brunch. You do brunch."

I take it as a beautiful sign of where our food culture is heading that at least this one meal, had in good company, is one of the things in life that's worth the wait.

CHAPTER 6

Diet Evangelism

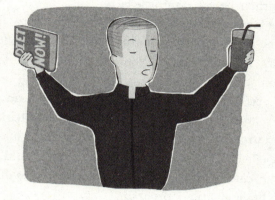

To hell with food. Not worth the trouble, not worth the time. That's the pitch for Soylent, a beige smoothie said to contain all the essential nutrients humans need to survive. One of Silicon Valley's most controversial innovations, it promises to spare you from ever having to bother with real food again.

The premise is, of course, concerning to start with—that you *have* to, not *get* to, eat three times a day.

Imagine replacing every meal with the same powdered liquid, every day, forever. It's not like on Monday you have the cheddar smoothie, and on Tuesday you try barbecue. Say good-bye to flavor as you know it.

Yet the company has raised millions in venture capital and sold millions of "meals."

When they first started preaching the gospel of their beverage, Soylent's founders hoped to raise $100,000 through a month of crowdfunding. They got it in two hours.

The inventors have been compared to young missionaries—insisting that the smoothie not only makes you more efficient, but also leads to clearer skin and a stronger physique.

Whatever diet comes on the scene, the people peddling it almost always have something in common: This new solution had been their personal miracle cure.

Soylent is merely one recent example of what I call diet evangelism: the predilection for not just latching onto the fad diet of the day, but of trying to convert friends, family, and the population at large.

What accounts for the proselytizing? Why do so many people swear by carb-free or gluten-free or the Mediterranean diet—and urge you to jump on board? Why do so many people feel compelled to tell other people how they should eat? And why is the Paleo diet all the rage among devotees of CrossFit, the mega popular fitness program?

How are men and women different with respect to dieting habits? Are peers or marketers more influential when it comes to adopting the latest weight-loss technique? What are the driving forces behind converts and preachers alike?

To understand all this, we have to first look at the origin of the tendency: What makes people diet in the first place? There's body image, for one. Thin has been in for decades, though in recent years we have added an emphasis on sculpted muscularity, for both the female and male ideals. (Think Michelle Obama's arms or Matthew McConaughey's abs.) So some people eat a certain way to achieve a certain body type. For them, food is a means to an end. They figure out which foods serve as the tools to achieve their goals: maybe ten almonds is enough to stave off afternoon hunger, or maybe it's a salad with raspberry dressing for dinner every day because it satisfies a nighttime sweet tooth.

A deeper and much-less-discussed reason for dieting is an underlying fear of death in this country. In general, we medicalize aging—from treating wrinkles with injections and creams to prolonging life no matter the tradeoffs. Most of us are uncomfortable talking about or even thinking about dying. It's often not until it comes time to care for a dying parent or relative that we really confront the idea of our *own* mortality. And when we do, it can involve IVs and hospital beds and long, expensive, agonizing procedures that are enough to scare the wits out of every one of us.

We are left feeling helpless, and researching the secrets to longevity and then following them religiously is the best we can do to channel our anxiety into action.

There is widespread fascination with what are called "Blue Zones," the five regions of the world where the highest percentage of people live to be one hundred years old. As a result of learning about the common habits of those communities, we up our fish intake or buy berries in bulk. Thoughts of longevity are the same reason many people drag their tired butts to the gym after a long day at work.

Researchers study a variety of correlations between lifestyle and the likelihood of death and disease—and we devour their results. Putting healthy things in our bodies, and moving our bodies around, can feel like delaying the inevitable. Or at least give us the peace of mind to sleep at night. After all, we've got to log those eight hours if we have any chance at one hundred.

So we turn to diets to try to *look* better and to *feel* better.

Obesity is now a global problem, as 62 percent of the world's 671 million obese individuals live in developing countries.

Rates continue to rise. But that doesn't keep it from being an *American* problem.

Thirty-five percent of American adults are overweight, and 28 percent are obese, for a total of 63 percent of the population over age eighteen.

By comparison, only 36 percent of Americans describe themselves as "somewhat overweight" or "very overweight," according to Gallup's Health and Healthcare survey. ("Obese" was not an answer choice; the other options were "about right," "somewhat underweight," "very underweight," and "no opinion.") Yet, in the same survey, 60 percent of American adults—56 percent of men, and 65 percent of women—describe their bodies as above their ideal weight. Perhaps it's all in the framing: Not-quite-optimal weight may represent hope, aspiring to reach a goal, whereas overweight might just feel discouraging.

On average, women in America feel further from their ideal weight than men do. In its poll, Gallup asked, "What do you think is the IDEAL body weight for you, personally?" Naturally, the numbers given varied depending on how much a respondent weighed at the time, but on average, 182 pounds was considered the ideal weight for men. The average actual self-reported weight was 193 pounds, for a difference of 11 pounds. The average ideal weight reported among women was 137 pounds, compared with an average actual self-reported weight of 157 pounds, for a difference of 20 pounds.

There is a difference between intention and action, though: Americans are twice as likely to *want* to lose weight as they are to actually *try* to lose weight. Respectively, it's about half versus a quarter of the population.

For people who are striving to reach a weight they deem ideal, what approaches are they taking? In the United States and Canada, 74 percent of those trying to slim down are exercising, 83 percent are turning to changes in diet, and 11 percent are using diet pills, bars, or shakes.

Among those changing their diets to lose weight, about one in four follow the low-carb, high-fat technique, about one in ten use Weight Watchers or another commercial dieting program, and one in five are following a different diet plan. About 40 percent are eating smaller portions, and about the same proportion of people are trying to cut back on processed foods.

Only 15 percent of customers of weight-loss products and services are men. Dieting among men was even more of a niche activity in the nineteenth and twentieth centuries, though, and for those who were into it, diets were positioned as a matter of efficiency: If you were lean, you were sharp, so you could perform better at your job; if you were lean, you were more fit, so you could perform better at sports. Yet recent trends like Paleo have moved male dieting further from the fringe.

Before we dive into the world of dieting today, and what accounts for all the proselytizing, let's step back and see how we got here.

A Brief History of Weight-Loss Programs and Products

Jean Anthelme Brillat-Savarin is best known for the saying "Tell me what you eat, and I will tell you what you are." But this French lawyer-politician was also one of the earliest slingers of low-carb. His 1825 book, *The Physiology of Taste,* pointed the finger at potatoes, sugars, and flour-based, or "farinaceous," foods, and warned that gorging on cakes and cookies would make a person fat and unattractive. He said anyone who eats that way will "die in [their] own melted grease." If that doesn't get you off the pastries, the angst about the melted grease will surely send you straight *to* them.

If you were already fat, he prescribed a strict regimen that involved drinking thirty bottles of seltzer water throughout a summer and wearing his patented "Anti-Corpulency Belt" twenty-four hours a day.

His book and his belt put Brillat-Savarin among the original self-proclaimed diet gurus in what we now call the weight-loss industry.

Diets go back as far as the ancient Greeks and Romans. Apparently they dieted for health reasons (or so their obliques would look good in the statues tourists would be ogling for millennia). During the 1600s and through the 1800s, weight-loss tactics ranged from avoiding sex to avoiding sleep and alcohol. Some doctors theorized that when alcohol was mixed with fat, it would light on fire.

There was also sprinkling your body with hot sand or salt, drinking fennel water, and one of my all-time faves, eating a bar of soap every night. It made you vomit, poop, or both, and yet was quite popular. And once Charles Goodyear figured out how to vulcanize rubber, people started wearing rubber undies to sweat off excess weight. But then World War I came in and broke up all the fun, since rubber was needed instead to, you know, build things.

A number of foods were said to have magical dieting properties. The plant caremyle, for instance, similar to licorice, was credited by James Fraser, secretary of Chelsea Royal Hospital in the 1600s, for helping him comfortably go sixty-six hours without eating. Charles II and his court enthusiastically endorsed it.

Various chemicals and nonfood items also became popular antidotes to excess weight: pills, poison—arsenic, for one, strychnine for another. Louise Foxcroft, a British medical historian, described in her book *Calories and Corsets: A History of Dieting over 2,000 Years* how laxatives were used for the "evacuation of the bowel." At a certain point in the 1800s, hormones and glands (especially the thyroid) became a big part of the conversation, leading to a market for related medicinal products.

And then of course, there was always eating naked in front of a mirror.

Inventive, you might say. Or maybe the word is useless? Shocking. Even dangerous, at times.

While history has seen a host of bizarre diets and weight-loss tactics, it was the Victorian era, the last two-thirds of the 1800s, when fad diets really took off. It was the time of waists that could be squeezed by a lumberjack's grasp, corsets, and other means of restricted breathing. (The irony of a corset? Well, it's a cage, which means you can hardly move. Not moving makes it a hell of a lot harder to get rid of whatever flesh that cage is designed to hold in.)

Probably one of the first well-known diet programs in the United States was the Banting System, a low-carb (high-protein) diet much like the one later introduced by Robert Atkins. First proposed in 1863, it remained wildly popular in the UK and America through to the 1920s. A similar diet, the Salisbury Method, called for lots of steak and cod, plus hot water—specifically six pints a day, sipped slowly.

Like the hot water sipping, a variety of weight-loss approaches have focused not on *what* you eat, but on *how* you eat. In the late 1800s and early 1900s, Fletcherism infiltrated American culture with a furor. This now-ridiculed practice of chewing hundreds of times before swallowing—complete with timers at dinner parties to cue a collective gulp—was totally legit in the medical community at the time. John D. Rockefeller and Franz Kafka were among the devotees.

Then along came cigarettes, and how could the 1900s have been the century of striving for slimness without Lucky Strikes? Advertisements urged women to reach for a Lucky to avoid the temptation of eating something fattening. A steady lineup of cigarettes was said to keep women from overindulging and, as one ad said, help "maintain a modern, graceful form."

The Modern Diet Landscape

There is clearly a wide variety of tactics for losing weight, and diets are one of the most common. According to *The Oxford Companion to American Food and Drink,* weight-loss diets fall into five main categories:

1. **Specific food prescriptions,** for example, eat just cabbage soup. Or, eat just meal-replacement bars. Or, eat just raw fruit. (In the movie *Notting Hill,* one of Hugh Grant's dinner guests proclaims that she is a fruitarian: She believes fruits and vegetables have feelings, so she will eat only those that have fallen off a tree or bush and are already dead. The carrots being served on the table have been "murdered.") These specific food prescriptions don't present a balance of food groups, so you end up deficient in lots of things deemed essential to human health—not to mention bored from eating the same thing all the time.

2. **High-protein, low-carb diets,** always with some new name, like Atkins, Zone, and Paleo. Without refined carbs and sugars, you don't get the blood sugar spikes, but you also miss out on the good complex carbs like fruits, vegetables, and whole grains. Plus, in trying to get an excessive amount of protein, many people eat an excessive amount of meat.

3. High-fiber, low-calorie diets, which basically rely on lots of vegetables that have a minuscule number of calories yet make you feel full. But, like anything in excess, there are problems with eating just barrels of vegetables, namely orchestral intestines and diarrhea.

4. Liquids! We all remember SlimFast, and today it's green juice and protein shakes. Convenient, for sure, except our bodies absorb sugars from foods in liquid form much differently from, say, a whole apple. Drinking our calories can lead to excess consumption because the satiety signaling is slower.

5. Finally, there's just **not eating.** Cultures have been fasting for various religious reasons for millennia, but often it leaves people feeling lightheaded and without enough energy to get through the day.

In sum, all diets are fraught with problems. They all have a way of throwing things out of whack. And what the diets also have in common is a kind of "you're in or you're out" group-think, a form of solicitation. They all involve "religion, health, fashion, and social and individual psychologies," as the *Oxford Companion* says, with a guiding logic that points to either doctrine or scientific studies to back up their case.

Dieting is big business: Americans spend between $20 and $40 billion a year on weight-loss products and programs. That includes diet books and drugs and even surgery, as well as specific eating programs like Weight Watchers. For context, we spend nearly $3 billion on Halloween costumes, $60 billion a year on pets, and $350 million on Halloween costumes *for* pets.

Today, celebrities can expect to earn anywhere from $500,000 to $3 million for endorsing a weight-loss program. Every week, another actress seems to be explaining what miracle herb or juice or fitness regimen is responsible for her overnight transformation from prego with twins to *Sports Illustrated* swimsuit cover model.

But beyond the money, the medical historian Louise Foxcroft reminds me, vanity is also a powerful motivator in Hollywood. If you're a big name on the screen, or want to be, it can boost your fan base and kick up your ego to know that millions of people will drink whatever elixir you promise will make them look just like you.

Beyoncé, for one, partnered with her personal trainer Marco Borges to launch a vegan meal delivery company, called 22 Days Nutrition. All the meals are non-GMO, organic, and gluten-, soy-, and dairy-free. The idea is that it takes twenty-one days to break an unhealthy habit. Beyoncé and her husband, Jay-Z, went vegan for twenty-two days during the winter of 2013, and they sure look good. So . . . Vegenaise for all!

(Beyoncé has since revealed that she does not personally eat a vegan diet, and that the company is actually good with more of a plant-based approach, which they've realized is more doable for most people.)

Again, the celebrity piece of diet evangelism goes way back. In the early 1800s, Lord Byron's ghostly look was the envy of quite a few Brits. Asked how he pulled it off, he revealed his secret was . . . vinegar. Yum-E. Every day he drank the stuff straight, alongside potatoes soaked in vinegar.

Given the cash cow of diet endorsement, it's easy to see why enterprising individuals have done what they have throughout history: Declare yourself an expert and start selling something, *anything*—a powder, a DVD set, a fat-sucking cellophane suit for all you care—to get in on a sliver of the spoils.

Just as celebrities go hand-in-hand with the weight-loss industry, so goes fraud. Part of that has to do with the fact that most of the industry isn't regulated by the federal government. Hundreds of products are marketed as dietary supplements, which are not subject to FDA approval, so there aren't any federal safety screenings or warnings about potentially dangerous side effects. Some prescription weight-loss drugs have received FDA approval, but in general, the FDA's website explains, "It is the company's responsibility to make sure its products are safe and that any claims made about such products are true."

But that's far from always the case, with reports landing on the FDA's doorstep of everything from stroke and seizure to death. In 2014 alone, the FDA recalled seven faulty weight-loss products, issued over thirty public notifications and other warning letters, and even sent some people to jail for peddling illegal diet products.

The FDA suggests that you arm yourself with the smarts to spot a fraudulent product by learning the list of warning signs, which include marketing through e-mail lists, promising quick results, using words like "guaranteed," and selling products as herbal alternatives to prescription drugs.

"Eating Season"

Almost everyone agrees that our big splurge months for food are during the holidays, beginning with Thanksgiving and lasting through the vacation week after Christmas. There are holiday parties and cookie exchanges, fruit cakes and stocking stuffers lying around the house. Then on January 1, everyone vows to join a gym, clear the cupboards, and stock up on plain yogurt. So the diet frenzy starts the first of the year, right?

Wrong. Myth-buster moment! It's actually the beginning of March. Our good friend Harry Balzer from the NPD Group told me that throughout his thirty years of studying American eating habits, a pattern has emerged in the yearly cycle that he calls "eating season." It's wider than the holiday binge we all typically acknowledge. It extends from Halloween through the Super Bowl. Yes, we might have a few false starts in January: There is a distinguishable uptick in dieting during the first two weeks of the year compared with the final two weeks of the year, which are clearly the drought period with respect to weight-loss attempts.

But then, with the Super Bowl just around the corner—and all of the grocery store displays for chips and guac, the ads for chicken-wing party packs, the feed-the-whole-gang pizza specials—it all falls apart.

Not that many of us actually *watch* the Super Bowl—well, a lot of us do, but more don't watch it than do, and by that I mean that over 200 million Americans just go about their day. But even so, the Super Bowl is a full-on feast in American culture. The buildup to the event also comes just a few weeks after Christmas as people are beginning to think about dieting (whereas, say, Fourth of July barbecues occur after a spring of having mellowed out a bit on the eating).

In a study at the Cornell Food and Brand Lab, researchers tracked grocery store spending among over 200 households from July 2010 to March 2011. Compared with the baseline period of July to Thanksgiving, people spent 15 percent more on groceries during the holiday period (Thanksgiving to New Year's). Three-fourths of the increase went toward unhealthy foods.

But the researchers were surprised that shoppers kept buying more *after* New Year's. Granted, a greater share was for healthy food, with a 29 percent increase of those foods compared with baseline, and a 19 percent increase compared with the holiday period. Yet, in the post-holiday period, people also *kept* buying the less-healthy foods they were accustomed to buying during the holidays. Total calories brought home each week increased 9 percent compared to the holiday period, and 20 percent compared to regular weeks.

Things start to shift right before Thanksgiving. Average household calories purchased peak during the Christmas season and the week before the Super Bowl—*and* the week before the week before the Super Bowl. Not only is the average grocery bill highest that week—at about $150—but so are average calories brought home. When we gear up for the big game, we don't exactly have green beans and rice cakes in mind.

Super Bowl Sunday is the "final blowout" of eating season, says the NPD Group's former chief industry analyst Harry Balzer. (Not to mention Valentine's Day. Hellooo, Whitman's Sampler.) It's actually at the end of February that Americans really get serious about losing weight, and the first week of March is the true peak of dieting in America.

These two reports shatter any notion that we put our mouth where our mouth is when it comes to New Year's resolutions.

Paleo

The Paleo diet, named after the Paleolithic era because the diet supposedly matches what people ate back then, springs from the idea that today's obesity and health problems are the result of eating too much processed food, particularly useless carbs. Hunter-gatherers in the Paleolithic era ate basically meat and plants. In case you don't know your Paleolithic from your Mesozoic (that was the one with the dinosaurs), we're talking about 1.5 million years ago.

Paleo has a massive following. Along with best-selling diet books and cookbooks for living the Paleo lifestyle, the Internet is swimming with testimonials. And Paleo preachers are out in full force in the blogosphere, along with podcasts and smartphone apps.

Robb Wolf, one of the most prominent, has a site that says, "Join My Tribe. Get your FREE Paleo Quick Start Guide plus my 24-part e-mail series on healthy eating and living." Just give him your e-mail address to get started. Of his many resources is "Robb Wolf's 30 Day Paleo Transformation" guide, with "real people, real results." One hundred percent money back guarantee. If these aren't the textbook warning signs for a fad diet, I don't know what are.

There's also a fascinating connection between adopting the Paleo "lifestyle" and having an all-consuming passion for the extreme fitness program CrossFit, which challenges people to beat personal records for various exercises using kettlebells, medicine balls, gymnastic rings, jump ropes, and such.

The exercises in CrossFit always seem to put people on that fine line between discomfort and excruciating agony. CrossFit—whose brand generates some $4 billion in annual revenue—was born in Santa Cruz, California, in 2000, and by 2014 had spread across the globe. Over 200,000 people sign up to compete in the five-week qualifier to compete at CrossFit Games, the annual shot at the title "Fittest on Earth." That, and a $275,000 prize.

Many CrossFit gyms in the United States promote Paleo eating, bring authors to speak, host Paleo weight-loss challenges, and share Paleo recipes. Robb Wolf estimates that between 90 and 95 percent of CrossFit affiliate locations endorse Paleo.

PaleOMG is really another Paleo preacher named Juli Bauer. Her popular blog and website includes CrossFit workouts and recipes, plus a diary of life on the road for her cookbook tour. Don't miss the section where she tries to convert you to not only Paleo living but also Boyfriend Jeans. I'm not sure what "Fashion Fridays" have to do with eating like a cave person, other than being an opportunity to show off her CrossFit-toned bod, but it's all there.

New York City has a delivery service called Kettlebell Kitchen that brings Paleo-compliant prepared meals to CrossFit gyms, and charges just $10 to $13 (reasonable, considering that won't buy you more than about three sips of a cocktail in most of the city's canteens). The Kettlebell Kitchen website assures you they aren't serving "Mastodon steak and shrubs." Instead, you get whole foods like meat, fish, nuts, and produce. Other dishes are pumpkin beef chili, with lots of nice herbs and vegetables infusing grass-fed ground beef, or bacon-wrapped pork (aka pork on pork).

CrossFit is hardly the only semi-cultish fitness and hobby subgroup out there. You've got your yogis who are often vegetarian or vegan, or your cyclists who eat GU packets, but few of them have such a close alignment between the eating and the activity as Paleo does with CrossFit.

So what's the connection? And what does it say about us?

Paleo eating reflects all three core American values: To start, there's the drive to be unique. Overall, fitness has become a more prominent part of American culture. Look at the growth in the markets for athletic wear or gym memberships. One of the most visible signs of how things have changed is the trend of women wearing yoga pants and running outfits while doing all kinds of activities not related to yoga or running. (Going shopping or getting coffee with a friend while wearing workout clothes suggests you're *on your way to* a spin class, or planning to go for a jog later, almost like "fixin' to.") But anyone can log thirty minutes on the elliptical. To stand out now in this more fitness-focused environment, you have to demonstrate superior metrics of human performance.

Second, training to reach personal records—and following a Paleo diet to feel best equipped in that endeavor—is the individualized, physical manifestation of our national value of progress. That deeply held belief that not only society but *I* personally can be better today than I was yesterday, and that tomorrow I can be better than I am today. All it takes to achieve those results is the third value: working as hard as you possibly can. Above all, many people swear they see the results in their CrossFit performance as soon as they start eating Paleo; they feel faster and stronger. A Paleo diet is the means to the end.

In this vein, there is something called lifehacking. The term "lifehack" means basically any tip, trick, or nugget of instruction that helps you "get things done more efficiently and effectively," according to the online lifestyle publication *Lifehack*. Lifehacking is dedicated to the reduction of "friction" in your life. It started in the mid-2000s and involves the automating or streamlining of everyday tasks. Think Gmail filters, out-of-sight, out-of-mind bill payments that happen automatically, and apps tracking calories, nutrients, and sleep patterns.

Lifehack offers articles on ways to make your life better, with headlines such as: "20 Beliefs All Happy People Share" and "7 Reasons Why Quitting Facebook Now Is Good for Your Future" and "Researchers Tell Us the Reason Why Some People Are Always Late" (I had to click on that one).

Paleo and CrossFit are feverish lifehacks: prescriptions for self-improvement.

For years now, "Paleo Diet" has been the top diet in Google searches, with the somewhat similar Atkins diet holding down number two and gluten-free at third.

Each year, *U.S. News & World Report,* famous for ranking colleges, produces a Best Diets list, rigorously selected by experts nationwide. The list includes "35 of the most popular diets," which to me is significant because it points out that our country has *more than* thirty-five different popular diets. (!)

Ready for the irony? Paleo ranks *last* on the *U.S. News* list. The rating, determined by a panel of America's leading nutritionists and public health professionals, is based on how easy a diet is to adhere to, and how nutritious, safe, and effective it is at helping people lose weight and reduce the risk of diabetes and heart disease. Pretty important factors, no? The concern with Paleo is that the diet shuns dairy and grains, which have their benefits, and promotes an excessive amount of red meat, which doesn't do anyone's heart any favors.

Paleo is ranked as the fifth hardest diet to follow: It cuts out entire, sweeping categories of foods and calls for grass-fed meats, which are expensive. The diet is so specialized you can hardly ever eat at a restaurant, and few people are able to sustain a habit of cooking every night.

"Experts took issue with the diet on every measure," said *U.S. News.*

Spreading the Good Word

It's nothing new that nearly everyone feels qualified to give advice about what to eat or what not to eat. Starting as early as the 1600s, doctors, intellectuals, chemists, and even politicians started offering their two cents on what the public should do to be healthy.

The reason seems to be that eating is something we all do. And after just a few weeks on a new diet, we feel compelled to pass it on to others—the good or the bad—especially to others struggling to find something that works for them. We're likely to take diet advice from our hairdresser, a neighbor, a colleague, or a friend. Even just a Facebook friend.

"By my casual glance of Facebook on a given day, I can tell who's on a given diet," says Traci Mann, a professor of psychology and the head of the Health and Eating Laboratory at University of Minnesota. "Isn't that weird? Why do I have to know this guy's Paleo?"

This is a branch of diet evangelism you might call "peer to peer."

Diet books are at the heart of dietary crusading—and always have been. Diet books are the means through which each new self-proclaimed expert hawks his formula to the masses. According to Louise Foxcroft, "a diet can be something of an odyssey," and many feel they need a guide on that journey.

Today there are more than 45,000 guides. That's the number of books Amazon carries on diet and weight loss. Moving over to the cookbook section, in Amazon's list of top twenty best sellers, only a handful are about things like barbecue or dessert or some type of exotic cuisine; *all* the rest emphasize their given set of recipes as the ticket to a healthier life, and four titles contain explicit reference to some variant of eating "light" or becoming "trim." Recipes and home cooking are of greater importance to people who are on a diet because, as mentioned, making food yourself gives you greater control over what goes into your body.

The first diet best seller of modern times was written in the mid-1400s by Bartolomeo Sacchi (known as Platina), an Italian Renaissance writer. Entitled *De honesta voluptate et valetudine* (On honorable pleasure and health), it was a book of practical cooking recipes that sought to marry the science behind food and health with the pleasure of eating well.

Another early diet book that sold well was *The Art of Living Long,* written by a man named Luigi Cornaro at the age of ninety-four. This Venetian merchant lived until he was 102 years old—at a time when the average life span was about fifty-two. He confessed to spending the first forty years of his life as an unmitigated glutton, then realized he must purge himself of his excessive eating habits. His book advocates self-control, twelve ounces a day of total food (he was partial to partridges and pigeons) and fourteen ounces a day of wine. Even better, he says, is consuming very little of anything at all. He seemed to take pride in his later years of making it through an entire day or two on a single egg yolk.

By the late 1800s, there was a diet book for just about every demographic. It was the dawn of the self-help genre. There was even a book that gave specific prescriptions for *gaining* weight. In *How to Be Plump,* written by T. C. Duncan in 1878, the premise was that some people, especially children, were missing out on the potential health benefits of having a certain amount of fat. Hard as it might be to recall—and even to realize about *modern* life in the United States—some people still don't get enough to eat. Undernourishment among kids was of great concern. Duncan describes how he became fat himself, accidentally, by eating lots of oysters. He also offers a prescription of plenty of sleep, "to give the system time to recruit" (fat, that is), and a pint of water drunk at four intervals throughout the day. It's especially important that the water not be too cold, or have sat in "the lead pipes or in a newly painted pail." In case that's the water you were thinking of using.

As the science on diet and dieting became more specialized and rigorous, and while more qualified experts challenged some of the nonsense being circulated, they also helped fuel it. Often a stamp of endorsement by a scientist gave bogus products and programs a false air of credibility.

Not *all* diet books were filled with utter quackery, though. Post-Renaissance food writers, for example, often emphasized plain, wholesome food, grains and legumes, and minimal meat and indulgences. Hmm, sounds a bit like the plant-forward camps of today. Vegetarian and vegetable-centric recipe books go back to the early 1700s. One argued that vegetable eating reflected sophistication, while meat eating reflected heathenism. (Having watched enough people delicately slice asparagus spears into thirds versus strap on a bib and typewriter their way across a baby back rib, I'd tend to agree.)

But often these more sensible approaches were peddled in ways that made them seem ridiculous. In the mid-1800s, Sylvester Graham, to whom we owe the venerable graham cracker, proposed strategies we'd consider healthy by modern standards: moderation, exercise, and dining with others. But he did so in a book written from the perspective . . . of a stomach. Along the way, he discussed his own bagpipe-like appearance.

Most of the diet experts throughout history have been men, while most of the diet*ers* have been women. Foxcroft explains why, historically, it was mostly women jumping on weight-loss bandwagons: "Society was unequal," she says. "There weren't as many opportunities for women, and most of their value lay in how they looked. Hundreds of years ago, the way to make a living for many women was to marry somebody. So you needed to look good." Today, she says, this has changed, though not as much as we like to think.

What has changed is the ideal body size and shape. Until even as recently as the early twentieth century, most women *wanted* to be full-figured. It signified wealth, health, even a kind of maternal glory. The American singer and actress Lillian Russell was among the best-known stars of the late 1800s and early 1900s to represent that standard of beauty before the war on fat took over.

During the 1900s, the number of media outlets, from women's magazines to TV shows, grew considerably, providing more avenues to spread the latest scientific breakthrough or pearl of diet wisdom throughout American culture. And then, decades later, we got the World Wide Web, which launched digital diet evangelism, and with it diet blogs and social media subcommunities for every school of food thought under the sun.

Historically, each new diet is presented as new and groundbreaking. But each proselytizer just regurgitates the same old stuff. There are only so many foods to dial up or dial back, only so many ingredients to grind into a powder or blend into a smoothie. All the diet brands follow a noticeable formula: often a personal tale, a great deal of self-experimentation, and a simple solution. Plus, commiseration.

You can imagine the basic plot as a Mad Lib: "Aw man, I've been there myself. I was down in the dumps, 10 to 200 pounds overweight. I had tried *everything* to shed the pounds: A and B and C, and nothing worked. I was ready to give up, but then, along came . . . D! It radically changed my life. Within 1 to 30 days/1 to 10 weeks, I lost 10 to 200 pounds/dropped 1 to 8 pants sizes, my sex life skyrocketed, and I feel gggreeeat! Here's my 3- to 9-step miracle plan. Instant results—*guaranteed*!"

Traci Mann says she understands "that if you want something that desperately, you'll keep trying things, even if they sound kind of like what you've tried before, but especially if it sounds different from what you've tried before. That's why you see [each one] cycling back about every twenty years or so." Once "everybody's tried it and failed," it almost has to disappear for awhile.

———

"Food is fashion," says Harry Balzer, and we must realize that "we wear our food like we wear our clothes." What we eat is an opportunity, several times each day, to make a statement about who we are. But again, like clothes we are suddenly willing to discard for something brand new, certain foods go in and out of vogue.

The whims of food as fashion are due to the influence of the marketplace. Balzer says that is far more powerful than any friend preaching low-carb at a dinner party. Or any kettlebell-lifter preaching Paleo at a CrossFit box.

He says the *quest* for health is the constant—what changes is the definition.

One day it's all about antioxidants, the next it's gluten. Words like these spring into the national vocabulary, with new product lines appearing on shelves, and celebrity endorsers carving out new followings. Balzer says these shifts in national eating behavior are so frequent, so dramatic, that we really need a flexible FDA nutrition label. Imagine if every few months or at least every year, the label changed with the latest nutrition research and related eating trends. It might drop cholesterol in the wake of the Dietary Guidelines Advisory Committee's report, add gluten given how many people have been avoiding it, and so on.

His idea makes you wonder if we will always latch on to new diets and health fads. While some in the public health profession might believe we're making gradual progress toward a stable set of widely accepted guidelines for how best to eat, Balzer considers that thinking naïve. The fluctuations are inevitable, he says. Might as well design products and labels and menus to change with the times, so people can locate the nutritional darlings and demons du jour.

———

Okay, beyond all of the marketing and sales pitches, does any of it actually *work*?

Three-quarters of people who try diets don't make it past a month. That's according to a study by Cornell Food and Brand Lab researcher Brian Wansink and his colleagues. Thirty-six percent last only a week or less. A mere 8 percent sustain a diet for longer than three months.

An analysis by University of California, Los Angeles researchers found that dieters can usually lose 5 to 10 percent of their body weight. But it almost always comes back. Looking at thirty-one long-term diet studies—by their measure, every study to date that followed people on diets for two to five years—the majority of people not only regained the weight, but also gained more weight than they had lost. Sadly, this is true for as many as two-thirds of people who go on a diet.

Here's the most shocking finding: One of the strongest *predictors* of whether a person will gain weight in the future is whether that person has dieted in the recent past. In other words, if a person has tried a diet before, that factor alone makes them more likely to put on weight.

It's important to distinguish diets in the sense of *going on a diet* from dietary patterns, ways of eating throughout a lifetime. Some people might feel that an extreme fad diet is what it takes to jump-start their shift to a set of more sensible habits that actually feel doable over the long run. So it's not that diets never work. It just means a lot of them don't work, overall they're difficult to sustain, and in many cases a person is actually better off never dieting in the first place.

Why Evangelize?

A big reason for the hucksterism may be about having an accountability mechanism. "I think people are more successful at dieting if they do it in a group," Foxcroft says. "The whole social media thing—if you publicize the fact that you're dieting, you're more likely to stick to it."

So while Louise Foxcroft, the historian, and Traci Mann, the psychologist, see the sermonizing as social reinforcement, Mann also considers it a *symptom* of adhering to a diet. She explains: "If you're serious about the diet, it takes over your thinking. Dealing with the diet becomes your primary focus in life. Because for a diet to work, even in a short-term way, that's what it takes. It requires this singular focus on it."

She supports this with evidence about the brain: "When you're on a diet, all kinds of changes happen—physically, physiologically, metabolism and hormones—but also neurological changes: People become more likely to notice food, and it has an increased reward value. It's harder to get those thoughts out of your mind. There's this neurological change that makes food and food-related stuff much more likely than normal to attract and hold your attention."

Knowing this makes me feel a little bit like a bully: Is Mann telling me that all the soapboxing isn't just for self-aggrandizement and profiteering—but that, neurologically speaking, some among us just can't help but be so fixated?

We've heard the social and the scientific explanations, but what about the cultural ones? Marion Nestle offered me this: "Think of it as a substitute for religion. I found God, God is good for me. God would be good for you, too. What's wrong with you that you don't find God?"

Dieting pits ideologies against one another. It's about adopting a belief system more than anything, a set of strict guidelines to keep you on the straight and narrow (or, I should say, straight and slim). It's also about purity and personal transformation. You see the many religious references like praying yourself thin, or books like *More of Him, Less of Me*.

Often there is a group element—found, for instance, on Facebook—but typically coming together in person for weekly sessions: *"I was drinking my kohlrabi juice every morning, but then, there was a birthday at work . . ."* Groans fill the talking circle. They all know what this means. She has strayed. She ate the cake, didn't she? *"So, I kinda, well, I had a piece of the German chocolate cake."* Sigh, disappointment. Comforting hands and words extend. But with confession comes absolution.

This is not to suggest that dieting actually replaces religion, but that it becomes another higher power that you rely on, almost like the Ten Commandments, Mann says. "People are zealots about their diets . . . the parallel is real."

Americans are not alone in their penchant for fad diets or in their diet evangelizing. But a few things that make us stand out are the long-time abundance, that excess of choice bestowed upon us by our vast and resource-rich land, and the disinterest in restraint that has, from our very founding, gone along with that. These, oh, and Hollywood: the engine of the fad diet industry.

Making Sense of It All

We're all trying to carve out our identities amid the sea of strong opinions. Myself, well, I guess I'd identify as a whole grains–obsessed, vegetable-oriented, fruitaholic, semi-flexitarian who counts calories for breakfast and lunch, then it's anything goes. On weekends, there are no rules.

I don't believe in juicing, and I go light on the spicy but heavy on the chipotle aioli. In theory I don't eat dessert because, you know, sugar is toxic and all that. But I've got a sweet tooth like none other, so I alternate between a chewy chocolate chip cookie once a week and ad hoc candy nibbles to no-sweets-whatsoever for seven- to ten-day stretches. While I don't eat much meat, I've got a soft spot for rabbit, preferably in a Greek stew called *stifado*. And . . . I ate a pigeon once. I know burgers are bad in too many ways to count, and they disagree with my stomach, yet I crave the taste and satisfaction of a homemade patty, on a sesame seed–topped bun with ketchup and tomato, grilled to perfection.

Oh, and I don't eat airline food. Talk about fifty shades of gross.

But goodness, here I am, spouting my own belief system. Am I unwittingly trying to convert you? I mean, I guess if I *had* to market my secret eating formula, it mostly consists of nuts and berries, so I could call it the Squirrel Diet. That would probably sell pretty well on Amazon, don't you think? I'd have to get Dr. Oz on board . . .

In all seriousness, we have to remember the consequences of the everyone's-an-expert mentality. Evangelists are typically evangelizing for financial gain, ego-boosting, and because being on a diet can produce one-track thinking. But consider the harm we might be doing by preaching, like stress and self-punishment at minimum. And it's even worse when the converting requires shelling out wads of cash for what is often unsubstantiated gobbledygook, and subjecting ourselves to the risk of even greater weight gain and health problems over the long run.

The nagging question for most people is still: What should we eat? Cutting through centuries of fad diets, more nutritional analyses and epidemiological studies than any researcher would care to count, the consensus is that Michael Pollan nailed it with his seven simple words: "Eat food. Not too much. Mostly plants."

The funny thing is, even the real-food eaters feel compelled to spread the gospel. Mark Bittman and Dan Barber, to name a few others. Even *they* can't just quietly eat their real food and let others eat their fake food. We're all guilty, it seems.

But the difference is that these suggestions are rooted in common sense, not extremes we can't maintain. They seem profound now because, frankly, having been assailed by so many extreme dietary doctrines over the years has dulled our ability to think for ourselves.

All those firm prescriptions shake us out of our default reaction to use common sense. It says Paleo on the label, so you eat it. Much like someone who drinks a Big Gulp of Coke every day with an afternoon cookie the size of a dinner plate and says, "What? I'm vegetarian."

Similarly, while many who go gluten-free do so for real health reasons, as I described earlier, others are being manipulated by companies capitalizing on our distorted assessment that *anything* labeled gluten-free is healthy. Because, in applying our national faith in innovation and progress to our diets, we are inadvertently relying on industry solutions. This renders our own skills and traditions and instincts and knowledge obsolete—enabling food marketers to leverage powerful misperceptions.

And stripped of our intuition about what to eat, we're left out on a limb. So all that preaching? Maybe from way out on that limb, we can't help but want a little company.

The Stoic philosopher Epictetus was born in the year AD 55, and even if only half the words in this quote are really what he said, the gist is brilliant. Of course, I think it's brilliant because it suggests he and I are kindred spirits, that he had had enough with all the diet evangelists running around the Roman Empire. He says: "Preach not to others what they should eat, but eat as becomes you and be silent."

CHAPTER 7

The Democratization of Wine

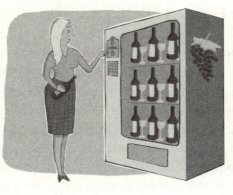

It was a bluebird California day in 1951 when Stanford junior Joe Coulombe was offered a glass of wine—from a jug!—by Bill Steere, a botany professor, while sitting on the Steeres' balcony.

Joe was courting the professor's daughter Alice. He was really more of a beer drinker and enjoyed throwing back a few with friends at Rossotti's, a roadhouse saloon nearby where patrons often arrived on horseback. No one drank wine in those days. And the first sip for this San Diego boy with Tennessee roots was a revelation. He grew to realize that California jug wine was how someone on a scanty teacher's salary could enjoy one of life's simple pleasures. Plus, since no one else was drinking it, a gallon of decent Chardonnay could be had for just a dollar.

Two years later Joe and Alice were married at Stanford's Memorial Church—and Joe Coulombe went on to become Trader Joe.

Over time, Joe's mother-in-law, Dorothy Steere, opened his eyes to a range of ways to enjoy good food on a tight budget. She was, for instance, the first person he ever saw cook with olive oil. And that's where he got the idea for the place Americans now say is their favorite grocery store. In a 2015 study on American grocery chains by the consumer research firm Market Force Information, Trader Joe's took the top spot for the third year in a row. The vision, Joe told me, was a store where "people who were overeducated and underpaid could find a certain richness on the table they otherwise could not."

That revelation on the balcony helped launch a wine boom in America. From its founding in 1967, Trader Joe's has been known for offering good deals on good booze. Americans now drink more than three times as much wine per person as we did when Joe discovered it in 1951. And we now consume by far the most vino since the Wine Institute began these recordings in 1934.

In 2010, for the first time, America beat France in total volume of wine purchased, a title we still hold. Granted, our population is nearly five times that of France, but the French used to outpace us in total consumption, too. They still drink far more per person; so by no means am I suggesting that we rival the French with respect to appreciation for the juice. But wine has become far more ingrained in American culture than ever before, and signs indicate that will only increase. The growth rate of wine is the highest of all the alcohol categories (beer, wine, spirits), and the firm International Wine and Spirit Research considers the United States one of the main drivers of their projected 4 percent growth in global consumption by 2018.

All these numbers reveal that wine has been brought to the masses. It's what I call the Democratization of Wine. Today, you can buy wine at CVS and Walgreens and Duane Reade, enjoy tastings at the airport, and sip a glass at some Starbucks locations. Wine vending machines have even started to pop up. The United States is the fourth leading producer of wine in the world, after Italy, France, and Spain, in that order. And wine is now being made in all fifty states (that's right, even Hawaii and Alaska).* We have a natural urge to support whatever our home state produces, and being exposed to wine production makes wine even more familiar.

"The industry is a little puzzled why wine has become so popular," says Robert Smiley, director of Wine Industry Studies at the University of California, Davis Graduate School of Management. Social media may play a part, his research suggests. Interest can spread peer to peer, with people posting photos of wines they like, or links to blog posts, events, tastings, and food festivals.

One person who saw this potential early on was Belarusian immigrant entrepreneur Gary Vaynerchuk. A lesser known member of the vanguard to democratize wine, he was groundbreaking in doing so *online*. I think of him as America's first Internet Personality with a Wine Agenda. Or, as *Mediaite* dubbed him, "The Social Media Sommelier." After transforming his father's New Jersey–based discount liquor store into the $60-million-a-year business Wine Library, Gary started a YouTube wine show in 2006. The goal of his Wine Library TV videos was nothing short of radical: to show you don't have to be a one-percenter to enjoy wine. And it struck a chord: His show has generated as many as 80,000 downloads a day, and today he has over a million followers on Twitter.

---

* All fifty states have approved appellations of origin for viticulture, which require that no less than 75 percent of the volume of the wine come from grapes grown in that appellation. I can't vouch for how much of this wine is actually drinkable, but Americans nationwide are at least making a go of it.

At an event I attended in New York in 2013, Gary said, "The second anyone gets even the smallest amount of knowledge about wine, they become a straight douchebag." He wanted to counter that, to make wine approachable. He was initially blasted by the wine establishment for dumbing down the art of wine tasting (he once smelled Conan O'Brien's armpit while explaining wine terms like "sweaty"). But Gary is now credited with helping embed wine in American pop culture.

Though better known as a social media and business consultant, he is one of the few wine critics to have helped break through class barriers. In 2009, *Decanter* magazine named him to their biannual Power List of the top fifty most influential people in the wine firmament.

Along with social media, wine's lower alcohol content has also likely helped increase its popularity. Psychologically, having a more tasteful way to drink in social settings may be part of the reason many Americans made the switch from liquor.

International Wine and Spirit Research predicts that the United States will remain the largest market from now till 2018 by a safe distance, and it considers millennials one of the main reasons behind the U.S. growth.

Young wine drinkers are fueling some interesting changes in the industry. For centuries wine came in bottles sealed with corks that needed special removers to be opened. The first big change was bottles with screw tops, which many wine buffs refused to accept. "Baby boomers have a lifetime of affiliating corks in 750-milliliter bottles with quality, and screw caps from Gallo or whoever with less quality," Smiley says. But not so for millennials. Today wine arrives in containers ranging from individual-size aluminum cans to plastic bladders holding four bottles' worth. "As you move down in age, they're more accepting," Smiley says.

This willingness to try new tastes and packaging is a great

example of the *benefits* of our culture's instability. So what else does our growing taste for the grape reveal about Americans? How does this wine craze connect with our concern for the environment, what's wrong with Skinnygirl wines, and who really brought wine to the everyman? There is a wide cast of characters, but we undoubtedly have three stars to thank: America's favorite grocery store (Trader Joe's), America's favorite wine store (Costco), and America's favorite imported wine (Yellow Tail).

Here's My Two Bucks

The snobby wine cliché is guys in tweed jackets and turtle-necks, sitting around a wood-paneled den, swirling the red liquid in a delicate glass, while sniffing and holding it up to the light to study the legs until it's just . . . Enough already . . . can we get our heads out of our—I mean *glasses,* our *noses* out of our *glasses!*—and move on with the tasting and enjoying?

In addition to being a form of entertainment for the elite and a symbol of sophistication, decent wine used to be prohibitively expensive. Very little wine was produced in the United States, and it was primarily imported from Europe, which increased its price. That also meant it was less available, except in big cities. But as the California wine industry grew in the twentieth century, not only were California wines just as good (and, as several European competitions showed, even *better* in some cases), they were also more available. And this had the ripple effect of forcing foreign winemakers to figure out how to get their product here at lower prices in order to keep up.

(I should note that decent affordable wine has been around for centuries outside the United States, as travelers to Europe know. In some Italian cities, I've found that wine is cheaper than water.)

Joe Coulombe was among the leaders in the good fight of wine for all. But before he could make wine widely available, it had to be of "acceptable quality," says the UC Davis wine industry expert Robert Smiley. "If it melts the enamel on your teeth, you're not gonna buy it again."

In 2002, Trader Joe's began carrying a wine under the label Charles Shaw that was produced by the Bronco Wine Company, which, according to *Business Insider,* makes 90 million gallons of wine a year. That's enough to fill more than 136 Olympic-size swimming pools. With wine!

Charles Shaw has won awards and raves from many respected wine experts. It carries the nickname "Two-Buck Chuck" because of its $1.99 retail price per bottle.* And, most important, people liked it. By the early 2000s, Charles Shaw became the fastest-growing wine label in U.S. history. That cheap price introduced wine to a new segment of consumers. Wine had long been attractive to a certain type of consumer who doesn't take "snob" as an insult but an aspiration. This was the opposite, though, and novice wine drinkers dove right in.

In early 2003, Charles Shaw claimed 19 percent of all wine sold in California. At the time, there were nearly 2,000 wineries in the state, so this was unprecedented. The label has at times sold a million cases per month. There are now at least 10,417 wineries in the United States—up from just 2,688 in 1999—and only a few see sales above a million cases per *year.* Since debuting the wine in 2002, Trader Joe's has sold over 800 million bottles.

"The wines have appeal for customers with even the most

---

* After over a decade at that price it went up to at least $2.49, though price varies by state.

discriminating tastes and have both transformed and appalled the staid and snobbish West Coast wine industry," writes Len Lewis in his book *The Trader Joe's Adventure*.

Charles Shaw has been called many things: "blue-collar wine," merely "potable," "functional," "a boozy come up," "quaffable," and even "Up-Chuck." *FoodBeast* described it as "wine roulette," noting it tastes like "depends," and no, not the adult diaper brand, but the variable flavor. Others consider it "not bad"—a connoisseur's way of saying, *"I've got three cases in my basement, but don't tell my friends who won't shut up about their 97-point Domaine Giraud Châteauneuf-du-Pape."*

Earning a catchy nickname and selling it exclusively at Trader Joe's helped solidify the wine's cult-like following: People tend to be terrible at remembering wine names. Raise your hand if you pick a wine based on how pretty the label is. Come on, you can admit it. The moniker Two-Buck Chuck went a long way in helping people remember Charles Shaw. Plus, you could only buy it at Trader Joe's, which also helped with the remembering. No more of that head-scratching moment after buying other wines: *"Honey, where'd we get that one red we really liked, you know the one with the little swing, with the butterflies? I wanna say it was from Napa maybe, or was it Sonoma?"*

You can't understand Two-Buck Chuck—and how it helped people jump from afraid to aficionado—without understanding Trader Joe's, and the ethos that underlies not only the seven varietals (or flavors, as some scoffers say) of their wine, but their entire operation.

It started with a small chain of Pronto convenience stores Joe purchased after attending the Stanford Graduate School of Business. Unable to battle the goliath of 7-Eleven, Joe reimagined his stores, expanding each one's floor space and adding a South Pacific theme to the décor and employee attire. Along with offering a variety of specialty food items, Joe made a point of buying wines at closeout prices from overstocked or financially strapped producers, selling them as great deals and introducing customers to a whole world of wines.

Five years after opening, the store introduced its first grocery product—granola— under the Trader Joe's private label, a strategy that underlies their loyalty and customer satisfaction ratings. They work with suppliers from all over to lock in high-volume purchases of items that are unlike anything else on the market, slap on the TJs logo, and sell them at bargain basement prices.*

It's like a stamp of approval from the company's curators, who sell only a fraction of the number of items at most supermarkets. The key is choosing top-notch products for that Trader Joe's private label. After all, if it's got your name on it, you want those items to fly off the shelves.

By the early 1990s, the company expanded outside of California, sweeping one state after another, and passing 400 total stores. In 2015, they opened over a dozen new locations. About midway through that rapid growth they introduced the game changer for the American wine scene: Charles Shaw.

Part of what makes Charles Shaw, like Trader Joe's itself, so widely appealing and so *American* is the way it shrugs at refinement, something we've done since at least the early 1800s. Back then, Americans mostly ate using knives, jabbing them right into a pot of food. That's according to the book *What's Cooking? The History of American Food* by Sylvia Whitman, who shares a note from a traveler to the United States from Europe, where forks and spoons were becoming customary:

---

* Pop Quiz: What's the most popular item sold at Trader Joe's? Speculoos Cookie Butter.

The traveler was stunned that even U.S. congressmen "plunged into their mouths enormous wedges of meat and pounds of vegetables perched on the ends of their knives."

Trader Joe's is privately owned and proudly closed-door with the press. They seem to have a who-gives-a-crap attitude, compared with other retailers who act far more buttoned up. Also, if the Hawaiian shirts, scavenger hunts for shoppers-in-training, and cow bells are any indication, TJs employees appear to be having *way* more fun at work. The company even injects humor into its fine print. At the bottom of the list of Customer Choice Award winners announced in early 2015, their webpage reads: *"NOTE: Since posting, the details of this item may have changed due to fluctuating market prices, federal regulations, currency rates, drought, pestilence, bandits, rush hour traffic, filibusters, clowns, zombie apocalypse, punctilious product developers. . . . Contact our Crew for current price and availability."* What's not to love?

Two-Buck Chuck, though still the customer favorite among all beverages at Trader Joe's, has lost its edge a bit in recent years. Sales have slowed, perhaps because of increased competition on the novelty front from craft cocktails, craft beers, and even a bloom of new ciders. Part of the slippage, though, is likely due to all the newcomers to the "super-value" category the wine helped create. Hundreds of new low-cost wines have emerged to tap this same snoot-averse slice of the market.

Australia's Yellow Tail debuted in the United States in 2001, sells for $5 to $8, and is the best-selling imported brand in the country by more than twice its closest rival. (In 2004, Australia surpassed Italy as the largest exporter of wine to the United States.) And affordable prices aren't Yellow Tail's only secret.

With its fruity, accessible flavors, Yellow Tail nailed "the perfect wine for a public grown up on soft drinks," wine industry consultant Jon Fredrikson told *The New York Times*.

Ditto for Barefoot, a top-selling wine from behemoth E. & J. Gallo Winery, aimed squarely at the abecedarian, maybe the college student or fresh entrant into the working world. It's on the sweeter side, and the price is well under $10.

Trader Joe's is far from the only place to buy affordable vino. Costco is actually America's top wine retailer.*

What the two chains have in common is selling wine in a decidedly no-frills way. As a wholesale outlet, Costco offers a hodgepodge of products at killer value in a giant, fluorescently lit warehouse. But most important, Costco sticks to their standard mark-up of no more than 15 percent above what the store pays, which keeps their wine prices down.

Cultural Transmission

Word of mouth has been a powerful force in establishing a more mainstream role for wine in our culture. Internet chat rooms, for example, are given at least partial credit for the rise of Charles Shaw. If people were suddenly talking about $2 wine at Trader Joe's, it meant they were talking *about wine*. And for a country where widespread wine consumption isn't in our roots, this was a boost to the whole enterprise. People were suddenly comparing Cabernet Sauvignon to Merlot, learning which wines were sweet, which were dry, which regions seemed to produce wines that tasted best to them, and which wines would go with whatever dish they were making that night.

It seems that women have led the charge in this respect. Think about it like this: There are few things more American

---

* Pop Quiz: What's the most popular item sold at Costco? Toilet paper.

than apple pie, right? But that goes for food. What's the most iconic drink? For men, I'd say it's standing around a grill in the backyard with a Budweiser in hand. Various cocktails have filled this spot over the years for American women (famously the cosmo, for one), but it seems that wine became a no-brainer for gabbing with the girls.

The data back this up: Wine is by far the top choice for women, according to Gallup polling, with 46 percent saying it's their preferred drink, versus just 17 percent among men. Nearly 60 percent of American men pick beer, and 20 percent pick hard liquor.

In American pop culture, female characters are more often drinking wine, and usually red. How and when they drink wine reveals a larger American tendency, which is to drink wine by itself, instead of with a meal, as Europeans most often do.

We'll order a glass at a bar, have a glass at home on the patio before heading to dinner, split a bottle with friends while chatting on the couch. It doesn't mean we don't *also* have it with dinner; it's just that, in classic wine culture, it's not often separated from food.

We see this in TV shows and movies all the time: Think of big-time lawyer Alicia Florrick (played by Julianna Margulies) on *The Good Wife,* with her nightly goblet by herself.

Eric Asimov of *The New York Times* has called the drinking of wine without food, and alone, "utilitarian." He observes that on *The Good Wife* and other shows such as *Scandal, Cougar Town,* and *House of Cards,* the women "gulp" and "guzzle," not "sip" and "swirl," the technique that is customary at even a beginner's wine-tasting outing. It's also religiously practiced by true wine connoisseurs but looks, well, snooty, to those who aren't.

Rarely are the characters on these shows wine snobs, as you can also tell by how they hold the glass by the bowl, not the stem. In these popular shows, wine is not the only thing women drink on-screen, but it's women who drink it. Men, on the other hand, usually drink whiskey or beer.

So while wine has risen in favor among both genders, why are women especially drawn to it? There are the fruity flavors, and the truth to the Latin phrase *in vino veritas* (meaning "in wine there is truth"), since loose lips certainly help with the gabbing. But more than anything, I suspect that women's greater preference for wine is driven by the belief that it's healthier than liquor and beer, and women tend to care more about that.

One of the more puzzling trends in this vein has been Skinnygirl, a line of diet wines and cocktails that has created a new market segment. The wines' label emphasizes that a five-ounce serving only has 100 calories. Sounds great, except there are just a few problems. The first is that it's a gimmick: The same serving of regular white wine has only 110 calories anyway. Red has only 120. So you're saving those calories for what, two pretzels?

The bigger problem may be how this affects us psychologically. You'll recall from chapter 4, about low-fat, low-calorie foods, that when we see labels like those, we tend to consume more of them compared with the regular versions, yet enjoy them less.

In general, consuming too much alcohol poses problems: It can increase the risk of certain cancers, damage the liver, and lead to acute physical risks like drunk driving and biking and walking.

For women in particular, having only two or more drinks per day—which is the case for 40 percent of American women—has been shown to increase the risk of breast cancer in large studies.*

* Remember though, as with any discussion of health risks, a host of factors such as genetics and lifestyle go into the mix in each individual's risk.

So where Skinnygirl goes astray is not only that it might accidentally lead to our drinking more than we mean to, given our hard-wired reactions to certain product claims. It's that it brings guilt into the mix when consuming something that's meant to be about pleasure. Skinnygirl wine is like the new nonfat cookie.

At the same time, the irony of this focus on the calories in wine is that, in *moderate* amounts, drinking wine is already considered healthy. ("Moderate" has been defined as one daily drink for women, and two for men.) In the United States, we can never just leave it at that, though. Allow me to illustrate.

Tom Standage, in his excellent book, *A History of the World in 6 Glasses,* shares a passage from a Greek play from the fourth century BCE. It refers to a *krater,* a kind of large vase of water mixed with wine, used at parties:

For sensible men I prepare only three kraters: one for health, which they drink first, the second for love and pleasure, and the third for sleep. After the third one is drained, wise men go home . . . the eighth is for breaking the furniture; the ninth is for depression; the tenth is for madness and unconsciousness.

I pass on this millennia-old wisdom to remind us of what everyone already knows: A little alcohol is good for us, and a lot isn't good for us or for those around us. Seems simple enough, except that knowing and doing are rarely one and the same. As we saw with protein, for example, as Americans we have a tendency to take something advisable, then go completely overboard with it.

The fact that the healthy Mediterranean diet includes wine in regular but moderate amounts is a major reason we collectively concluded that wine is good for us. And along with *that* has come a borderline obsession with plant compounds called polyphenols, especially resveratrol. It's found in the skins of red grapes (among other plants), and its antioxidant properties are thought to fight aging and disease. But the attention has led to its sale in the United States as a supplement. Not only are the health effects of the supplements unclear, they aren't regulated. So you don't always know what's in the bottle.

Moderate alcohol intake appears to be good for the heart and blood pressure, as confirmed by dozens of studies, consistently decreasing risk of cardiovascular disease among both men and women by between 25 and 40 percent. It also appears to reduce the risk of type 2 diabetes and overall mortality (mostly because cardiovascular disease is the leading cause of death). But popping pills of resveratrol won't do the trick. Neither will drinking barrels of red wine every night.

Hear it from Harvard: Eric Rimm, a professor at the medical school, says the benefits are not much different by type of alcoholic beverage. Harvard's Nutrition Source website says: "What you drink (beer or wine) doesn't seem to be nearly as important as how you drink. Having seven drinks on a Saturday night and then not drinking the rest of the week isn't at all the equivalent of having one drink a day. The weekly total may be the same, but the health implications aren't." This suggests that the protective effects *could* come from the ethanol itself, which might help our arteries by increasing good cholesterol, or HDL.

But as is often true in science, though a little disappointing, the research has produced mixed results, and more is needed to tease all this apart. As a country, our interest in health and wellness sometimes outpaces our collective knowledge about health and wellness.

Whatever the drink may be, we have to take the more holistic view and remember that it's not just the potential physical ben-

204 ▶ DEVOURED

efits of moderate alcohol consumption but the social and psychological ones. Also known as: fun! Whether unwinding at the end of a stressful day at work or having a night out with friends, these get-togethers contribute to well-being in real ways.

Despite all that's unknown about health and alcohol, Rimm can say with certainty: "People who drink moderately live longer (and happier!) lives."

And I'll drink to that.

Beyond the potential appeal for health reasons, Americans' interest in wine transferred from the upper classes across all spectrums of our culture. As a result, it has become diversified and lasting.

The fashion world has a standard "trickle-down theory," which says that each social class is influenced by the one above it. Richard Wilk, the Indiana University Food Institute co-director and professor of anthropology, explains how this same thing applies to what we eat: "Food that's elevated trickles down and permeates, but as it becomes mainstream, the avant-garde drop it. That's how fashion cycles work in modern industrial consumer society."

But there's another type of cultural template, which Wilk calls a "style sandwich." This happens when you have people at the top—socioeconomically, that is—eating something, and people at the bottom eating it too, but the folks in the middle aren't having it.

"Wine for a long time was associated with immigrants from southern Europe, or the very rich [as part of the American adoration of French food], but it really wasn't something for ordinary people," says Warren Belasco, the leading food scholar and professor emeritus of American Studies at the University of Maryland, Baltimore County. "My parents in the fifties, living in the suburbs, it was beer and scotch, never wine." As we know, that has changed.

Today, Wilk's sandwich is looking a little different. On the one hand, you have wine trickling down from the upper echelons, having become firmly middle class. To distinguish themselves, the elite are making wine at home or buying limited-release cases from some boutique winery, or joining clubs to gain access to the smallest, most precious producers, who, along with their wine, provide perks like multicourse dinners amid the vineyards.

At the same time, you've got the bottom part of the sandwich, the bargain items swimming to the surface, also reaching the mainstream, and the elite want in on that, too: As reported in *The Trader Joe's Adventure,* it became fashionable to bring Two-Buck Chuck to even very chic dinner parties. In places like Woodside, California—one of the wealthiest zip codes in America, where Teslas and $5,000 bicycles share parking spots at the country market with horses guided by women in English riding apparel—you'd see empty bottles of it filling the bins on recycling day.

Another example of the flow of influence from the bottom up is bourbon. Wilk says, "Artisanal bourbons are big in Indiana: You can go to a bourbon tasting, do a flight of different bourbons; there are bourbon blogs. It's really interesting, because [bourbon] used to be very low status."

There are even data to back up his observation. According to Nielsen, a consumer research firm, whiskey has been growing in popularity across all generations.

This highbrow/lowbrow interplay throughout American culture is fascinating: the women who buy all their swimsuits at Target but their handbags at Burberry; the readers who subscribe to both *Us Weekly* and *The New Yorker.* To illustrate how prominent this relationship really is in American society, *New*

DEVOURED

York magazine's regular "Approval Matrix" plots cultural news on axes of despicable versus brilliant and highbrow versus lowbrow. It includes witticisms like "Gmail adds 'undo send' option. Breathalyzer not included." That one is considered a brilliant lowbrow item. In the opposite quadrant, you get despicable highbrow items such as "A trio of tourists crashed their drone into the roof of Milan Cathedral."

Another way that wines have become more embraced by the masses is seen on the outside of the bottle: Think of how wine *labels* have changed, and how they differ based on price. Yellow Tail, with its playful wallaby on the front, was the first to use an animal on its label, and that led others to follow. Between 2003 and 2006, 18 percent of new, financially viable wine brands had a label featuring an animal, according to a study by Nielsen. The trend known as "critter labels" has died down some, but any walk through the wine aisle can still give you the sense of being at the zoo, watched by rows of insects, birds, and other pastoral creatures. It's part of a larger, ongoing sign that many winemakers don't take bottle art too seriously anymore, and instead see it as an opportunity for fun and creativity. A far cry from the traditional cursive type, the sketches of chateaus, and the sensitive portraits of Roman philosophers.

I first noticed this new direction in bottle art a few years back at a California winery called Sort This Out Cellars. They're constantly coming up with new labels, and the more creative renditions have included comic-book-like illustrations, for instance a silk-screened spider web across the bottle for "Elvira's Macabrenet," and 1940s- and 1950s-inspired magazine covers such as "Oh My Gosh! Grenache."

Some people are appalled by the changing standards. On

the website LocalWineEvents.com, a novelist and wine label designer named Roman Payne, who lives in France, laments how casual American culture is in general, with all the sporty clothing, for one. "I hate to even mention aloud the names of modern wines that insult the millennia-old art of wine-making, with horrible names on them such as 'Bad-Ass Cabernet,'" he writes. "Uttering such a name in a written article is a violation of my artistic, and my literary, taste."

What Sets Us Apart

All this discussion of social strata reminds me, we're due for another quick pit stop at Merriam-Webster. The word "democratize" has three definitions:

- ▸ to make (a country or organization) more democratic;
- ▸ to make (something) available to all people;
- ▸ to make it possible for all people to understand (something).

This family of meanings is invigorating. It makes me want to fly Old Glory out on my porch. (That is, of course, if I had a porch. Times are tough in the San Francisco rental market, and porches are even tougher in a city that averages sixty degrees in summer.)

Back to wine, though. We've seen how it has become more available to people. At least to those of legal drinking age. But to understand the first and third definitions, we have to look at what used to prevent wine from being more democratic or possible to understand.

One thing we know about eating is that taste trumps all. Whether you want someone to eat healthy, or eat less of something or more of something, you have to lead with flavor. But whether or not something tastes good can vary from person to person. Still there are many wine drinkers who look to critics to help them sort good from bad. They do so in the hope that they will enjoy wines as much as the consumer guides do.

Robert Parker, an American, is the world's most influential wine reviewer. He is responsible for the 100-point rating system used just about everywhere, and for making and breaking wineries as a result.

There has been a burgeoning shift away from the Parker rating system because, if I had to guess, it's not very democratic to let one man's nose and tongue set the course of an entire industry.

Part of that shift has been calling out annoying winespeak for what it is: annoying. Wine writers have a tendency to use words that are confusing, and define them with other words that are still confusing. *Wine Spectator,* for one, explains that a wine might be considered "awkward" because it is "clumsy," "flabby" because it lacks "backbone." Better yet: "foxy" when a wine is particularly "grapey." The only word that comes to mind for me is: Huh?

Other common descriptions include "anise" and "barnyard," along with my favorite, "hint of leather." Has anyone honestly taken a sip of wine and thought, *Wow, you know, that's so funny—this tastes* exactly *like that belt I ate last night.*

Another part of this shift is that even Parker, a self-proclaimed Francophile, has acknowledged the rising status of California as a wine producer. He has said America has a leg up *because* of our receptiveness to different kinds of wines. Increasingly, we want to decide for ourselves what tastes "good" instead of relying on critics; we don't want to stress out about training our palates to appreciate what has been deemed the highest caliber or worthy of our money. We might see a bottle posted on Facebook from a friend and give it a try, or read a wine blog touting a new label, but Robert Parker's point scale is not the deciding factor.

In the early 1800s, Americans outdrank nearly everyone. They drank more alcohol than citizens of all the European countries save for the Scots, the French, and the Swedes. Across every region and race and gender and class, early American society was about little else. In *The Alcoholic Republic: An American Tradition,* author W. J. Rorabaugh writes:

> Americans drank at home and abroad, alone and together, at work and at play, in fun and in earnest. They drank from the crack of dawn to the crack of dawn . . . Americans drank before meals, with meals, and after meals. They drank while working in the fields and while travelling across half a continent. They drank in their youth, and, if they lived long enough, in their old age.

To put it mildly: They drank all the damn time.

We've settled down a bit since then, or perhaps the record-keeping has gotten more precise in other countries, but in any case, for per person consumption among all countries, here's how the United States stacks up:

▸ Total alcohol: 48th

   ▸ Eastern European countries sweep the top, as do European countries in general, though Australia and South Korea are also high.

▸ Tequila: 1st

   ▸ Mexico is 2nd.

▶ Whiskey: 3rd

    ▶ France and Uruguay are the top two, respectively.

▶ Beer: 14th

    ▶ Again, it's Europe across the board and Eastern Europe especially, though Venezuela makes the top ten.

▶ Wine: 56th

    ▶ The Vatican is the highest by far, and again European countries claim all the top spots. The UK drinks about twice as much as we do per person. Even other countries that produce a lot of wine, as does the United States—Argentina, Australia, and New Zealand—are well ahead of us for consumption.

Clearly, wine is still far from our national drink. Among adults in the United States who drink alcohol, 2014 Gallup data showed that 41 percent say they most often choose beer, 31 percent say wine, and 23 percent say hard liquor. We in the United States consume over seven times as much beer as wine.

Our nation's wine capital is, well, our nation's capital: Washington, DC. (This taste for wine may have to do with DC's Francophilia, as we remember from chapter 5, on brunch.) The New England states are also high for per capita wine consumption, along with Nevada and California. Mississippi and West Virginia are the least enthused. According to the Wine Market Council, 60 percent of American adults don't drink wine at all. To be fair, 36 percent abstain from alcohol altogether. (The proportion of American adults who drink, about 64 percent, has remained roughly the same over the seventy-five years Gallup has been tracking it, hitting as high as 71 percent in the latter part of the 1970s, and as low as 55 percent in 1958.)

What really sets us apart with respect to wine, though, is our open-mindedness. That trait applies to Americans in general, but research shows that millennials are even more adventurous with food and beverage choices than our already willing-to-experiment parents and grandparents. So while baby boomers may make up the largest chunk of wine drinkers, millennials are far more interested in wine than previous generations were at our age.

How has this fact changed the industry?

For starters, about 25 percent of young American wine drinkers will do so . . . using a cup and a straw. That's according to a recent survey that Libran Research & Consulting conducted on behalf of E. & J. Gallo. Personally, I can't help but love the Sofia Blanc de Blancs from Francis Ford Coppola Winery, which comes in a mini-can with a cute little bendy straw. All I can say is: We grew up on juice boxes. It's not much of a leap.

That Capri Sun must have left quite the taste in our mouths, because we also prefer sweet wines. In the Libran survey, moscato was nearly twice as likely a choice as any other varietal, and we're 12 percent more likely than older drinkers to buy it.

Prosecco, sparkling wine from Italy, has been growing substantially in popularity in the United States, in part because millennials are seeing wine more as something for every day, whereas prosecco used to be associated only with special occasions. Clearly, soda too has left its mark on our palates.

As a country, not being tied down by rigid rules and expectations means we have the willingness to reinvent the way we eat—and drink. While this mind-set makes our food culture unstable, it also presents a blank canvas.

Wine and the Environment

One of the most democratic things about wine in America has been the outpouring of creative new vessels in which to drink it. It's also another example of how younger drinkers are taking the industry in some intriguing directions.

Just as we'll applaud the boot during Oktoberfest, joyously drink sake in little ceramic cups, and even attend football games wearing beer helmets, there's a whole sector of innovative packaging for wine. Many of the inventions make wine drinking more affordable and more environmentally responsible. In the age of BuzzFeed and listicles, let's use a list of superlatives to tour some of the standouts of America's alternative wine-packaging movement.

Best for . . . a Boozy Walk in the Woods: Bandit

Like a milk carton, sort of, this Tetra Pak wine container is great for backpacking because its squishiness helps with the Tetris challenge of packing the backpack, and unlike schlepping out a hollow bottle afterward, you can fold the empty carton flat. Bandit's packaging is full of fun facts to make you feel warm and fuzzy inside (or is that the wine talking?): award-winning vino, check; good for the planet, check. Manufacturing the package material involves a much lower carbon footprint than using glass bottles. Transporting the cartons is more fuel efficient because they're much lighter and "space efficient" in a cargo container. That's because of their tall, rectangular shape instead of a bottle with the skinny neck and that weird inverted nipple at the bottom. Bandit touts the fact that it takes fifty-two semitrailers to carry a million empty wine bottles, versus just two for a million empty Bandit cartons. All that, and their standard container holds a third more wine than a bottle.

Most of the leaders in the nontraditional container movement argue that the money they're saving on packaging and shipping means they focus on good grapes and good wine-making. They're not compromising on quality. For the skeptics, you know you're in good hands because the winemaker is the same guy, Joel Gott, who is behind the namesake label from Napa Valley sold in stores and restaurants out of standard glassware. In the words of Bandit, "It's what's inside the bottle that counts."

Best for . . . Sneaking into the Movie Theater:
Underwood

Gary Vaynerchuk must have been smiling the day he first saw Underwood, the wine in a can. Yep, you read that right. The company's marketing is all about ditching the stuffiness. Or, as they call it, the "fussiness." A product of Union Wine Company, Underwood launched it in Portland in 2013 with a "Pinkies Down" campaign.

If there's one thing Oregon is not, it's pretentious. Instead of a tasting room, Union has a mobile tasting truck. Their website says, "Wines for Everyone." The point is that the people who produce the wine should be able to afford to drink it. You can get a four-pack for just $24, and the math on this one will blow your mind: There are more than two glasses' worth in each can. People are often concerned at first that the aluminum might not taste so great, but a liner serves as a barrier between the aluminum and the wine, similar to other canned drinks. See for yourself. Especially with the white wines, it's rather refreshing out of a cold can. I even have friends who stuff these in their purses before heading to a movie theater. (I hear the Pinot Gris pairs well with popcorn.)

There's a similar canned wine called Turn 4, Cab or Sauv Blanc in a container that's unusually tall and slender. At first glance, I thought, *Eureka: It's the tall boy of wine!* But it turned out to be an optical illusion since it holds the same amount as a standard can.

As Underwood has demonstrated, changing the marketing of wine is also key to making it more mainstream. It can't just be about gourmet food and elite social functions. E. & J. Gallo's head of marketing, Stephanie Gallo, told *AdWeek* that lately they too are having a bit more fun with the juice, making it "less intimidating." They had their Barefoot wine sponsor the World Series of Beach Volleyball. (Both, of course, involve bare feet.)

Best for . . . Keeping It Classy: Copa di Vino

This is wine . . . already in the glass. The taste is decent and the container is irresistible. A community revival project from a small town in, again, Oregon, Copa di Vino developed a soft plastic, ergonomically appealing, single-serving cup—with a lid. Much as I hate to admit, there's something elegant about it being so similarly shaped to a traditional wineglass. Now, because it's a single-serving container, my eco-friendly alarm is sounding a bit, but the flat lid does make it stackable, which helps reduce the transportation burden on the environment. There's a foil cap, like on applesauce containers, to prevent spoilage, as can sometimes happen with cork. It's 187 milliliters, or one glass, and you can even reseal it to drink the rest later. Better still: Reuse it, put homemade tomato sauce in it, or make it your daily water bottle.

Best for . . . Hosting a Party, or the Hump Day Solo Drink: Bota Box

It's hard to beat Bota's intersection of (relatively) high quality with bang for buck: Each box has four 750-milliliter bottles' worth of wine, or three liters, for about $17. That's twenty five-ounce glasses. Quick: Invite everyone you know! Drinks are on you, at no threat to your credit score. The real magic lies in the spigot. Before you say Franzia, allow me to assure you this is a *very* distant cousin of the cough syrup in a bladder. It's won contests and stuff for how it tastes.

This device suits my generation's spontaneity: Rather than be hemmed in by the ticking clock of a whole bottle of wine, you pour yourself exactly the amount you want, at the time you want it, and kick back, because it lasts over a month after you've opened it. As anyone knows who has received the last-minute text, *"Sooo sorry to bail, but I [insert excuse for got a better offer],"* we like to keep our options open. Make "game-time" decisions. And Bota Box is the perfect complement to that lifestyle.

(My hunch is that this new social norm is one of the main reasons behind the declining prominence of that great institution known as the dinner party. Who wants to splurge on top cuts of meat, clean the whole house, and cook for days only to have half the guests cancel the week of? And this is not just a millennials thing but an all-adults thing, as described in *The New York Times* piece "Guess Who Isn't Coming to Dinner." The Hartman Group's data show that the average American adult only attends 3.6 weekend parties *per year* at someone's house. Many Americans seem to feel it's easier to meet friends at a restaurant instead—one you all confirm via group text that morning, no less.)

But back to Bota Box. Just think of all the packaging you save. It's a BPA-free plastic pouch nestled inside a paper box made of fiber that's mostly been recycled once before and can be again.

Americans and the Environment

A product's recyclability is not just a niche concern: It's a distinctly American way of looking at the environmental impact of humans. Americans are more likely than the global average to recycle. But that's about the only area of environmental responsibility where we stand out for the better. Hang with me here for a second; after the guilt trip, I promise there's a silver lining.

The National Geographic Society, in partnership with a research firm called GlobeScan, produces a Greendex report surveying 18,000 consumers in eighteen countries about their attitudes and behaviors related to the environment. It touches on topics like housing (i.e., water and energy usage), transportation, and items you buy, including food. The two organizations started producing the report in 2008, and Americans haven't fared too well when it comes to sustainable behavior. Every single time, we have ranked dead last. I know, I was shocked too.

Interestingly, developing countries outperform most developed countries, with India and China ranking highest, and Canada and Japan rubbing elbows with us at the bottom of the pack. The United States is one of the only countries whose behavior has become *less* sustainable since 2012. We consume a lot of resources overall, in part because we really like disposables—disposable diapers and contact lenses and razors and Ziploc bags, to name a few. And take-out containers don't grow on trees.

Perhaps one reason we rank so low is that we're among the least likely to experience what is called "green guilt." Only one in five of us said we feel guilty about our environmental impact.

What's behind these figures? Again, it's our individualism.

For example, we also rank last for taking public transportation, walking, or biking, instead of driving. We rank among the highest for driving a car or truck by ourselves. To some extent, we can blame the infrastructure—our cities are designed for cars, as many, *many* people have lamented. City planners are hard at work to make our subway systems, sidewalks, and bike paths more attractive to appeal to more users. But our habits are also driven by values. We feel it's our right to drive our own cars, leaving at exactly the time we wish to leave, listening to exactly the music we wish to listen to, with the air conditioning set to our personally optimal temperature.

On the plus side, we are *great* at recycling. And it's probably because we rank highest in our faith in an individual's power to help the environment. Case in point: We also rank high for consuming energy-efficient appliances and insulating our homes. Sure, we may be more likely than people in some other countries to feel we can *afford* to make those investments, but it's also that we think those changes will make a difference. Individualism may have its negative consequences, but it also means we see great potential impact from discrete personal actions when added all together.

Here's the silver lining: With the many new approaches to wine, America is on its way to being an eco-friendly standout for once. California is leading a movement on sustainable wine-grape growing and wine production, and this has huge implications because the state produces 90 percent of all wine made in the United States. Sixty percent of all wine consumed in the United States is from the Golden State, meaning three of every five bottles we drink is a California wine. Many of the innovative packages, as well as wine on tap at restaurants, conserve resources on labels, glass, foil seals, and so on, while preventing oxidation, which is the main concern. Perhaps because of millennials' mobility—we try on cities and jobs and apartments with whimsy, not settling down or buying homes as early as our parents did—we aren't terribly concerned about *aging* wine. So if it tastes good, doesn't cost a fortune, and helps the environment, why not?

To celebrate the eightieth anniversary of the end of Prohibition, *Time* magazine made a list of "80 Reasons Why Drinking Alcohol Is Great." There's a provocative history lesson in reasons 30 through 34:

30. A well-timed drink helps you chill out. Take the trusty advice of beer brewer (and President) Thomas Jefferson: "Beer, if drunk in moderation, softens the temper, cheers the spirit and promotes happiness."

31. Actually, all of our forefathers want you to drink. George Washington opened the nation's largest whiskey distillery in 1797.

32. John Hancock was an alcohol dealer.

33. Lincoln was a licensed bartender and owned his own tavern.

34. Wanna know who supposedly didn't touch alcohol? Hitler. Just saying.

One of the traits we sought to shed from our British roots during the American Revolution was the snootiness. We're the country of the T-shirt and jeans. So it's exciting to think that lowering the snobbery of wine—in the wine itself, and in how we market and deliver it—can also boost its sustainability.

In the United States, we're encouraged to explore, free to fail. But fail quickly and move on. It's the battle cry of the

American entrepreneur. There are many admirable European values: On the whole, Europeans are less focused on money, more on family. They care about stability and tradition. But that leaves them less open to new ideas. In Europe, there's more stigma associated with failure, according to *New York Times* writer James B. Stewart. For example, he says the penalties for bankruptcy in Europe are far more serious than in the United States, where he calls them "simply a rite of passage for many successful entrepreneurs." I admit, we probably shouldn't take *too* much pride in that particular example, but with greater risks, we tap into greater levels of creativity. And ultimately, that gives us a shot at greater rewards.

Sure, we might be inclined to ditch a given food fetish rather abruptly, avoiding the burden of letting it become too deeply associated with our identity, but our food ways also benefit from our open-mindedness.

Wine likely won't replace beer. But it *could*. We can embrace wine despite our history as beer lovers. Because in the United States, we take pride in not doing what our parents did. Given the great pluralism we embrace here, it's not so much about pushing out beer to make room for wine, but welcoming a more prominent tile for it in the mosaic of our national drinking culture.

CHAPTER 8

The Age of Stunt Foods

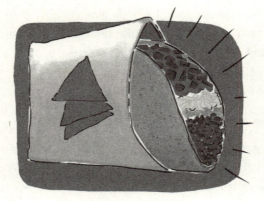

It's midday on a Friday, and I'm in Orange County, California, sitting around a table with four women gabbing about food. No one is eating except me.

Typical, I think to myself.

But this is not some sidewalk bistro in Laguna Beach, and these are not the ladies who lunch. We're at a semicircular counter in a windowless room in a nondescript white office park that's home to one of America's largest fast-food giants. And my lunch mates are some of the masterminds behind one of the most successful fast-food products in history: the Doritos Locos Taco.

The table is inside the "innovation forum" at Taco Bell headquarters, a pseudo-classroom with a kitchen used to simulate a restaurant. Like the rest of the building, this room has the vibe of a Virgin America airplane. Bright menu panels line the back wall, and two amphitheater-style rows of purple cushioned chairs face large television screens above the table and demo kitchen. The squeaky-clean, stainless steel kitchen is stocked with heaters and timers, plastic drawers of taco shells, and stacks of to-go containers. These food scientists and marketing gurus may not be eating, but I'm about to become one of the very first outsiders to bite into the third flavor of the Doritos Locos Taco, "Fiery DLT."

When the original nacho cheese DLT debuted in March 2012, its sales figures were as eye-popping as its neon orange shell. It quickly became the company's most popular menu item of all time. It hit the 100-million mark in an unprecedented ten weeks. (Granted, times were different, but it took McDonald's ten *years* to sell its 100-millionth burger during the 1950s.) Before the taco reached its six-month birthday, every third person in America had had two DLTs. To date, Taco Bell has sold more than a *billion* Doritos Locos Tacos, at a rate of a million per day throughout its first year.

You may even know it as the taco that helped "save America," as *The Daily Beast* put it, because the growth in Taco Bell business led to the creation of 15,000 new jobs.

Certainly food innovation is nothing new—the food industry calls it "differentiating." But the DLT and its brethren from other chains are a unique breed. Are they fast food? Of course. Junk food? Well, absolutely. Yet these concoctions are so absurdly, unabashedly decadent that we need a new category. At the close of 2010, *Gourmet* writer Jennifer Wright declared the launch of KFC's Double Down—which features two chicken filets with bacon and jack cheese in between them—and products like it the "rise of stunt food." But if that was the rise, we are now at the full-blown mania. Call it Stunt Foods 2.0 or, to borrow from food product development expert Barb Stuckey, the era of "Shock-and-Awe."

The fast-food ecosystem used to be fairly stable and well defined: burgers here at McDonald's, pizza there at Pizza Hut, fried chicken at KFC. But that has changed.

In 2012, as the DLT was sweeping the country off its feet, Burger King took its bacon sundae nationwide, Baskin-Robbins deconstructed an ice cream cone into "nachos," and Cinnabon applied its trademark spiral for baked rolls to a personal pizza. The years since have seen even more unimaginable gastronomic offspring. Among others, we saw Chili Cheese Fry Burritos at Del Taco, Pop-Tart ice cream sandwiches at Carl's Jr., and bacon-egg donut sandwiches at Dunkin' Donuts. Pizza Hut started wreathing its pizzas with mini cheeseburgers in the Middle East, then in the summer of 2015, did the same thing with mini hot dogs here in the United States, sending a wave of hype across the country.

These inventions all owe a creative debt to the almighty KFC Double Down, which, health-wise, has twice as much sodium as a Big Mac—and 25 percent more than the daily limit—but is similar calorie-wise to many fast-food mainstays. The Burger King bacon sundae has a similar number of calories—around 500—as a grande Starbucks Mocha Cookie Crumble Frappuccino and slightly less sugar (61 versus 69 grams, a smidge more than two Snickers bars' worth). There are differences in ingredients and sourcing to consider in the health equation, but all are indulgences. What's unique about the Double Down, the bacon sundae, and the like is their flagrance.

Clearly, there are plenty of us who have come to accept—even to relish—fast food as pure indulgence. The nutrition police be damned.

Stunt foods are about *celebrating* decadence, rather than hiding it. Some of the promos for the DLT simply said in big block letters: "GIVE IN." A few years back, Pizza Hut ditched the internal name for a new pizza it was about to debut, "Stuffed

Italiano," in favor of "Crazy Cheesy Crust." In its press release, it called the innovation an "explosion" and invited customers to "let loose" with their next order.

So what to make of all this? Is it as straightforward as an innate desire for novelty? Or could it be a sign of a brewing backlash against the daily health-food agitprop—a metaphoric flip of the bird to Michelle Obama and all the others telling us how to eat?

From a marketing perspective, why do these work? Why, good people of America, are we such suckers for stunts?

Inside the World of Fast-Food Menu R&D

The stunt-foods trend came about because of two forces within the fast-food industry. The first is an imperative for research-intensive product development—"menu R&D" in industry speak. Product development is certainly nothing new, but the pressure to satisfy customers' desire for new food experiences has been heightened.

Paired with stiff competition from fast-casual restaurants (like Chipotle and Panera Bread), fast-food chains that have been around for decades may start to look, well, like they have been around for decades. If you don't innovate, you fold. Compared with those of the 1990s, menus at fast-food restaurants now have twice as many distinct items, according to market research firm the NPD Group.

It's no longer enough to merely invent new products. Now you have to provide shock value. Nutritional train wrecks that are this over-the-top used to exist mostly at state fairs—fried

butter on a stick, for example. But now these types of unbeliev-
able combinations are being sold at national fast-food chains
where people dine on a regular basis.

And in this new world order, all the lines are blurred. Consider the hamburger-looking ice cream sandwich at Carl's Jr.,
which mixed dinner mentality with dessert reality. Menu items
like these cross meal categories, or qualities from meals and
snacks. To win over consumers with the Doritos Locos Taco,
the innovation team would learn they could not use a run-of-
the-mill corn taco (standard dinner fare). Instead, a successful
hybrid would have to offer distinct *chip* qualities, putting the
eater in a decidedly snack-oriented frame of mind.

Meanwhile, the increasing influence of social media has also
driven these companies to pursue stunt foods. This has made
many fast-food execs question the power of traditional advertising and instead court the free attention reaped when a product goes viral. Put those two forces together, and the incentives
are clear. Start with an idea that's too absurd to ignore—then
use serious science to bring it to life.

How did the Doritos Locos Taco come to be? Did Taco Bell just
sprinkle some orange powder on a plain old taco shell? Hardly.
Doritos is a billion-dollar brand. "Nothing gets to call itself a
Dorito unless it walks like a Dorito, talks like a Dorito, and
tastes *exactly* like a Dorito," says Barb Stuckey, chief innovation officer at Mattson, a company that helps clients develop
new food and beverage products. "That makes [merging with
another food concept] very unwieldy. You've got a gold standard you have to meet. I guarantee it was the furthest thing
from easy."

The union of Frito-Lay and Taco Bell took place in early
2009 at Taco Bell headquarters, the LEED-certified "Restaurant

Support Center" in Irvine, California. Frito-Lay was among the companies invited to participate in an "ideation session"—a calculated attempt to collaborate.

Earlier that year, Taco Bell's CEO at the time, Greg Creed, had posed a challenge to his innovation team: Reinvent the taco. *Rock* the industry.

Taco Bell's chief product marketing officer, Stephanie Perdue, and senior brand marketing manager, Kat Garcia—who together "shepherd ideas from paper to drive-thru"—combined this edict with the consumer insights they were gathering from focus groups. "We really saw our consumers' palate changing," says Perdue. "Millennials want flavor." So with the Doritos Locos Taco, they were targeting a group of millennials they call "thrill seekers." They wrote up a memo describing that target customer ("all about their wants and needs," Perdue says) and put out a call for ideas from select brands.

Inside the innovation forum, after vendors presented thirty ideas, Frito-Lay was the clear standout. "They are so clever with their seasoning—what they can get your brain to think your mouth is experiencing," Creed told me, in his thick Australian accent. (Among other things, he says "TACK-o," not "TOCK-o.") He also told me about a time he flew down to Plano, Texas, to visit Frito-Lay headquarters. His eyes lighting up like a little kid's, he gushed that one of the chips he tried there "tasted like a hamburger!"

Frito-Lay and Taco Bell were a likely match: Frito-Lay's parent company, PepsiCo, used to own Taco Bell. In 1997, Yum! Brands, Inc. (formerly Tricon Global Restaurants) walked out on PepsiCo, taking Taco Bell, KFC, and Pizza Hut with it. But PepsiCo and Yum! have remained cordial over the years, close even. (Ever notice that only Pepsi products are available at these chains?)

Kentucky-based Yum! is the largest fast-food company on

the planet, with more than 41,000 restaurants in more than 125 countries and territories. Having struggled to increase domestic sales, Yum! has increasingly looked overseas. It now earns over 75 percent of its revenue outside the United States. It opened 156 new locations in India in 2014 alone, and in China, averaged about two new locations per *day* through 2015.

Taco Bell, for its part, is America's leading Mexican-themed fast-food restaurant. It serves nearly 37 million customers a week, across 5,600 restaurants. But in 2009, it needed a boost.

At the time, décor at many traditional fast-food outlets had begun to look downright clinical. Menus felt bland, out of touch with America's increasingly daring palate. So chains including Taco Bell started taking a few cues from fast-casual restaurants and began revamping stores and menus. Some even offered free Wi-Fi to foster a Starbucks effect, along the lines of a he-who-lingers-spends strategy.

The collaboration session hosted by Taco Bell also likely stemmed from a more basic perennial reality: "The moment you open a retail establishment, it's getting old," says the NPD Group's Harry Balzer. Satisfying the human desire for novelty is at the core of the food industry. And today, the number of new food products is higher than ever. Yet, 80 percent of all new product innovation fails, so it's risky for both reputation and profits.

And while Taco Bell was facing these usual challenges and changes in the fast-food landscape, they were also approaching a major anniversary in 2012: the big 5-0.

It's easy to see why it was time for them to redefine themselves.

Stunt foods share certain characteristics. Many are the result of crossing two familiar brands—which makes good business sense: Rather than inventing something from scratch and having to explain what it is, preexisting brand recognition and product familiarity go a long way in getting people to try something that sounds crazy. Our desire for novelty is tempered by our need for familiarity.

"If you don't have to spend the money to tell people what a Dorito is, you're halfway there," says Stuckey.

Brand partnerships have been popular in fast food for years, perhaps most memorably beginning with the McDonald's McFlurry, using ingredients like Oreo, Snickers, and M&M's.

Yet a company may be protective of certain elements of its brand. "So instead of McDonald's putting Kraft cheese on their hamburgers, they want to put McDonald's cheese on their hamburgers," Stuckey says. "Because they don't want to give up any positive associations to Kraft—they want to keep that for themselves." Other companies resist cobranding altogether, concerned that it "dilutes their brand message," she says. But intertwining Doritos and Taco Bell felt natural, almost inevitable.

Yet it was a long road from boardroom brainstorm to nationwide sensation. Product development took twice as long as usual.

At first, Taco Bell sprinkled some nacho cheese powder on a regular shell and called it a day. They presented it to focus groups, acknowledging it was still in its early stages but explaining that they were eager to know how consumers felt.

It was a disaster. What they felt was disappointment.

"Out comes this hand-seasoned yellow shell, and it's kind of like you're totally bummed out," says Steven Gomez, a food scientist who worked on Taco Bell's DLT team. " 'This was the best idea ever, and this is what you guys give me!?' "

The taste and texture were totally off.

"The hardest thing anyone does in the food business is reverse engineer something so it tastes like something else," says Stuckey. From twenty-plus years in the business, from Kraft to Whole Foods Market, she has learned that getting a product 98 percent there is usually doable. But "closing the gap," nailing the final 2 percent of a product's essence, is extremely difficult and expensive. So expensive, in fact, that often, "it costs more than it's worth."

Off-the-charts ratings for the concept from consumer testing gave Taco Bell the wind at its back to press on.

"All of the technology that went into this were *dreams,*" says Erin Peffly, also a food scientist from the DLT team at Taco Bell (a career path she credits in part to the night she watched Alton Brown explain the thermodynamics of popcorn, prompting her to ditch premed for food science). Peffly, Gomez, and the thirty or so other members of the innovation team went through nearly two years of technical challenges.

They worked with Frito-Lay's technologists and flew back and forth between Plano and their Irvine office for a stretch. They confronted questions like how much seasoning to use, what the right color would be, and what to do about the fact that Doritos are triangles and taco shells are circles.

Maintaining Doritos' "tooth-rattling crunch" was crucial, Gomez says. But so was finger residue. "One of the equities of [Nacho Cheese] Doritos is you get orange seasoning on your fingers and you lick it off," says Gomez. That's part of the experience. "Although that's great for Doritos, we have to make taco shells all day along with other products. We can't let that transfer over [onto other items that customers order]."

So they hunkered down again, brainstorming solutions for the fingerprint problem. Maybe their restaurant crews could use tongs to grab a shell each time someone ordered a DLT. In the end, it came down to kindergarten basics of cutting and pasting: The breakthrough was a "taco holster" made out of cardboard. The shells are shipped separately in long stacks, so the paper sleeve would allow each shell to arrive at the restaurant in what Gomez called a "nice little snug package," preventing seasoning from spreading.

The holster proved a crowd pleaser in ways they hadn't even intended. The sleeve prevented the shell from cracking and kept the messy taco intact, while also serving as a kind of bib. "Consumers started saying, 'And it even comes with . . . this thing you can eat out of, that catches the ingredients that fall out of the taco,'" Gomez says. Plus, it was as if each taco now had its own miniature billboard, an opportunity the marketing team would later seize on.

During my visit to the innovation forum at Taco Bell headquarters, when I asked how the seasoning step works, my perky hosts fell oddly silent. Their eyes darted around at each other, as if they'd forgotten their lines.

"The cheese dust fairy," Peffly said.

Right. The cheese dust fairy.

In reality, Taco Bell worked with Frito-Lay to tweak existing manufacturing lines, and Frito-Lay licensed some technology and built new lines from scratch.

After years of work, the big day finally arrived in March 2012. Like many lucky newborns, the DLT came into the world embraced by fans who needed no more reason to love it than the fact that they loved its parents.

As for the name, Doritos *Locos* Taco, why did they go with "crazy"? One glance at the color should make that pretty obvious. And, like any celeb couple's kid, growing up with a weird name comes with the territory.

Once the idea for a stunt food has been hatched, bringing it to the table in real life can involve as many scientists as a government task force. Fast-food chains' R&D rosters include people with degrees in culinary science and nutrition, but also chemistry and industrial, packaging, and mechanical engineering. R&D teams also rely on prototypes and operations tests, focus groups, and market tests.

The challenges include addressing everything from sogginess, dryness, and breakage to uneven distribution of ingredients. And any fast-food item needs a system in place to keep the thing hot—and tasting fresh—until the customer gets it home. Altogether, months and even years can pass between conception of an idea and birth of a product.

Take that Chili Cheese Fry Burrito. At its headquarters in Lake Forest, California, Del Taco has a sensory lab where it conducts preference tests—asking consumers to rate different items that appear in chutes—and matching tests. During the latter, expert tasters sit in booths with red and blue lighting (which eliminates preferences triggered by visual cues) and try to detect differences between versions of a product. The biggest problem with the burrito was the ratio of dry and wet ingredients. That is, they had to merge wet chili with dry starches— crinkle-cut fries and a tortilla—without producing either a swampy mess or a chalky log.

Plus, as with all fast food, there's the issue of portability— how would the product hold up in transit? So they tested the burrito at five-minute intervals. "I've got to guarantee the product is as hot and fresh and just as flavorful forty minutes after I've prepared it as it is five minutes after I've prepared it," says Mike Salem, former senior director of research and development at Del Taco, who is now vice president of product marketing at Papa Murphy's International.

From the perspective of a food marketer, the problem with pizza has always been the crust—the part of the product that many eaters throw away. Nearly twenty years ago, Pizza Hut answered that challenge with the Stuffed Crust Pizza, which, according to the company, added some $300 million to total sales. Since then, Pizza Hut has experimented with all manner of other crust enhancements. The spring of 2013 saw the release of the Crazy Cheesy Crust Pizza, with pockets of cheese that turn the crust into a decadent detachable appetizer. The pie took about a year to develop, director of culinary innovation Dominique Vitry said in an e-mail, with most of the work going into the blend of cheeses.

After trying out fifty-plus variations, Pizza Hut chose a combination of five cheeses because "once we went below that number, we lost the 'wow.'" The R&D team then tested the color, texture, and "ooey-gooey" stretch on 1,280 slices. The company even performed driver simulations: carrying the completed pizza over railroad tracks, back roads, and busy streets to ensure that it would arrive in a noncrazy condition.

Interestingly, not all fast-food innovation is high tech. One of the more creative mash-ups, and another example of co-branding, was the Strawberry Pop-Tart Ice Cream Sandwich from Carl's Jr. After a month-long trial period in Southern California, the company rolled out the $1.49 delicacy chain-wide in July 2013 to rave reviews. "The pastry-to-ice cream ratio is spot-on, giving a gleeful juxtaposition," wrote *The Phoenix New Times*. Comedian Jimmy Kimmel wondered: "Is Carl's Jr. reading my dream journal?"

So what's the secret? It was quite simple: "We freeze the Pop-Tarts first," Carl's Jr. marketing honcho Brad Haley wrote to me in an e-mail. "That way they cut cleanly without crumbling"—the sandwich uses half a Pop-Tart on each side—"and they also don't melt the ice cream." Then they put a big scoop of vanilla ice cream between the halves, package the treat, and refreeze it. At 320 calories, it's one of the healthier desserts on the restaurant's menu. (Carl's Jr. also sells a 720-calorie Oreo shake.)

To be fair, Americans aren't the only ones into ingenuity with regard to food; other countries produce over-the-top novelties and products to grab attention, too. A recent invention from Argentina called DestapaBanana is a sort of wine opener device that removes the core of a banana—imagine a long straw—and replaces it with the liquid of your choice, namely caramel or chocolate. And KFC UK developed edible coffee cups. That's either good news for the environment (fewer cups sent to the landfill) or bad news for public health (the cups are made of sugar paper and heat-resistant white chocolate).

One major difference between us and other countries is the influence American food chains have around the globe. I'm talking about Domino's (the world's largest pizza delivery chain) sweeping India to make it the second-largest market outside the United States. I'm talking about the 66,000 units overseas just among the ten largest U.S.-based fast-food chains. And in 2013, for the first time in France's history, its regular food receipts were overtaken by fast-food receipts. Sales aren't coming just from McDonald's—which has the overall largest international presence at 119 countries across six continents. They're coming from local eateries, clearly having been influenced by Mickey D's and the like, that are serving microwaveable processed meals and foods on the run.

Stunts and Social Media

Burger King's bacon sundae sprang from the chain's innovation team scanning Pinterest and other sites to analyze how consumers were using bacon in creative ways. Del Taco launched its Chili Cheese Fry Burrito after it realized that customers were making the concoction themselves in the restaurant; at least one franchise reported that customers were asking the counter staff to make it for them special. (Ironically, says Salem, formerly of Del Taco, getting the idea for the burrito from customers actually made them more difficult to please because the food scientists had to "emulate the product as the consumer had created it in their minds.")

And that granddaddy of the stunt-foods movement, the KFC Double Down, had Internet help out the gate. Between the blogosphere brouhaha and YouTube videos—in which thousands of people watched other people go to test-market KFC locations and try the sandwich, bragging, "Bet you wish you lived here!"—the Double Down earned more buzz during testing than any other menu item in the company's history. So much so that KFC announced the product's nationwide arrival before it was even available. In the April 2010 press release, Javier Benito, executive vice president of marketing and food innovation at the time, explained the unusual move: "We want fans to have time to arrange their schedules in advance for a visit to KFC to try this legendary sandwich." The release also boasted that the chicken chain would be donating "unneeded" sandwich buns to food banks.

"Things like the KFC Double Down and [Burger King] bacon sundae are only *partly* meant for consumption," says Stuckey. "They are in large part media stunts. . . . With KFC, imagine how much free publicity that Double Down generated just because it was so outrageous."

It was 2012 when I spoke with her, and she added, "Burger King has had really difficult times financially over the last five years. It's almost like a Hail Mary pass, because they don't have anything to lose."

When it came time to debut the DLT, the Taco Bell marketing team went full throttle, launching its "biggest marketing effort in recent history."

There were, of course, ads galore, but most of their efforts involved more innovative, interactive ways of acquainting consumers with the DLT. Music and a new emphasis on discovery anchored the campaign. Taco Bell offered samples at music events and slapped the taco holsters with QR codes linked to exclusive music video footage. Taco Bell announced a short-term opportunity for tweeters of hashtag #DoritosLocosTacos to be featured on digital billboards in Times Square and on Sunset Boulevard.

The month before the launch, Taco Bell announced a new tagline of "Live Más," proclaiming a shift from "food as fuel" to food as experience and a way of life. It explained in its press release that the tagline "celebrates getting more out of life, encouraging exploration and discovery beyond food." Producing a neon-orange food species was certainly an apt time to promote trying new things.

In launching and sustaining the DLT craze, Taco Bell was as maniacally active on social media as the teens it targets. Once the nacho cheese dust had settled from the debut of the original DLT, customers began asking for Cool Ranch flavor, and Taco Bell started teasing it online. In January 2013, it posted an image to Facebook of a taco and a bag of Cool Ranch Doritos with the caption "anything could happen in 2013." Among the company's most liked Facebook posts ever, it garnered more than 133,000 likes. Taco Bell even created "Taco Speakeasies" in New York, Dallas, and Los Angeles, where fans could use social media to "unlock" the locations of places to try the new taco. During testing for another of Taco Bell's shock-worthy stars, the waffle taco, one Instagram photo snowballed into 4 million social media impressions—for a product still confined to five test restaurants.

The natural hype makes you wonder how much Taco Bell needed the highly orchestrated hype. It's a taco made of Doritos—the minute people hear it or see it, they talk about it.

And curiosity goes beyond talk. Stunt foods get even the least likely among us in the door. Once the DLT was born, countless reporters, bloggers, and even *New York Times* food writers went to see for themselves. Following a feature on the history of the taco shell in light of the DLT debut, *The New York Times* dining section published a verging-on-sincere review of these tacos, analyzing the spice allocation and "topography" of the Dorito shell versus chip, the philosophical identity crisis of the crossbreed, as well as the relative amounts of orange fingertip residue. NPR called the orange dust "the fat man's cocaine" and mused about what substance the shell comes from ("Dorito Sheetrock," perhaps). The Huffington Post took the time to conduct eight experiments inserting Doritos into other fast-food items, like sprinkling ground Dorito powder on Dunkin' Donuts.

Even at a conference I attended among culinary elite, when the presenting speaker asked for a show of hands of who had tried the Doritos Locos Taco, a third or more went up.

When it comes to gawking, analyzing, and yes, *eating,* stunt foods—we just. Can't. Help ourselves.

The Health-Food Agitprop Rejectionist Movement

In the world of deciding what to put on menus, what and how to feed people, there are essentially two camps: Team Michelle Obama and Team DGAF. (That's "Don't Give a Fuck.") In one corner, we've got legislators forcing restaurants to post calorie counts, junk food brands voluntarily reformulating their products to contain less salt, sugar, and artificial ingredients, and chains using antibiotic-free meat. To muddy the waters, former McDonald's execs are now running Lyfe Kitchen, a fast-casual restaurant chain that touts sustainable sourcing, animal welfare, and across-the-board health.

On the other side of the ring, we have the conscientious objectors of the whole obesity conversation. Food scientists and marketers, they spend their dollars and days contriving flagrant—albeit imaginative—novelty foods. Amid parental pleas to stop marketing junk food to children, these industry reps have instead fortified their foothold among kids by innovating both what and how they sell. Are they bad people, plotting ever more harmful ways to hook us? What they are most definitely is *business* people. "They don't sit there and say is it healthy or not," says Hank Cardello, the former Coca-Cola exec turned food industry health consultant. "They try all kinds of concepts, and they're just looking to find the right formulas where they can sell some product."

While many parents and public health professionals argue that these companies' marketing machinery makes us defenseless (particularly children), Balzer and Stuckey argue that it's *because* we buy these ludicrous iterations that food chains will continue designing them. Balzer and Stuckey say people incorrectly think the food industry wants to make us fat. "That's not true," Stuckey says. "If vegetables and water are going to sell, that's what they're going to put on their menu." But as we know, it just so happens we're drawn to foods engineered with plenty of salt and sugar and not-so-good fats.

So yes, the DLT can easily post record sales in the midst of a pervasive national conversation about diet and health. And stunt foods aren't going away any time soon. Baseball fans can surely attest to that, if the Fried S'mOreo at the Texas Rangers' stadium and the pulled-pork parfait at the Milwaukee Brewers' stadium are any indication. Through its runaway success, the

DLT has emerged as the standard-bearer for a whole platoon of new food species.

Consider a few of the more recent examples of mash-up mania:

Fried chicken chain Church's Chicken announced in late 2014 that for the month of December it would be stuffing its iconic biscuits—of which it sells 160 million a year—with Oreos. For their Oreo Biscuit Bites, they took crumbled Oreos, which is apparently America's favorite cookie brand, mixed them into their biscuit dough and topped the bites with vanilla icing. Keep in mind that Church's had never touched its honey-butter biscuits in fifty-two years of selling them, likely for fear of mutiny.

Papa John's got in on the fun with Frito Chili Pizza. This one, I'd have to say, gets almost no points for creativity, given that Frito pie (which is typically made with chili) has been around for decades. This pizza takes a Papa John's pizza of cheddar and mozzarella cheese, tomatoes, and onions, tops it with ground beef and chili sauce, then, after it's baked, adds a bunch of Fritos. Pretty simple. As part of NPR's "Sandwich Monday" satire, a team featuring comedians from the show "Wait Wait . . . Don't Tell Me!" described the pizza as "blurring the line between 'recipe' and 'spilling your Fritos in exactly the right place.'"

The NPR team went on with this dialogue of analysis between two staffers:

Ian: I look at this and half of me sees "pizza," half of me sees "place a hamster would live."

Peter: I love it. I don't care what's in it. I'd eat any of you people, with enough Fritos on top.

Two more chime in:

Eva: My late grandfather used to eat a bowl of Fritos every night as a special treat. I'm sad he's not around to die again from eating this pizza.

Mike: This is so much better than Papa John's pizza topped with free toes. A significant improvement.

Little Caesars couldn't be left out, so in early 2015, they debuted a deep-dish pizza with bacon wrapped around the crust as a sort of picture frame. Made with three and a half *feet* of bacon per pizza.

"People are *so* sick of hearing about what healthy foods you should be eating, and how we are a nation of obese people," says Stuckey. "When one of these chains comes out of left field and introduces something so shockingly indulgent, it's like a release from the onslaught of fearmongering about our health."

As we feel increasing pressure to eat healthier at school, work, and home, "restaurants are going to become the last bastion of decadence," Stuckey says. When health is a daily refrain, the desire for a night off only feels more urgent.

So when fast-food chains produce stunt foods like Chili Cheese Fry Burritos—or in the casual-dining realm, when they offer specials like Olive Garden's Never Ending Pasta Pass for unlimited pasta, bread, salad, and soft drinks for seven weeks straight—they resonate with many people.

Jack in the Box created a Munchie Meal combo, only available from 9:00 P.M. to 5:00 A.M. It bears a head-spinning menu structure: Your order comes with two tacos, Halfsie fries, which are half curly fries, half regular, and a 20-ounce drink. All for just $6. But then, since that's not the "meal," you pick your choice of four entrées. This seems a little like saying, *"Buy an air freshener and this excellent radio system and a set of*

*floor mats—oh by the way, which car would you like to include
with that?"*

A subset of the customer segments that are the least interested in healthy eating, or even a strand of behavior that might
flare up occasionally among all of us, is a kind of backlash
against the daily deluge of feel-good healthy eating PR. Among
the most entrenched, they actively reject the movement toward
healthier lifestyles and see it as paternalism at its worst.

In talking about that deep-dish pizza at Little Caesars, the
one with forty-two inches of bacon lining the perimeter, Darren
Tristano, executive vice president of the food research firm
Technomic, told *USA Today,* "It's a rebellious show of strength
by many consumers to show that the health and wellness traction is like car tires spinning on ice."

Some people have had it with Gwyneth Paltrow and her
recipes for beet-cilantro "native juice" detoxes and cauliflower
black bean bowls. They're tired of hearing their doctors whine
about risk factors and watching Michelle Obama parade through
yet another school garden. They're outraged by soda taxes and
want the anti-GMO freaks to quit their yapping. And no, they
don't want to order off the Guiltless Grill menu at Chili's.

Why Do They Work?

The story of the DLT, and of the stunt-foods phenomenon at
large, reveals two startling realizations about who we are.

1. At Odds with Ourselves

Weekday mornings just after sunrise, seventh-grade literacy
teacher Natalie Jones watches as students gather on the basketball court before class begins at her school in East Palo Alto.

They come clutching items from the taco truck parked in front of campus or from fast-food joints on the way: French fries, soda, Munchies Flamin' Hot Snack Mix, to name a few. Ms. Jones just shakes her head. She's an educator, not a nutritionist.

But she's continually stunned by how her thirteen-year-olds start their days, and by the bizarre new "foods" to which they introduce her. At the start of the 2012–2013 school year, her students were especially crazy about Taco Bell's Doritos Locos Tacos. So she became something of an expert on the America-saving taco.

A quick show of hands revealed that half of Ms. Jones's students had tried the DLT, and the rest chimed in with jealousy. "Feels like I'm lost in a Doritos taco land," said one. "*Sooo* good I can taste it right now," said another. "It's the 'certified bomb'!" Given what Ms. Jones has observed as typical morning fare, the next result came as no surprise: About a third of the experienced students had eaten the tacos *for breakfast*.

Do stunt foods reflect ingrained, immutable differences between Americans? A fundamental divide between consumers who care about eating healthy and consumers who couldn't care less? Or do they reflect contradictory impulses within *all* diners? That is, the desire to be "good" or "bad" at different times and on different days and for different occasions and different meals?

This question was a total setup, obviously, because the answer is . . . both.

As a people, we are health seeking on the one hand, while indulgence seeking on the other. Some of us are, fundamentally, one way or another. We will probably be that way for life. Other people might go back and forth over time, and still others of us go back and forth within a given week, day, and even meal.

So when DLTs and Double Downs and whatever's coming down the pipeline next enter the picture, they appeal to those consumer groups we discussed earlier, the Eat, Drink & Be Merrys and the Magic Bullets. (Think: Ms. Jones's students.) Stunt foods are pretty much guaranteed to be winners with those consumers all the time. With the other groups, it's more complicated.

"Embrace that consumers are irrational," writes the Hartman Group in summing up one of its key takeaways from a quarter-century of studying consumer behavior. "Consumers lead messy lives that are full of contradictions. People will eat at McDonald's even though they're cooking with organic food at home. They used to smoke cigarettes after jogging. No longer are we analyzing specific data points; we are reconciling how consumers say they live to what consumers really do day to day."

Another quirk that explains the popularity of stunt foods is what Stuckey calls "the hot fudge sundae and the Diet Coke." She says, "If you have the salad, you might let yourself have a pumpkin spice latte with whip cream for dessert."

Indeed, the data support this. Hank Cardello conducted some research with the Natural Marketing Institute on indulgent products like soda, candy, and salty snacks. While the Well Beings certainly consumed less of these products, the amount they consumed was still substantial. So it turns out, when you dig a bit deeper into that cohort, he says, "underneath the pile of twigs and berries in the pantry, you've got some Oreos in there."

While it may *feel* like we are all eating healthier than ever—or are at least more fixated than ever on eating healthier—the numbers speak for themselves: On top of DLT sales figures, consider that eight in ten Americans eat fast food monthly or more often. Half eat it at least weekly. These numbers have barely budged in over a decade.

Or you hear that kale consumption has increased 475 percent since 1994, and you think,*Wow, we must really be changing our ways.* But then you look at the data, in this case supplied by the NPD Group, and realize that we went from 0.4 percent of Americans eating kale at home at some point during a two-week period to a whopping 2.3 percent. (Similarly, you'll hear that Sriracha intake tripled between 1984 and 2014, and take that as a sign that we all must be a bunch of foodies. Well sure, but the increase was from 2 percent of the population to 6 percent.)

While food companies keep inventing new indulgence foods, they also know that lots of people care about health. (Or at least tell themselves they do as they walk in the door of an eatery. What happens *after* they catch a whiff of fresh-baked chocolate chip cookies is another story.)

In truth, there has been a fundamental shift in the food industry in recent years—driven in part by millennial diners—when it comes to transparency about ingredients, sustainable sourcing, animal welfare, and labor and fair wages. There has been an expansion of both the supply and demand for healthier foods offered in fast, convenient, reasonably priced meals. In many cases, though, don't give these food companies too much credit for tossing fruit cups and oatmeal on the menu. They know full well that the majority of people aren't going to order those things. They aren't their big money makers, either. But at least they can point to them as examples of covering all their bases and offering healthy food *choices*. Stuckey calls this "eliminating the veto vote." The potential veto comes, presumably, from someone trying to eat healthy in a group that wants fast food. "And that may be the same consumer, weekday versus weekend."

2. Experiential CV

Inherently, we crave exploration and experimentation, culinary adventure and discovery. This second revelation, and the most compelling, is a pattern of consumer behavior called an "experiential CV." This idea is offered up by Anat Keinan, an associate professor of business administration at Harvard Business School, and Ran Kivetz, a professor of marketing at Columbia Business School. They conducted a series of studies demonstrating that, across a variety of settings, there is a strong preference for collectable experiences, from vacation destinations to dessert choices.

Just as we collect wine corks or shot glasses, coins or seashells, we collect life experiences. In the same way that résumé builders accumulate educational milestones and job experiences, checking off items on our bucket list of personal experiences seems a way of measuring how full a life we're leading. It's also about projecting a self-image of having done a lot of exciting things. And for many people, an important component of that experiential résumé is trying new foods.

Given what we saw with their Live Más campaign promoting "food as experience," Taco Bell must have read up on Keinan and Kivetz. Oddly enough, it's this experiential résumé hypothesis that makes me kind of *appreciate* food companies—just as I would thank a chef in an outstanding restaurant for providing such a rich and unique culinary experience—for giving us opportunities to live . . . interestingly. *Try Doritos Locos Taco. Take a picture and tell friends about having tried said item. Count yourself among those who have tried one.* These food chains are just trying to help us check things off on our bucket list. (Granted, they do so by adding items we didn't even know we wanted on our list in the first place, or items that didn't even exist six months ago or definitely ten years ago when we first made our list.)

So it's partly about telling friends and about the self-image, but it's largely about the satisfaction of having possession of an experience. Having done a thing—having eaten a bacon sundae, just as having gone zip-lining or skydiving—is an experience we get to own for life. Stash it in our personal archive. Consuming experiences is in large part about consuming *concepts*.

Let's say you go on safari. Unless you really get hooked, once you have possessed that concept of riding out in a van looking with binoculars for animals, you probably feel sated. It will satisfy you for a short while, then you're on to the next craving. *Hmm, come to think of it, I've never hiked Machu Picchu, have I?* In other words, we have an insatiable appetite for new ideas, and by extension, for new meal concepts and ways of interacting with food. Most stunt foods won't hold our attention long enough to become menu mainstays. But we'll always be primed for the next one.

We seek novelty. It is and it isn't that simple.

The credit we can give ourselves about how to live full lives falls apart when these experts explain that the tendency holds even when we recognize that the concept or experience is actually less pleasurable. In Keinan and Kivetz's studies published in 2011 in the *Journal of Consumer Research,* participants were given a set of scenarios, several involving food, and asked which would be more pleasant and memorable, and which they would choose. Although only 11 percent believed that staying in a Quebec ice hotel instead of a Florida Marriott hotel would be more pleasurable, 98 percent thought it would be more memorable and 72 percent said they would choose it. Choosing between an exotic restaurant and a familiar restaurant, only 4 percent rated the exotic restaurant more pleasurable; 92 percent would consider it more memorable, and 70 percent would choose the more exotic.

So we seek out ways to add wild, Instagram-able food experiences to our résumé of tastes—even if the tastes themselves aren't much to write home about.

Why is this urge so powerful? And is it human nature, or American nurture? "We propose that such choices are driven by consumers' continual striving to use time productively, make progress, and reach accomplishments (i.e., a productivity orientation)," write Keinan and Kivetz in their paper. "We argue that choices of collectable (unusual, novel, extreme) experiences lead consumers to feel productive even when they are engaging in leisure activities." They explain that a "productivity orientation," constantly "accomplishing more in less time," is something characterizing much of Western society in recent decades but most prominently the United States, the true standout as a "nation of clock watchers."

So it turns out that consuming collectable experiences is actually about feeling productive. It's another reflection of our prioritization of work and progress. Of our need to produce outcomes. As discussed earlier, we've never had a very healthy relationship with leisure or pleasure. It feels . . . lazy, somehow. We don't know what to do with ourselves.

I must admit, the DLT actually does taste good, in the temporary way that something like orange chicken at Panda Express "tastes good." But the decent flavor in the DLT can be attributed to its not really being that different from Taco Bell's regular hard taco—you only slightly taste the nacho cheese flavoring of the taco shell, and mostly it tastes good because it has the identical composition of sour cream and beef and cheese and salsa oozing all together that their longstanding beef taco has.

But the *concept* is new, and that's what we're "consuming" in our minds. While we applaud ourselves these days (and should!) for eating cricket-flour protein bars and "anything that moves," as Dana Goodyear's book by that title suggests, on a mainstream level we are only daring within limits. The DLT is radical and bizarre, no doubt, but it's still the marriage of two familiars. We like adventure within the conventional.

Leave it to Harry Balzer, the man who may understand us better than anyone, to put it to us straight: "We are all explorers," he says. "But we never leave the sight of land."

More from the Stunt-Food Kingpins

As with all new product creation, the nature of stunts is that they often fail. Most stunt foods don't become permanent fixtures on the menu. But the Doritos Locos Taco was the rare stunt that did the opposite of fail—it took the country by storm. And it continued to keep us rapt well past 2012. (In May 2014, the CEO of Taco Bell at the time, Greg Creed, was promoted to CEO of all of Yum! Brands. Coincidence? I think not.)

Taco Bell came out with new flavors like Cool Ranch, Fiery, and Spicy Chicken Cool Ranch. Throughout 2013 and 2014, every week it seemed like someone else emerged in the news claiming to be the taco's true inventor.

In the wake of the Doritos Locos Taco's success, Taco Bell and Frito-Lay even turned the chip-flavored taco *back* into a chip. The media responded with headlines like "Snack Food World Collapses In Upon Itself" and "Frito-Lay Messes With Our Heads." To the dismay of some consumers and the gratitude of others, bags of these Doritos were sold for a limited time only.

And since then, both Doritos and Taco Bell have been busy churning out a wide range of novel concoctions.

In July 2014, 7-Eleven unveiled Doritos Loaded, a sort of triangular mozzarella stick, served warm, with a crust flavored with Doritos Nacho Cheese. Remember the close ties between Yum! and PepsiCo? That fall, the Internet lit up at news that PepsiCo was testing a new product on select college campuses, called Dewitos. As in, Doritos-flavored Mountain Dew.

In early 2015, Taco Bell began testing a donut hole covered with icing—and Cap'n Crunch's Crunch Berries. (Side note: As with Doritos Locos Tacos, don't give them *too* much credit for across-the-aisle collaboration: Cap'n Crunch is made by Quaker Oats, which is a division of PepsiCo.) Never mind that there's no apparent connection between cereal-coated donut holes and Mexican food. These came less than a year after Taco Bell waded into breakfast waters, coming on strong with the waffle taco, AM Crunchwrap, and Cinnabon Delights, of which this Cap'n Crunch version is a spinoff.

Amid this truly loco foodscape we inhabit, a final consideration is that much of the reason people responded to and ate Doritos Locos Tacos was that they were there to begin with. We've seen how stunt foods come to life, and why we fall for them, but why they exist at all is due to the space created for them to enter. That is, as a culture we continually look to the food industry to devise new and tantalizing concoctions. Science and innovation are America's bread and butter (if you'll excuse the phrase), our prized global exports. So we're apt to embrace those traits in everything from the Mars Rover and Facebook right on down to our pizza crusts and taco shells.

I'm not against innovation as a concept in the food world. In fact, I'm thrilled to have entrepreneurs at the table.

And I'm not even necessarily altogether against stunts. Take a Pizza Hut move from 2014: a sixteen-foot rotating cannon that launched pizzas. That's right, a real-life Teenage Mutant Ninja Turtles pizza thrower. Who among us doesn't have a soft spot for TMNT? I'm fun. I'm down.

But did you notice that none of the examples of stunt foods happened to be, say, "jicama sticks with insane magic yogurt dip!" or "spinach salad now with brand-new epic dressing!" For the most part, they were novel forms of fried dough, or un-heard-of combinations of dough and meat and cheese.

To be clear, I'm not blaming us for liking these things. We know the cravings for certain foods are hardwired. And I like cheesy salty goodness as much as the next guy. When we hold the mirror up, though, we see that the premium we place on progress, our willingness to let science be our guide to eating too, keeps fueling mash-up mania.

I admire a certain level of creativity when it comes to food, the spirit of ingenuity and innovation that defines our nation, and the idea of living life to the fullest through an experiential résumé. But stunt foods and their hold on us somehow rub me the wrong way. I might be a tad more excited about their next incarnation if they didn't make me feel like such a *sucker*.

CHAPTER 9

Cheesepocalypse

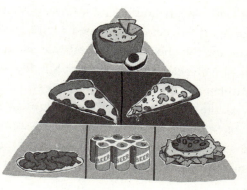

On January 7, 2014, Kraft Foods issued a warning about a Velveeta shortage. It was, as *Advertising Age* magazine wrote, "just as the dip season kicks into full gear."

I know, this may be the first time you've heard of "dip season." But keep your focus on the more alarming part: This warning came just twenty-six days before . . . the Super Bowl.

Two days later, Velveeta's Facebook page carried this message: "We are incredibly humbled and appreciative of the outpouring of love and support for the Liquid Gold of Velveeta." It also said, "Please know that we are working tirelessly to get more Velveeta on store shelves as soon as possible and that this was in no way a 'publicity stunt.' We always want Velveeta where it belongs—in your hands, in your homes and in your stomachs."

Details on what caused the shortage were hard to come by, but it seemed to be a manufacturing hiccup that delayed shipments to stores. And only one-pound boxes of the product were affected.

Kraft launched a website, Cheespocalypse.org, entitled "Velveeta Cheesepocalypse Watch: Guiding America Through the Cheesepocalypse of 2014." News headlines during this time included "#Cheespocalypse: Surviving the Super Bowl without Velveeta" and "Kraft Could Face a Cheesy Meltdown with Velveeta Shortage." Velveeta even issued a cheese sauce coupon to compensate for the shortage. Around that same time, there was a recall of Velveeta Cheesy Skillets Singles, which Kraft said was "unrelated."

As funny as the Cheesepocalypse campaign is, the real joke was on us: Most consumers purchase the two-pound boxes, which were as available as always. More important, Velveeta isn't even one of the most popular snacks we eat on Super Bowl Sunday.

It turns out, Velveeta doesn't "index high," according to the NPD Group. This means it isn't something people eat a great deal more of on Super Bowl Sunday compared to any other Sunday. Sure, this second cousin of cheese, twice removed, is used to make queso, which is indeed something some people like to eat on game day. But not in quantities meriting quiiite this level of freakout. By contrast, if there were, say, a chicken-wing shortage, NPD's Harry Balzer predicts, there'd be "riots in the streets." Why? Because chicken wings are the day's best-selling dish: 1.25 *billion* consumed on that day alone.

Pizza and beer also top the list of "high indexers." More pizza—about twice as much as average—is sold on Super Bowl Sunday than on any other day of the year. Beer, obviously, flows like Niagara Falls. Not unrelated, one in sixteen Americans will call in sick the next day—also more than on any other day of the year.

What do our food traditions related to the Super Bowl show about who we are? Why do we feast as if it's our last meal?

To understand all this, we'll explore the marketing wizardry of once-a-year specials, the behavioral economics behind this time of hoarding and postponing diets, and the history of the big game.

Plus, how sounding the alarms about "shortages" of foods like Velveeta—humble items turned Super Bowl "staples"—is just the latest way food marketers have both created and capitalized on the peculiar eating habits of the day.

The Super Bowl in American Culture

The first Super Bowl took place in 1967. It was the championship game between rival leagues, the American Football League (AFL) and National Football League (NFL). In 1970, the two leagues merged, but the Super Bowl remained.

Fifty million people watched that first Super Bowl game—and that was when the U.S. population was about 200 million. Even then, most American households had a TV, though it had only a handful of channels. As the popularity of the NFL and the Super Bowl rose, companies that make and sell TVs and home entertainment systems convinced American consumers that the Super Bowl was a great reason to give their living rooms a makeover.

In 2015, a record 114.4 million viewers watched the Super Bowl showdown between the New England Patriots and the Seattle Seahawks. For comparison, by then the U.S. population was 320 million. And what do you know: WalletHub reported that 7.5 million households had reported an intention to buy new TVs for that year's game.

The number of Americans who care about the Super Bowl was high from the start and has grown significantly, to the point that nearly half the households with TVs now tune in. If that doesn't seem like a hefty portion of the population, let's put things in perspective: The all-time-highest rating, or percentage of U.S. households watching anything, was the series finale of *M*A*S*H* in 1983, at 60 percent.

Nine out of ten of America's most-watched events on TV have been Super Bowls. An extra 80 million or so more Americans watch the Super Bowl than watch an average NFL game. Still, *regular* NFL games are also among the most-watched broadcasts in the country. Which is to state the obvious: Americans love football.

Why do Americans love football? I . . . really can't say. It probably has something to do with men not hugging one another enough.

Why do Americans love the Super Bowl? That one I can take a stab at.

You've got this championship game happening every year, and a bunch of homes decked out with elaborate entertainment systems with wide-screen TVs, and all of this led to a whole new fixture in American society: the Super Bowl party. It became one of the most universally appealing activities on the calendar. Friends and family huddle in someone's den, order in delicious food or make it themselves, drink lots of beer, and even build "snackadiums," aka stadiums made out of snacks. So my take is that Americans love the Super Bowl because some of them like football, most of them like day drinking, and all of them like feasting.

One of the most defining aspects of the Super Bowl turns out to be one of the most defining aspects of American food culture at large: our predilection for eating in the comfort of our own homes. In other countries, like the UK, fans are apt to congregate at a local pub to watch the game with their buddies. But nine out of ten Super Bowl viewers watch from home (either in their own living room or at a party hosted by friends or family).

And it's not just bros who are watching: 46 percent of Super Bowl viewers are female. According to *The Washington Post*, more women watch the Super Bowl than the Oscars, Grammys, and Emmys combined. (Individually, these each earned 37 million, 25 million, and 12 million total viewers, respectively, in 2015. Again for perspective, *Seinfeld*'s last episode in 1998 brought in 76 million viewers.) But the Super Bowl is about so much more than the football, for both men and women. By some estimates, less than half the people watching the game are there for, well, the game.

The day's festivities wouldn't be what they are without all the commercials. During 2013's game, we watched fifty-one minutes of ads, and sixteen minutes of actual playing time. We watched another twelve minutes of the half-time show. (And 2013 was the year of the blackout, so we watched that for another thirty-four minutes.)

The peak viewership moment the following year, 2014, wasn't during the game itself. It was the half-time show starring Bruno Mars. It pains me to admit that the most-watched moment in 2015 was at the end when my team, the Seattle Seahawks, suffered a cataclysmic loss. The decision not to have Marshawn Lynch, arguably the best running back in the league at the time, run the ball from the 1-yard line on second and goal with twenty-six seconds left, has been deemed by some as the worst play call in Super Bowl history. But I digress.

The Super Bowl is so cemented in American culture that, as reported by WalletHub, one in five Americans would rather skip the wedding of a close friend or family member than miss seeing their team play.

Even from the early days, companies have spent hundreds of thousands of dollars on Super Bowl commercials. A half-minute spot during Super Bowl I cost the modern equivalent of $266,000, and that price has gradually crept up through the decades. The price tipped into million-dollar territory in the late 1980s, and today you can secure your thirty seconds of air time for a cool $4.5 mill. The price has especially taken off during the last ten years, with a 75 percent increase.

Why do ads cost so much, and why do the ad slots routinely sell out?

For one, we know that people actually *watch* ads during the Super Bowl. People also tweet about Super Bowl ads and talk about them the next day, giving the ads greater longevity in the Twittersphere, blogosphere, and social conscience than ads shown during pretty much any other time.

The real payoff for companies may not be sales resulting from the spots but a bump in stock price (for those that are publicly traded), according to researchers at the University of Colorado Boulder. That doesn't happen the day after the Super Bowl, when presumably people go out and buy whatever they saw in the ads. It happens at the time the ad buy is announced, and in the weeks leading up to the game when the ad is hyped in the media. The leaks of little teaser clips on YouTube are all part of their master plan.

Hollywood sees a major return on Super Bowl ads. That's the finding of a study by advertising researchers at the University of Wisconsin–Eau Claire. On average, promoting a film during a Super Bowl between 1998 and 2001 resulted in *twice* as much total box office revenue—and twice as much in the film's first week and weekend—compared with the average film not promoted during the game.

The biggest reason for the high price tags is the sheer number of eyeballs staring at the screen. Think about it like this: When the game started in the late 1960s, there were only a few channels, so you had a lot of people watching the same thing at the same time.

Over the years, more households got TVs. (Many people even put one in each room of the house, including the bathroom, so as not to miss any of the action while taking one of countless pees—the 110.7 million gallons of Super Bowl beer have to go somewhere . . .)

With so many channels now—and not only the hundreds provided through a cable package or on-demand, but also Netflix, Amazon Instant Video, and other Internet streaming services—viewership has become more and more fragmented. The cultural hallmark of the mass-audience live television event has become increasingly rare. Which means, today, there is simply no other marketing opportunity like the Super Bowl.

The Super Bowl's Most Iconic Foods

We eat more on average per person on Super Bowl Sunday than on any other day of the year except Thanksgiving. Why is that? And if it isn't Velveeta, what *do* we eat?

In recent years, chicken wings have surpassed pizza as Americans' favorite Super Bowl food. Of the 48 million Americans who order takeout for the big game, the National Restaurant Association has reported that about two-thirds consider chicken wings a "must-have." These are doubly good days for pizza chains that also offer chicken wings, namely Pizza Hut and Domino's Pizza, which sell 5 and 2.5 million wings, respectively. Domino's has been selling wings since 1994, a few years after fellow fast-food chains McDonald's and KFC got into the biz.

Nearly eight of every ten American adults would identify as a person who eats chicken wings. That's what participants told Harris Interactive polling service in early 2013, on behalf of the National Chicken Council (which represents 95 percent of all chicken sold in the United States). Surprisingly, wing popularity does not vary much by geography or gender: 77 percent of women eat wings compared with 82 percent of men. And, because people who work in food professionally can't help but make food puns, the chicken council's chief economist and market analyst at the time, Bill Roenigk, said in a press release: "We also know that [chicken wings] are nonpartisan and politically independent. That is, there are really no extreme left wings or extreme right wings." Such a universally appealing product kind of makes me want to quit this writing shtick and take up with the chicken producers of America.

For those 80 percent of us who eat wings, ranch dressing is the preferred dip, followed by barbecue sauce, hot sauce, and blue cheese, in that order. *These* preferences do vary a lot by region. Northeasterners, for example, lean the most toward blue cheese and steer clear of ranch.

While pizza may have lost its title as the Super Bowl's Number One Food, that Sunday is still the year's single busiest day for pizza restaurants. All told, 12.5 million pizzas go out the door. Pizza Hut, for its part, sells about 2 million pies on Super Bowl Sunday. That works out to 16 million slices. Domino's Pizza isn't far behind, at roughly 11 million slices. Compared with a normal Sunday, that's 80 percent higher sales volume.

After Super Bowl Sunday, the highest days for pizza sales are New Year's Eve, Halloween, and the night before Thanksgiving. (!) Other popular times for pizza are New Year's Day (more football) or Valentine's Day (feed the babysitter).

With this, just as coopers in Kentucky are doing big business with the rise in the American bourbon habit, box makers have their work cut out for them to keep up with the national appetite for pizza, which is especially pronounced during the stretch of holidays from October to February. Starting around December, they ramp up their box production by about 10 percent to get ready for the Super Bowl.

A single company makes all the boxes for half of the takeout pizzas sold in America. It also supplies all the boxes for Pizza Hut, and many for the three other largest chains (Domino's, Papa John's, and Little Caesars). Based in Georgia, the company is called Rock-Tenn, and it operates twenty-four hours a day, seven days a week, producing 400 pizza boxes a minute. That's nearly seven boxes a second.

Pizzas used to be carried in those thin cardboard boxes you often see bakeries using for cakes, or on cardboard discs covered by paper bags. In the 1970s, corrugated boxes came on the market, and they did a much better job of optimizing the texture and temperature of the pizza. The boxes keep heat in and let some steam out through an interplay of corrugated flutes (the squiggly stuff between two flat pieces), slits between the lid and the side walls, and the finger hole vent.

The Super Bowl is also the second-biggest weekend of the year for grilling, surpassed only by the Fourth of July. A remarkable 62 percent of people who own a grill will use it that Sunday.* That's a pretty big deal when you consider that the Super Bowl takes place in *February*.

---

* I imagine some of those grills are being used to grill hamburgers, but be careful what you read: A widely repeated stat about the Super Bowl is that 14 billion hamburgers will be consumed. The population of the United States is 323 million, so every American would have to eat at least 43 burgers in one day for this to be true. With the stat about 1.23 billion chicken wings, this averages out to about four per person, which is still high but at least plausible. One could imagine that many people won't eat any wings at all, and many people will eat more than four wings, whereas the burger figure is just inconceivable.

If the chili smells good enough and the cake is decorated like a giant football, some of us will go to the trouble of finding utensils. But for the millions who cook instead of ordering takeout for Super Bowl parties, finger foods rule the day: nachos, meatball subs, pulled pork sliders, deviled eggs, and yes, dips galore. Spinach dip, artichoke dip, bacon-cheese dip, seven-layer taco dip . . . take-the-only-thing-left-at-the-grocery-store-and-mix-it-with-cream-cheese dip.

As for beer consumption, I'll just tell you that more than 49 million cases of beer are sold for the Super Bowl and leave it at that.

So what explains the over-the-top spreads and full-throttle feasting? Let's tour a few possibilities and see what we think.

You could argue that what's behind our relationship to the Super Bowl as gorge fest is the consumerist culture that pervades our country, the same explanation behind Black Friday. This is the stance taken by Warren Belasco, the pioneering food scholar who also edits the international journal *Food, Culture & Society*. He says, "Whereas other holidays have the obligation of mutual gift giving," this is about treating yourself—a "pure pig-out." Especially with all the commercials, he says, "It's a celebration of America's *broader* consumerism" in every aspect of our culture, not just food.

At a total bill of $5.6 billion, Super Bowl consumption does not discriminate: We consume snacks and drinks, but also flat screens and sofas, hats and jerseys. And for some fans, tickets. Ohh, the money we will spend on a seat. In 1967, tickets were only $12. In 2015, the average price was $4,833.25. But heck, if you can rack up thousands of dollars in credit card debt on Christmas presents for *other people,* why shouldn't you spend as much or more on yourself?

Of course, some people find that the Super Bowl stresses them out when their team's chance at glory is on the line, so they eat for comfort. Marketing researchers at INSEAD, a business school just outside of Paris, studied the relationship between what we eat and when our favorite football team loses. They looked at more than 3,000 days of eating among over 700 participants during two regular NFL seasons and found: "On the Mondays following a Sunday National Football League (NFL) game, saturated-fat and food-calorie intake increase significantly in cities with losing teams, decrease in cities with winning teams, and remain at their usual levels in comparable cities without an NFL team or with an NFL team that did not play."

Saturated fat intake especially fluctuates, increasing nearly 28 percent after losses and decreasing 16 percent after wins, compared with normal eating habits. We eat even *worse* after a defeat when the team we lose to is evenly matched, when the loss is nail-bitingly close, and when we live in a city whose NFL fans are more committed (read: Pittsburgh).

The theory is that a loss reflects badly on our sense of identity, bruises our ego. If our players are losers, by extension, we must be losers too. But this research applies only to what we eat the day *after* an NFL game occurs, and our usual Super Bowl feasting begins hours before kickoff. Plus, the French are apparently susceptible to this too—the same study found similar unhealthy eating patterns among French soccer fans who had to watch a highlight reel of their team's defeat. It's still possible that we're nervous about the outcome of the game, so we stress snack while it's happening and not just the day after.

But I argue that we stuff ourselves because the Super Bowl is a full-on holiday in America. It may not be officially recognized as one, but the research shows that we operate under a completely different set of rules and norms related to food on holidays than on normal days. And the Super Bowl not only follows those patterns, but in many ways shows the rest of the holidays how it's done.

The Super Bowl as National Holiday

Super Bowl Sunday marks the end of "eating season" in America, as we discussed earlier. It's that final blowout—one last shoveling before swimsuit season.

"The Super Bowl . . . has always exemplified America at its best, America at its worst, and more than anything else, America at its *most*." These are the wise words of the sports writer Michael MacCambridge in the foreword of Bob McGinn's book *The Ultimate Super Bowl Book*. Marketers and ad geniuses helped make the big game what it is today, but it was a spectacle from the start. It took a page from the entertainment guide to college football bowl games, with bands and cheerleaders and over-the-top half-time shows: Super Bowl I brought "men flying around in jet packs," MacCambridge writes, and followed the next year with football monster floats, then two years after with "the daily double of hot-air balloons taking off from inside the stadium (and, in one case, crashing into the stands and injuring a beauty queen)."

Whether we're unbuttoning our top pants buttons on Thanksgiving, dragging pillowcase overflowing with candy along the sidewalk on Halloween, or scarfing chicken wings on Super Bowl Sunday, the latter is as much a national holiday as the rest because it represents America at its most. Regardless of its lack of any official designation (de jure, to use the fancy Latin term), there are clear signs that the Super Bowl occupies de facto holiday status in American culture. Just look at the wreckage the day after.

Kronos, a workforce management company, found that 4.4 million Americans show up late to work on the Monday after the Super Bowl. More than a million call in sick. This happens for most of the same reasons it does after Thanksgiving or

Christmas: too much. Too much of all the things that peak on this day, from the beer to the guac, the pies to the wings, and the chips and the dips.

And it's often a specific *kind* of sick. The best description I've read of the symptoms is by author Kingsley Amis in his novel *Lucky Jim:* "He lay sprawled, too wicked to move, spewed up like a broken spider-crab on the tarry shingle of morning. The light did him harm, but not as much as looking at things did; he resolved, having done it once, never to move his eyeballs again. A dusty thudding in his head made the scene before him beat like a pulse. His mouth had been used as a latrine by some small creature of the night, and then as its mausoleum."

Sound familiar? If you're still not convinced, ask a hospital's ER department—the Monday after is packed. The ailments are usually blood pressure spikes, stomach issues, and other emblems of excess. (Antacid sales also increase the next day, by 20 percent, according to 7-Eleven.)

It's Monday not Sunday that's swarmed because people want to enjoy the rest of the Super Bowl party before bothering to see a doctor. Visits to the emergency room decline among male patients during big sporting events, according to a study published in the *Western Journal of Emergency Medicine*. In other words, while this pattern is especially pronounced the day after the Super Bowl, it's a pattern seen across a variety of major matches.

The proof is also in the productivity plummet. Thanks to our collective distraction the day after the Super Bowl, our economy takes a billion-dollar hit, as estimated by the global outplacement firm Challenger, Gray & Christmas. On the plus side, all that post-game analysis in the break room is good for something: Morale gets a 20 percent boost, according to another workforce firm, Glassdoor.

So why not spare everyone the indignity of calling in "sick," the time and agony invested in brainstorming excuses or trying to muster enough mental clarity to make it through the day? Enter the grassroots movement to declare the day after the Super Bowl a national holiday. In 2008, nearly 16,000 Americans signed a petition urging everyone to lean in to the reality of the day. Proposed names for the holiday have included Super Bowl Monday and National Sports Day.

More than merely adding his signature, Marc Kinley—vice president of nMotion Technologies, who helped launch the website SuperBowlMonday.com in advance of the 2006 game—gives his employees half the day off.

Another petition was started in 2013 by Josh Moore, head of the fantasy football website 4for4.com. You can find it on the official petition website of the White House, We the People. Moore and his supporters wrote that the 2012 Super Bowl was not only a huge television event throughout the country, but "one of the largest location-independent gatherings of American people to date."

The arguments are to reduce drunk driving and other bad things on Monday resulting from the night before, but also to promote camaraderie among Americans and "honor the most popular event in modern American culture." The petition needed another 80,000-plus signatures for the Obama administration to have to take it seriously, but the point remains.

To all this, I say: They're on to something! Because the bottom line is that the Super Bowl unites us. Well, at least it unites many of us. A lot more of us than just about anything else does. There's a lot of tension in this country, about big, messy issues. Politics, immigration, climate change, education, inequality. No other event transcends boundaries of race and religion, gender and region in such a way. It's why it's such an integral part of American *food* culture, too. It's why the food we eat on this day reveals so much about who we are as a nation.

Fake Shortages

A shortage is a powerful marketing tactic that obscures reality. That's why Cheesepocalypse was such a success for the Velveeta brand, noticeably boosting sales, even though the product isn't really the Super Bowl favorite it claimed to be.

"Think about toys at Christmas, or beanie babies," says Richard Wilk, the Indiana University anthropology professor and director of the Food Studies Program. "There's nothing that gets people excited as much as scarcity in the marketplace."

As a graduate student, Wilk worked on a study called the Tucson Garbage Project. From 1987 to 1995, archaeologists at the University of Arizona sifted through thirty tons of waste from landfills across North America. What they learned was baffling: When foods are pricier and harder to come by, people waste *more* of them. That seems backward, doesn't it? During a nationwide beef shortage at the time of the study, prices rose. People purchased cuts they didn't ordinarily buy, and in high quantities (apparently out of fear that things would only worsen). Curbside garbage bins revealed packages of beef *still sealed* from the supermarket! A year later, a sugar shortage hit, and residential waste of sugar and sweets doubled. Wilk attributes much of this paradox to "the hoarding impulse." And surely Kraft Foods knows that impulse applies to game-day Velveeta.

So every year as the Super Bowl rolls around, the stocks of something else seem to run dry—and the news of the short supply makes us go nuts to have it.

In 2009, it was avocados, which posed a threat to the great Super Bowl guacamole tradition. In each of the last ten years or so, we have consumed between 92 and 240 million avocados on Super Bowl Sunday. Even if we don't use the peak amount for our calculation, this is equivalent to every person in the country, on the same day, grabbing a friend and splitting an avocado. To wrap your mind around what that many avocados actually looks like, picture a football stadium with avocados filling the field from one end zone to the other. Each year for the Super Bowl, the Hass Avocado Board's marketing team calculates the height this theoretical pile would reach based on which stadium the game is being played in. That pile has ranged from about 18 to 46 feet tall. And remember, we're talking about a little fruit that can fit in your hand, and just the amount consumed *on* Super Bowl Sunday.

All of which is to say: It was a big deal in 2009 when the California Avocado Commission warned of the lowest avocado crop in twenty years. They cited wildfires and high temperatures and subsequent water rationing. Was the drought in California serious? Definitely. (Though not as serious as it became in the years after, which was orders of magnitude beyond the worst in history.)

But in this particular case, there was some false alarming going on: The irony, as *Smithsonian* magazine reported, is that "about 75 percent of the avocados shipped within the U.S. in the weeks leading up to the Super Bowl came from Mexico." And most of the remainder from Chile. Why? California's avocado season is usually just beginning around the Super Bowl. (Farmers there wish the big game would land around early March instead.)

In 2014, just as was the case in 2009, 85 percent of avocados sold in the United States were grown outside the United States, with Mexico as the world's largest avocado grower. *The Christian Science Monitor* reported in 2009 that avocado exports to the United States have transformed the central Mexican state of Michoacán, halting immigration and contributing the second-greatest share of income for the state behind remittances from Mexicans living in America. It is said that Hass avocados are so lucrative in Chile that they go by the name *oro verde,* meaning "green gold."

Mexico's stronghold dates back to the North American Free Trade Agreement in the 1990s that allowed winter avocado imports into the United States. Before that, most avocados in the United States were consumed in places where they could grow, California or Texas. Ever since, though, avocado consumption has grown dramatically. The UN Food and Agriculture Organization reports that, since 1993, consumption of avocados has more than doubled around the globe, and tripled in the United States.

One part of the shortage scare that's actually true is that global supply is having a tough time keeping up with demand. Given how water-intensive the fruit is to grow, there's something of an arms race happening among growers in Chile and Mexico to address constraints on water. In Chile, farmers are digging deeper wells and working hard to protect their access to existing wells, and in Mexico researchers are studying a genetically engineered avocado that would require less water.

Avocado marketers are the envy of many a produce promoter. In 2000, Americans ate a mere eight million pounds of avocados during Super Bowl parties, but today, the two are interchangeable. As the Huffington Post has reported, only "the avocado has so completely—and so quickly—attached itself to this utterly unrelated sporting event. As recently as 13 years ago the avocado wasn't the football juggernaut it is today. It has been a relentless and cunning campaign to victory, achieved in part through marketing muscle." The tenfold increase can be attributed to the Hass Avocado Board, formed in 2002 to promote its fruit. It managed to persuade the major grocery store chains to stock avocados in January. Then it went gangbusters with recipe contests, TV ads, athlete endorsements, and sweepstakes.

Scott Horsfall, former head of the California Kiwifruit Commission, tried to attach kiwifruit to Groundhog Day in a similar fashion, because, as he told the Associated Press, "kiwis and groundhogs are both fuzzy." Somehow the pairing didn't gain traction. The same goes for the USA Dry Pea & Lentil Council's efforts to unseat the avocado. The council's annual marketing budget is a mere $100,000 to the avocado industry's $37 million.

Avocados From Mexico has emerged as an unprecedented player not only in the produce industry but in the Super Bowl industry. In 2015, Avocados From Mexico released the first-ever Super Bowl ad on national television for a fresh produce item.

One of the nice things about associating your brand with the big game is the year-round customer loyalty it can give you. While avocados are, of course, consumed in foods like sandwiches and salads, the number one use is guacamole. You eat chips and guac on game day, have fun with friends, and then that positive association sticks with you throughout the year. To bring home this message during the January 2015 playoffs, Avocados From Mexico ran a PR campaign called "No Guac, No Game."

In 2013, the National Chicken Council alerted customers to a wing "shortage" due to high corn and feed prices. It was everything the NPD Group's Harry Balzer had warned: Headlines such as "Possible Chicken Wing Shortage Looms Ahead of Super Bowl" appeared on Fox News; "Super Bowl Crisis? Chicken-Wings Shortage Looms" could be found in *Business News Daily*. Demand for wings that year reached "an all-time high," the chicken council said in a press release. Higher corn and feed prices were blamed on a drought and the requirement that 40 percent of corn grown in the United States be turned into ethanol. Production of chicken wings was limited to 1.23 billion wing segments that year, 12.3 million fewer than during the Super Bowl the year before.

But it also turned out to be a false alarm. Why? Basic economics. There wasn't a *shortage* in the usual sense of the word—running out—just more demand than supply. That meant, no surprise, higher prices.

You see, the trouble with chickens is they have only two wings. Yet, wings are the part of the chicken that is in highest demand. You still have to raise a whole chicken to get the wings, so the supply of wings is limited by the supply of chickens. (Wing industry giants are said to long for a six-winged chicken to boost processing efficiency.) When the demand for wings exceeds the demand for other parts of the chicken, wing prices go up. That's what happened in 2013 and what seems to happen each January. Prices peak in the buildup to Super Bowl Sunday and are sustained by a steadily high demand during the NCAA basketball tournament throughout March. In 2014 the pendulum swung: American farmers had plenty of feed because costs of corn and soybeans were down. Yet fewer total birds were slaughtered, so the wholesale price of wings went up 30 percent from 2013 to 2014.

The way it works is that most wings are disjointed, with meaty first and second joints being sold in the United States, and a third joint, a thinner piece called "the flapper," being exported to Asian countries. A single wing is typically split into two pieces, or segments: the "drumette" and the "flat."

Chicken wings appeared in U.S. markets because of the trend in the 1980s away from whole cooked birds to boneless, skinless breasts—which was part of the fat scare that took place at the same time as the whole SnackWell's cookies and "nonundelow" boom discussed earlier. The wings became a byproduct of chicken producers singling out the more coveted breasts, and they sold the wings at low prices. Restaurants and bars latched on because of the bargain, and they noticed that serving wings with salty or spicy sauces sent beer sales soaring. Beer was already firmly intertwined with football, so it was a natural next step. Plus, wings are one of the few foods that are both shareable for groups of friends and family, yet also customizable to the individual, thanks to the various dips.

A key factor at play in these fake shortage cycles is clickbait, the web content designed to generate ad revenue. Running a headline that says, "Avocados to Cost More Because More People Want Them" is a lot less attention-grabbing than "Super Bowl Save—Grocers Avert Guacamole Shortage," the headline that ran in February 2009 on SF Gate.com, for example. Ditto for the media hype we've seen in recent years for inadequate supplies of Nutella (hazelnuts) and kale. There is always going to be heightened demand leading up to the Super Bowl, and we see why the media plays along, so this scare tactic is likely to remain an annual tradition.

Foods of Privilege

Even healthy eaters cheat sometimes. That goes for the most diligent among us. But we especially cheat during the holidays.

We ditch the usual rulebook—Halloween and the aforementioned willingness to eat one anothers' bottom of the barrel, Thanksgiving food coma inductions, Christmas parties spent grazing cookie trays and downing festive cocktails with abandon. Think about being on vacation; the same set of reactions applies: *I work so hard. I deserve a treat.* All our calorie counting and guilt ladling, all our *striving* goes out the door. For this reason, the holiday food business is good business.

"[Candy companies like Hershey's] have a better understanding of human nature than probably most philosophers," says Nicholas Fereday, the executive director and senior analyst at Rabobank focused on food trends. He adds: "Candy is in a privileged category, and the same goes for a Super Bowl party—you don't go there to be healthy."

In 2013, a Taco Bell ad mocked any loser who would show up at a Super Bowl party with a veggie tray (akin to "punting on fourth and one"); silly health freak, you're supposed to bring a Doritos Locos Tacos variety pack! The Center for Science in the Public Interest kicked up a shame storm on Twitter, Taco Bell pulled the ad, and said health freaks . . . went out and bought DLT variety packs.

Amazingly, carrot sticks do make the list of the Super Bowl's high indexers as well. My only explanation is that they must be vehicles for all those dips. Those and the wildly creative structures that some Super Bowl fans construct, snackadiums: Think gingerbread houses where the bricks and mortar are meatier and cheesier. Incidentally, Kraft posted its own step-by-step instructions on Pinterest for a stadium calling for a *pound* of Velveeta to fill the "field."

What does it mean to be in a privileged category? It means consumers don't hold your product to the same health and quality standards as they do other foods. I recently bought some Easter candy at Walgreen's, those speckled malt balls shaped like eggs, which I used to love, and I was stunned to see that they contain partially hydrogenated oils, or artificial trans fat. For the most part, trans fat has been dramatically reduced from the food supply given near unanimous agreement about its hazards to health. Yet holiday candy gets a free pass. Clearly, no one purchasing Easter egg malt balls is buying them because they've given the nutrition panel a good scan and thought, *Yep, looks like a wholesome buy*. I'm buying them, frankly, because they remind me of my childhood.

The privileged foods in our culture are the ones that are about creating memories. Treating ourselves. Satisfying our cravings. For those tall orders, salad doesn't tend to do the trick. But why is that? Because of the foods that have become associated with special occasions.

"The marketing of some of the companies like Frito-Lay have just got this down to an art form; they know exactly how to press all the right buttons," Fereday says. He describes an event he attended where most companies spoke of the shifting consumer demands and the need for healthier products, greater transparency, greater nutritional value and calorie quality. "But then, PepsiCo and Hershey's, who operate in another universe or planet, are appealing to another eating occasion, so they just don't care about health and wellness. Super Bowl Sunday is all about having fun, and the fun element of food is what they play up now with their products. No one is trying to say this is a fortified Dorito."

Fun is the engine of a force so powerful it's hard to overestimate its effectiveness as a marketing strategy. That is: nostalgia.

Because food marketers know this, they make a point of being present at events like birthday parties and the holidays, planting lifelong associations in our minds with our happiest, most fondly remembered times. This is why Avocados From Mexico succeeded in making "guac" NFLese for "party."

"Nostalgia is kind of a cheap trick but an effective one," Fereday says. Food companies manage to make certain connections intuitive, like cake = birthday wishes; pizza + beer = good times with your buddies.

Cheesepocalypse was a classic example of nostalgia at work. Velveeta has been around since 1908. And despite having been forced by the FDA to change the way it identifies itself on its box, from "Pasteurized Process Cheese Spread" to "Pasteurized Prepared Cheese Product," many people still have a soft spot for the stuff.

When you think back to Super Bowl Sunday, you remember cannonballing your Tostitos Scoops into the salsa bowl. You remember high-fiving your buddies, Bud Light in hand.

"Everyone knows that what's fun for you is what would have been called junk food," Fereday says. "Entertainment with your mates. It's the story of excess and indulgence, like twelve-foot subway heroes you see in the adverts."

Nostalgic sentiments tend to be shared by people with a common history. Part of that has to do with geography. For example, Rabobank's Nicholas Fereday was raised in the UK. He says, "You can keep your Reese's Pieces—they mean nothing to me. But if you put a Cadbury Creme [Egg] in front of me, it would be gone in a minute."

Shared history also stems from your generation. Different cohorts share nostalgia for the same foods because they grew up with the same trends. As we see with cereal, this is playing out in fascinating ways among millennials. Food companies will do whatever it takes to earn the food dollars of the largest generation ever. One approach is bringing back products after long(ish) droughts.

In the game of conjuring fuzzy feelings of our childhood, Kellogg's, Post, and General Mills are heavy hitters. Cereal consumption is high when you're a kid, falls as a teenager, then picks up again as you get older. So cereal companies like to find ways to remind people of their old favorites in hopes of bringing them out of the breakfast sandwich habit and back to their bowls.

French Toast Crunch, which was sold from 1995 to 2006, became widely available again in January 2015. A spinoff of the enduring Cinnamon Toast Crunch, this sister cereal consists of mini toast-shaped corn bites that taste like maple syrup. "You asked. It's back," boasts the box, which includes a quiz to test how 1990s you are—did you dance the Macarena, did you secretly prepare for Y2K, and so on. Targeting those children of the 1990s (millennials), who are now adults making grocery decisions for themselves, is a tactic that works very well: Consumer research shows that adults remain extra fond of brands and products whose ads they were exposed to as children.

"The consumer brain is a bag of concrete mix before a person turns 13," writes trend analyst Derek Thompson in *The Atlantic*. "Anything you can slip in the soft blend is likely to harden, along with our neural networks, by the time we become a money-spending adult." Chipper mascots like the Trix rabbit don't hurt with that cementing.

In 2013, to reach adults with Honey Nut Cheerios memories, General Mills released an ad playing "Must Be the Honey," a song that featured blinged-out Honey Nut Cheerios boxes and music from the beloved 1990s rapper Nelly. He even wears a gold chain necklace that says "Heart Healthy." The same year, General Mills released ads for Lucky Charms specifically aimed at adults, reminding them how much they liked the taste as a kid. Lucky Charms saw a 3 percent increase in sales in fiscal year 2014.

M&M's Crispy returned in January 2015 after a ten-year hiatus, just barely long enough for us to miss it. It's like when famous athletes "retire" and then make a big splash about returning just one season later. That same year, Dairy Queen announced that by a "landslide" fan vote, it was bringing back the cotton candy Blizzard flavor it had discontinued.

There was even a Reddit thread devoted to reminiscing about

discontinued food products. It garnered more than 14,000 comments, such as: "They still make Oreo O's in South Korea. I remember seeing a seller on eBay who will sell them to you. God speed my friend. :)" People shared tips for jerry-rigging some long-gone favorite foods, as in a recipe for "homemade Ecto-Cooler," or, if you're missing Dunkaroos, buy a tub of Betty Crocker cake frosting and dip Teddy Grahams in it.

Moving over to the soda aisle: Coca-Cola announced in September 2014 that it had brought back Surge, the citrus-flavored, nuclear green soda similar to Mountain Dew that had been off the shelves for twelve years. Coca-Cola partnered exclusively with Amazon to sell Surge, and the retailer ran out of the drink just hours after the announcement.

Originally launched in 1996, Surge resonates well with the millennials it targeted through its rerelease. The drink has been gone since 2002, likely because high-caffeine sodas fell out of favor and energy drinks hadn't yet come on strong. What happened in 2014 was a social media campaign called "the Surge Movement." Thanks to crowdfunding, the group was able to install a billboard near Coca-Cola headquarters in Atlanta. The billboard read: "Dear Coke, we couldn't buy SURGE, so we bought this billboard instead."

Across all of these examples, having removed the product in the first place is what made it so compelling for consumers to have it back. Taking the product away puts food companies in the position of *"Well shucks, guess we better listen to the people."* It's exactly like the fabricated Super Bowl shortages, where you combine the power of nostalgia with the perception of limited supply.

Oscar Mayer ran a magazine ad in 2015 with a mini ham sandwich bun, sketched to resemble a Christmas ornament. The ad reads, "The taste of the holidays, without having to get the decorations out of the attic." It goes on: "Slow Roasted and Carved Thick. Oscar Mayer Carving Board gives you all the taste of the holidays, without all the hassle. It's *Holiday, Any Day* Food. It's *Oscar Mayer*."

There are, in my opinion, few food brands more *American* than Oscar Mayer. So the ad was bound to resonate with consumers. As I said, it's good to be in holiday foods. But it's even better to be selling your regular food as if it *were* the holidays, throughout the year. Namely, spring, early March, when this ad ran. Hmmm, what did we learn from Harry Balzer about precisely what time of year that is? Ah yes, the *end* of eating season. When the holidays, which extend for nearly half the year by some measures, are over. By then the Super Bowl is a month in our rearview mirror, the Valentine's Day chocolates have long ago been obliterated, and it's just the St. Patrick's Day hangover still on the horizon.

At this point in the year, nearly a quarter of all Americans are on a diet. The ad hits us when we're vulnerable. Your thought bubble immediately goes to: *I'm two weeks into this miserable juice cleanse, I'm all out of free passes to play in the supermarket, and now you're telling me I get to lay down the holiday card any time I want!?*

So nostalgia is one reason we react differently to foods associated with holidays.

The other reason is scarcity in the marketplace. Selling products for limited times during holidays and certain seasons are part of a family of techniques related to scarcity. That portfolio includes fake shortages like those around the Super Bowl. More precisely, these techniques leverage a *perceived* scarcity. Put another way, they capitalize on that social phenomenon whose term is almost as clever as Cheesepocalypse: FOMO. Fear of Missing Out.

Limited Time Only

There's a saying you've probably heard a hundred times at the tail end of a radio spot or TV commercial: " . . . *but hurry in—they're available for a limited time only!*"

"Like the McRib sandwich they do once a year at McDonald's, it's like a pleasureful indulgence that pops up for a few weeks and then goes away," says Hank Cardello, the former Coca-Cola marketing exec. "These are items they use to goose their sales."

In November 2014, for a limited time only, Dunkin' Donuts rolled out a croissant donut (piggybacking on the cronut craze started by the Dominique Ansel Bakery in New York City). It became one of Dunkin' Donuts' best-selling bakery items of all time. They announced in early 2015 that the croissant donut is here to stay. And the platform has expanded with new flavors.

As we remember about stunt foods, limited-time offers, or LTOs, aren't typically the healthiest options. "Healthier items are not often viewed as a treat, something special," Cardello says. "It's a different headset. It's the rules committee showing up and telling you you have to eat these things." He expects this divide to remain until we see more from the likes of Bolthouse Farms. They're putting real marketing muscle toward making healthier foods equally appealing and enjoyable. Making healthy food *fun* even.

In the category known as CPG, which stands for consumer packaged goods, food manufacturers are constantly coming up with new products. For instance, Cherkees—chips merged with beef jerky—and Chollives—the same idea except with green olives. But CPG seems to reserve a special focus on innovations that leverage the holidays, seasonality, and nostalgia.

Gearing up for the holidays in 2012, Pringles ventured into

dessert flavors, presenting pumpkin pie spice, white chocolate peppermint, and cinnamon and sugar. The next year brought pecan pie. All were limited-time offers. And, since limited-time offers are great for consumer testing, Frito-Lay must have learned that the first two flavors were flops, while sales of cinnamon and sugar were strong enough to bring back in 2013 alongside pecan pie.

When Nabisco released caramel apple Oreos—*its* way of celebrating fall—it created a sense of extra urgency by selling them exclusively at select Target stores, just as Coca-Cola did with Surge on Amazon. This move adds not only a time constraint, but a geographic constraint, generating buzz for the brand. You had Canadians, for instance, asking Target Canada on Twitter if the Oreos were available at *their* stores.

But of course, the rock star of seasonal LTOs is the almighty pumpkin spice latte from Starbucks. It's the company's most popular seasonal beverage of all time. The latte first debuted in the fall of 2003 and was an instant hit. It has reached such a level of fame that, like DLT for Doritos Locos Tacos, it goes by a shorthand, PSL.

In the fall of 2014, on his show *Last Week Tonight*, John Oliver said he has had it with "the coffee that tastes like a candle." The famous (infamous?) latte is the archetype of, more broadly, the Pumpkin-Flavored Everything Craze.

Americans spend more than $300 million a year on pumpkin-flavored products. Oliver noted that every year, for a reason that is inexplicable, pumpkin spice food products grow more "omnipresent." Products have included pumpkin-pie-flavored Pop-Tarts, pumpkin-spice cream cheese from Philadelphia, pumpkin gum from Extra, pumpkin-pie-flavored vodka from Pinnacle, and pumpkin-spice Jell-O, to name just a few. I have yet to see one that is *not* a limited edition.

Pumpkin gets marketed for its health benefits, which is

great, if it weren't for most of these products' complete . . . lack of pumpkin.

The American public has been starting to notice, though, and after more than a decade flying under the radar, Starbucks announced in 2015 that it would be switching to real pumpkin. Only in America would it be headline news that a pumpkin spice latte will now actually contain pumpkin.

My other beef with these products is they almost never taste like what they promise. The white chocolate peppermint Pringles, for one, actually tasted like toothpaste. All of these companies take advantage of our soft spot for thinking of happy times and looking for nice ways to celebrate the seasons. They take the shortcut—luring us in with the cozy image of the thing we're pining for, without actually putting the thing *in* the product. (The pumpkin-pie-flavored Pop-Tarts also appear to contain some pumpkin, but it's buried among forty-one other items in the ingredients list.) The true taste of pumpkin is something we'll hardly ever know because our taste buds are being assailed by faux products.

Trader Joe's has really made its mark going all in on pumpkin innovation. Gothamist counted thirty-five items available just at one Trader Joe's store on a single trip in October 2014. Some of their unique offerings are pumpkin pie mocha ice cream, pumpkin cornbread croutons, pumpkin biscotti, Pumpkin O's cereal, and iced pumpkin scone cookies. The difference is that at least many of their products actually contain pumpkin. That, and the store does sell real, whole pumpkins.

"We tolerate pumpkin spice because we like the fall," Oliver said on his show. "It's the best season, because you get to stop thinking about how weird your legs look in shorts." But anything that reminds us of autumn would do the trick; he for one would rather drink a cable-knit-sweater spice latte.

————

I used to love going to the Half Moon Bay Art & Pumpkin Festival each fall. You stop by pumpkin patches along the way and eat pumpkin pancakes and pumpkin chocolate chip cookies, pumpkin sausages and pumpkin churros, warm pretzels with pumpkin sauce, and pumpkin seeds. You drink pumpkin-flavored Jack-o-tinis and pumpkin beer. It smells and feels like fall.

Craftspeople there sell lots of things, but more than anything they sell pumpkin-shaped tchotchkes. People wear pumpkin earrings and, yes, cable-knit sweaters (embroidered with pumpkins). It's home to the world's third-largest pumpkin, wouldn't you know, at 2,058 pounds. Traffic is hellish, but you're so full of autumnal warmth and fuzziness, you couldn't care less.

What gets me about seasonal LTOs is that they feel like adulteration. These brands position themselves as merely celebrating the unique pleasures of the holiday season. But, just like fake shortages during the Super Bowl, they throw us into a spending frenzy with their warnings to stock up now or risk missing out.

But there's a difference between savoring a food because it is legitimately available for only a short period of time—say, fresh Copper River salmon—versus being suckered into buying something out of fear of regret. Because, in reality, who's to stop you from baking pecan pie long after the limited-time-only pecan pie Pringles are off the shelves? Try roasting the heck out of a pumpkin and throwing it into your coffee pot instead of waiting in line for a PSL. And just because the Easter malt eggs are no longer being sold at the drug store doesn't mean that spring is over for me.

I get a kick out of the Super Bowl—the game itself, the ads, the halftime show, the way it connects us as a country, and especially the idea that we live in a place where we can create a holiday from scratch. Even if that holiday status does trigger the feeling that it's time to chow down till we can't see straight.

But I could do without all the stress brought on by the marketing magicians. The fabricated frenzy. Trust me, you can still have one hell of a Super Bowl party without wings, *or* guac, *or* Velveeta. Surely the Rock-Tenn pizza box makers have our backs.

We have to see through it all. To quote Jon Stewart, "Something about this Velveeta shortage feels a little—what's the word I'm looking for—bullshit." We're often like puppets pulled by marketers' strings. So it might make a difference if 114.4 million of us went ahead and called them on it.

CHAPTER 10

The Story of Spaghetti

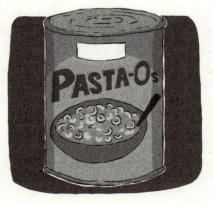

Missoula sits at the base of a beautiful valley in Montana where five mountain ranges and three rivers converge. From 1941 to 1943, 1,400 Italian nationals and 250 Italian "aliens" were interned at Fort Missoula. While Japanese Americans were interned in far greater numbers during World War II, there were also several camps around the country that held Italian and German Americans—some of them U.S. citizens.

This particular camp was men only, and author Jerre Mangione, who toured the camp while working for the Immigration and Naturalization Service, wrote that some men considered it "cruel and inhuman treatment" to be deprived of women all that time, and therefore a violation of the Geneva Conventions. But the internees made the best of it: They organized Fort Missoula like a small city, complete with a hospital, bakery, tailor shop, and school. With plenty of time for recreation, they swam in the swimming pool and put on operas in the theater that were attended by many in the greater Missoula community.

A photo from that time shows some of the men huddled around a table covered with mountains of pasta, breadsticks, and meat. They hold glasses full of wine, raised in a toast. The caption reads, "Do you think this is a concentration camp?"

There in the Rocky Mountain heartland, these men relished the food that would eventually touch every corner of this country. Across the Atlantic, American GIs were getting by on Chef Boyardee—and developing quite a fondness for it. The seeds of America's widespread love affair with Italian cuisine were being sown.

Americans would so enthusiastically adopt these internees' native foods—which at the time were foreign enough in the United States that a reporter had to explain what "peet-za" was—that it's now inconceivable to imagine "American cuisine" without them. Whether delis nationwide are selling panini, or the likes of The Cheesecake Factory and Applebee's are featuring pesto and arugula, or we're making ravioli from scratch or installing pizza ovens in our backyards—Italian food is ubiquitous in America.

To see how we got here, we'll journey through the evolution of America's relationship with Italian food: from the early 1900s, when social workers tried to assimilate Italian immigrants, lamenting that their insistence on fresh baked bread was subversive and their garlic disgusting; to the rise of canned spaghetti during World War II; to the 1980s when Olive Garden rapidly appeared in every corner of the country, defining "Italian food" in the minds of countless Americans; to today, when, as author John F. Mariani's book title suggests, Italian food has "conquered the world." That circus of a store called Eataly, the largest Italian marketplace on the planet, has locations not only in Chicago and New York but also in Japan, Brazil, and the United Arab Emirates. Eataly's popularity in the United States signals a growing appreciation for Italian cuisine in general *and* a growing understanding of the country's different regions and their various specialties. For instance, there are sardines from Sicily and black truffles from Umbria; citrus from Amalfi and pesto from Genoa; the soulful ragu of Bologna; the buttery risotto of Turin; and the minimalist *cacio e pepe* of Rome.

As a nation of immigrants, we have always been open to the cuisines of any number of countries. France had a good run for a while. Currently, we're lapping up the fare of India, Thailand, Greece, and beyond. And Chinese and Mexican have been firmly established in American food culture for decades. These two, along with Italian, are America's top three global cuisines (though these rankings are debated depending on the source).

Italian has become so deeply embedded in American culture that we hardly notice it anymore. *Chicago Tribune* reporter Christopher Borrelli wrote in 2011, "While every third cookbook these days espouses Italian, and every other new restaurant offers branzino, we actually take for granted just how pervasive Italian has become." At home, cooks are using Italian-style ingredients and techniques. And there are more restaurants serving Italian food in the United States than any other international food. The National Restaurant Association no longer lists Italian food as a "trend" because it's too ingrained, and Americans have not just adopted it but adapted it—and made it their own.

Where did spaghetti and meatballs come from? When did everyone suddenly start eating pesto? And what *is* it about Italian food that has made it so exceptionally, universally adored?

Pizza and pasta are relatively cheap. The flavors of Italian food aren't too spicy, and kids like it. But there's much, much more to it.

An Abbreviated History of Pasta

There is much debate about the "true" origin of pasta. Did Marco Polo bring it from China, or was it nomadic Arabs who ferried it west? Did the Italians invent it themselves? One thing is certain: Noodles have existed in Asia for thousands of years. But the birth of Italian pasta can effectively be traced to the 1100s, when dried noodles were traded throughout the Mediterranean. Because of its long shelf life, dried pasta could travel across international borders. First, though, it had to become understood as a distinct type of food, separate from noodles, separate from other wheat products, and also separate from fresh pasta, which grew into haute cuisine at the time.

So what *is* pasta, exactly? How is it different from noodles? Pasta is unleavened dough made by mixing water or eggs with semolina flour, which is milled from ground durum wheat. The dough is extruded through a machine into more than 300 different shapes. You've got angel hair and fusilli, farfalle and penne, lasagna, manicotti, fettuccine, and (one of my top picks) *strozzapreti*—little twists whose translation has something to do with strangling priests. Not to mention the array of shapes filled with creamy fillings.

The durum is the key distinguishing feature compared with other kinds of noodles. It's ideal for processing into pasta because of its high gluten content, which makes it durable. Its moisture content is low too, which means it doesn't expand or bulk up in the machine while being extruded. The last step in making dried pasta is the drying, of course, which is preferably done at a low temperature for a long time, but in industrial processes is usually done at a high temperature for a short time.

As its production became more industrialized, pasta trickled down to the lower classes, and by the eighteenth century, dried pasta was a staple in Naples. Along with Parma becoming a key center of pasta production and canning, Naples rose as a major food hub, cultivating and processing tomatoes and olive oil, as well as turning Sicilian wheat into pasta. These areas had formerly been major cultivators and exporters of citrus, but California and Florida came on strong in the 1800s in the citrus and nut categories. That led many Italian growers to either emigrate in search of new work or turn to these other products.

Naples is credited with mastering the idea of cooking pasta "al dente," which literally means "to the tooth." This involves cooking the noodles until they push back a little against the tooth when bitten, beyond the point of crunchy but still firm and pleasantly chewy, which stood in contrast to the historic practice of cooking the noodles to a pulp. The al dente habit spread throughout Italy.

The first evidence of Americans eating pasta dates to 1800. It will come as no surprise to anyone keeping score of their Founding Father MVPs that Thomas Jefferson—after declaring that all men are created equal, greenlighting the Lewis and Clark expedition, kick-starting the Library of Congress through his *personal* book collection, and founding a college during his retirement—was also a pasta pioneer. We have him to thank, in part, for spaghetti and meatballs. Well, sort of.

Like any self-respecting Renaissance man, Jefferson had spent time in Paris. In his case, as ambassador from 1785 to 1789, he'd gotten hooked on pasta. Some scholars say Jefferson brought the first pasta-making machine to America, after sending a friend on a very special mission while that friend was visiting Naples: Learn how pasta is produced. Jefferson even requested that his friend buy him a personal macaroni press. Other writers—such as Dave DeWitt, in his book *The Founding Foodies*—call this notion "fakelore," so . . . who knows. But it's safe to say that Jefferson helped popularize pasta in America by serving it at Monticello and the White House.

Recipes for baked macaroni soon started appearing in American cookbooks. There is a recipe for macaroni and cheese in Mary Randolph's *The Virginia Housewife,* published in 1824, which some consider the first truly American cookbook; it is certainly the first regional American cookbook. By the 1830s, mac and cheese was a common dish, with pasta and tomato sauce appearing a few decades later. (Cheese has been an accompaniment to pasta from the beginning. Another burst of genius from the early days was to take cheese-dusted pasta and sprinkle some cinnamon on top.)

The first pasta factory in the United States was built in Brooklyn in the mid-nineteenth century by a French immigrant named Antoine Zerega. To operate his new factory, he toyed with horse power, then steam, then electricity, ultimately finding great success. Zerega even took it upon himself to climb on the roof to dry the pasta. (Bird poop, anyone?) His operation is considered the birth of the American pasta industry.

For a long time, Russia was the top durum wheat grower around, but the United States had a couple of Dakotas to spare, and it turned out that wheat grew pretty well there. By World War I—when Russia suffered a breakdown in food supplies and distribution—the United States had become one of the leading wheat growers on the planet. But then they had to figure out what to *do* with all their wheat. (Sound familiar to the portfolio of corn derivatives used in just about every product in the supermarket today?) So we get turned into a nation of macaroni eaters. It took a few decades, but American producers eventually succeeded in transforming a formerly foreign food into an everyday product, both laying the infrastructure for pasta packaging and mass production and disseminating the marketing materials and recipes for how to cook it.

We went from eating very little pasta to downing nearly four pounds per person per year by 1930 (versus fifty pounds in Italy). By the mid-1980s, it was eleven pounds (versus sixty in Italy), and nineteen pounds as of 2012, the latest data from the International Pasta Organisation (versus fifty-seven in Italy). The United States ranks seventh worldwide in per capita consumption of pasta. Italy eats twice as much as the second-highest-ranked country, Venezuela, followed by Tunisia, Greece, Switzerland, Sweden, the United States, Iran, Chile, and Peru in the top ten.

Jefferson may have introduced pasta to some lucky diners in his elite circles and was certainly ahead of the curve in his taste for the dish, but it wasn't until the mass immigration of Italians from 1880 to about 1920 that pasta became what we know it today—a staple of American cuisine.

The Evolution of Italian Food in America

Harvey Levenstein is a historian and contributor to the book *Food in the USA: A Reader*. According to him, it takes two generations for immigrant groups to assimilate to American tastes. He also writes that, historically, even though we did incorporate some foreign ingredients and cooking techniques into our standard ways of making and eating food, this occurred "in ways that did not disturb essentially British palates."

The most notable exception, he argues, is Italian cuisine. The Italians were the largest of the droves of immigrants to set foot on Ellis Island between 1880 and 1921. And they brought with them a determination to preserve their traditional preferences in the face of assimilation. They were not the *only* group to have done so—sushi sales and burritomania today surely confirm that. But Italians were the first to pull it off.

From the story of spaghetti and meatballs, there is much to be learned about what leads people to change behavior. To form habits and routines, to go from never having tried a food to folding it into one's weekly repertoire. From the story of spaghetti and meatballs, we see the roots of America's adoption of global flavors into the "essentially British palates" that long defined our food culture.

Few things are more evocative of Italian American food than spaghetti and meatballs. It's *Lady and the Tramp* and Buca di Beppo; it's "Uh-oh, SpaghettiOs" and babies and kitchen walls plastered in noodles and red sauce. So how did spaghetti sweep the States?

Between 1870 and 1970, more than 26 million Italians left, heading to other parts of Europe and both North and South America in search of work. That's equivalent to the entire state of Texas emptying out over the course of a century. (Except that about half of those people eventually returned to the Old Country.) In 1850, there were fewer than 4,000 people of Italian heritage in the United States. Because of severe poverty in the rural south of Italy, it became increasingly common to emigrate to the United States after 1880, and by 1920, 5 million immigrants from Italy lived here. Those who came were mostly peasants and artisans (actual craftspeople, mind you, not "artisan" as we use the word today about everything from Tostitos chips to Starbucks breakfast sandwiches). Two-thirds were men. Most settled in Eastern cities, namely New York, Boston, Philadelphia, and Baltimore, and some in the Midwest in Chicago and Detroit.

In total, the Italian population abroad was about a quarter of the population *in Italy*. There wasn't a single city left on the Italian peninsula that had more Italians living there than New York City or Buenos Aires.

All of these Italians abroad created substantial markets for imports. Italian immigrants were often better able to afford their native products in the United States because they earned more money living overseas than did Italians living in the home country.

The two largest groups to leave Italy from 1880 to 1921 were from Campania (where Naples is located) and Sicily. Because these immigrants came in large numbers, the cuisines they brought with them became the most influential of the Italian immigrant groups. Along with that, the necessary infrastructure was set up for imports, so their products were more widely available, in greater variety, and at better prices. These regions' cuisines were characterized by tomatoes, onions, olive oil, cheese, and garlic, and as a result of their size and influence, we have taken these flavors to represent *all* Italian food.

It's important to note that "Italian" food is somewhat of a misnomer to start with—inhabitants of Italy's North and South barely wanted to share the same borders, much less eat the same dishes. This is because Italy unified only in 1861, at a time when nine of every ten Italians—including the first monarch, Vittorio Emanuele—could not speak the "national" language, the dialect of Tuscany. Italy as a whole had existed for only a few decades when the first large wave of immigrants arrived in America in the late nineteenth century. So, calling this group of immigrants "Italians" was in itself creating a whole new category, just as it was creating a new category of "Italian American."

For a long time, American social workers, educators, and nutritionists tried to persuade Italian immigrants to adopt American food ways. Garlic got a bad rap. The smell was considered a lack of fealty to the United States, a sign of Italian immigrants' unwillingness to relinquish foreign customs. The same was true of the habit of seeking out freshly baked bread, versus the American way of buying it the day before for the next day's breakfast, which was considered more . . . proactive? The reformers were also worried about the immigrants' grocery bills: the expense of importing olive oil and buying small blocks of special cheeses, among other things. Vegetables, popular in Italian households, were considered nutritionally useless in those days, given their high water content. All their growing and canning seemed like a lot of wasted effort.

The tomato—at the heart of southern Italian cooking—was vilified throughout the 1800s because of a fear that it was poisonous. Stories were often told of European elites getting sick and dying after eating the fruit. It took some time to realize it wasn't the tomato's fault, but the dinnerware: Pewter plates were fashionable among the wealthy, and the poisoning was actually due to lead. The tomato's high acidity leached lead from a plate. The tomato's name was further sullied in the late 1880s when a study concluded that it was linked to cancer.

Add to all this the concerns among many Anglo-Saxon Americans about using lots of herbs in cooking, as Italian methods did, and the Italians' food was firmly out of favor. There were theories that spices were overly stimulating and that consuming them caused people to also consume excessive amounts of alcohol. Plus, many Italian dishes mixed meat with grains and vegetables in a single pot, causing gasps and sighs among the nutrition authorities. Experts cautioned against combining foods for the supposed havoc it wreaked on the digestive system.

But the Italian immigrants could not have cared less about the reformers. They left seats empty at the American-style cooking classes offered in their neighborhoods. Many refused to visit the hospital because they found the food there so intolerable. (Doctors were stymied.) They had their own thing going, and they were sticking to it.

So how did the Italians manage to drag their cuisine out of the gutter? They Americanized it. They did so both for themselves—given that certain traditional ingredients were difficult to come by, while other new ingredients were available in abundance—and as a way to elevate their home country's status in American society.

Much has been written about the differences between what Italians actually ate in the Old Country and what "Italian food" was and has become over time in the United States. Poor immigrants from southern Italy went from spending three-quarters of their income on food in Italy to one-quarter in the United States. So for many, it meant trying foods in the New World that they couldn't afford in the Old World and incorporating new foods into their cuisine. Sugar and cheese and other things traditionally considered holiday or Sunday-only foods in Italy became available on a regular, even daily, basis. For instance, it was fairly rare in Italy for peasants to eat pasta; instead, their diets centered around polenta and bread.

In America, Italians not only ate more pasta themselves, but had great success selling it to Americans. Italian cuisine did fairly well in the 1870s and 1880s, namely at some of the most chichi New York restaurants like Delmonico's, but by the turn of the twentieth century, France was winning the fashion war. Upper-class diners were shifting from American and English dishes to "Continental" cuisine, which had a French bent. At the time, it wasn't so much about keeping up with the Joneses but with the Londoners and Parisians. As John Hooper writes in his book *The Italians,* it wasn't until relatively recently that

"Italian cooking came to be recognized as something other than a poor second to French, even by the Italians themselves."

At the time, most Italian immigrants living in American cities were packed into slums and performing menial labor to make ends meet. So when introducing Italian food on upper-crust menus in the early 1900s, it had to be done with the reassurance of sophistication. You saw dishes like "spaghetti Italienne," with the French spelling. French chefs were, for a time, conduits between Italian dishes and American diners.

To be sure, gains were modest at first as traditional recipes were certainly altered to appeal to American palates. The tomato sauce in one spaghetti recipe axed the traditional garlic, heaped on the sugar, and even called for Worcestershire sauce. To further underscore that these were baby steps, consider the old American customs of boiling pasta to a soggy mush and mixing tomato sauce with beef broth. Today we enjoy pesto, amatriciana, carbonara, and many others, but for a long time, a simple marinara sauce carried the torch.

The first pesto recipes in the United States that I'm aware of were published in the 1940s in *The New York Times* and *Sunset* magazine. Pesto didn't really become popular until the 1980s and 1990s, though, once fresh basil was widely available in grocery stores. Home cooks started toying with different combinations, too, realizing that pesto is a brilliant blank canvas, lending itself to virtually any union of herb and nut. Today we see kale and walnuts, mint and pistachios. A recent favorite of mine is carrots and hazelnuts. Veering from Parmesan is fair game as well, and manchego and pecorino are especially suitable.

There had been canned tomatoes since the 1840s, and especially during and right after the Civil War. Dried pasta emerged midcentury as well, so it was only a matter of time before someone realized you could sell the pasta already *in* the canned sauce. Genius! In the 1890s, the Franco-American brand—of SpaghettiOs fame—started selling canned spaghetti (emphasizing the company's Frenchness), and Campbell's and Heinz entered the market in the 1920s, producing equally underwhelming iterations of canned spaghetti. The sweetness and ultra-mild flavor made these products childhood favorites for countless Americans. As a result of this popularity, American producers started selling kits for Italian spaghetti dinners. These consisted of a can or bottle of tomato sauce, spaghetti, and that object of Warhol-level Americana: the green, cardboard cylinder of Kraft Foods grated "Parmesan" cheese. It too deserves a slice of the credit for propelling the widespread cooking of spaghetti throughout American homes.

A key transition point for the status of Italian cuisine in the United States was World War I, when Italy was a U.S. ally. This led many Americans to look more favorably upon the people they'd viewed as smelly slum-dwelling assimilation resisters. A second key factor was a nationwide conservation campaign led by the U.S. Food Administration. Staples like meat and wheat were needed to bolster the war effort, so millions of families signed a pledge to observe national days of cutbacks, including "Wheatless Wednesday" and the origin of today's popular "Meatless Monday," which was revived in 2003 as a public health campaign.

So instead of balking at Italian recipes for their lack of meat, Americans seized an opportunity, oddly enough, to be patriotic. By 1918, it was common to see articles with Italian recipes in women's magazines, bearing headlines like "Meatless Days Have No Terror for Our Italian Friends of California," as *Good Housekeeping* wrote alongside guidance for making spaghetti and ravioli. The piece went so far as to say, "Ravioli, favorite dish of our Italian ally, should be served on every American table." Food prices rose during wartime, furthering the appeal of cheap, simple Italian dishes—like mac and cheese—among American families. Dishes had been passed on for generations among poor Italians making do with what was available on slim budgets in the Old World. And now, the meatlessness of many of their dishes was among their greatest assets in the New World.

Another reason the influence began to run the other direction in the mid-1920s was an act of Congress—the Immigration Act of 1924—that brought a halt to the great faucet of Italian immigration. With fewer newcomers to deal with, less attention was placed on Americanizing the ones already here. This opened the way, in essence, for them to simultaneously *Italianize* us.

By around the 1910s, many Italian immigrants had discovered California and its familiar Mediterranean-like climate. The transcontinental railroad meant red wine from the Golden State could be had in big cities in the East. And people got over their fears about tomatoes, which became a familiar item for most Anglo-Saxon Americans. That familiar taste was one part of the cuisine's appeal to Americans, who started coming in sizable numbers to restaurants run by Italian immigrants.

Cafeterias were an approachable kind of restaurant for the middle class, extremely popular in the 1920s, as were spaghetti houses. Both cropped up around the country, serving spaghetti to the masses. They helped extend Anglo interest in Italian dining beyond those cities with large populations of Italians, such as New York and San Francisco.

But there was another key factor: Large, coastal cities where large populations of Italians happened to settle were also "the important cities for the dispersal of culture in general," as Mediterranean culinary expert Clifford A. Wright told me.

Over time, Americans became captivated by the glamor of Italian culture as a whole. In recent decades, as "celebrity chef" turned into a unanimously recognized type of figure in American culture, we've turned to icons like Giada De Laurentiis, Lidia Bastianich, and Mario Batali for that cool factor.

But food industry marketers have also leveraged Italian food's just-right level of exoticism. You'll see products like Nabisco's "Tuscan Herb Flatbread" crackers, or dishes like Tuscan Chicken at restaurants and in American cookbooks. Despite the fact, as Wright says, that you won't find Tuscan Chicken in Tuscany. "But it's become such a catchword that even now, we can start naming Italian regions as a marketing tool—Tuscan this and Tuscan that," he says. "It indicates to the person using it that they're sophisticated. And what's so curious is Tuscan food is about the least interesting food in Italy. It's like deciding that the most important food in America is from Nebraska."

In 1929, the Great Depression hit. Many countries felt they had to protect their own economies, which resulted in increased trade barriers and prices on imported goods. This led to a boost in domestic production of items that were in high demand among Italian immigrants: The United States significantly increased its production of pasta, canned tomatoes, and cheese (emulating, though not perfectly, the aged hard cheeses of Italy such as Parmigiano-Reggiano).

One man in particular benefited from the economic opportunity of making Italian food in the United States rather than importing it. That was Ettore Boiardi. An immigrant from Piacenza, Italy, he became known as Chef Hector in New York. As a teenager, he headed the kitchen at the Plaza Hotel, and by age twenty, was the lead caterer for President Woodrow Wilson's wedding. Before his thirtieth birthday, he had moved to Cleveland, found a bride, and opened a successful Italian restaurant.

The next part sounds a little like the microwave story from the second chapter—too cute to be true—but I'll be a good sport and tell you that Chef Hector's spaghetti and meatballs was so popular he started selling it in milk bottles. Combining canned tomatoes and pasta in a single can, the "Chef Boyardee" brand was born in 1928. (The official history on the brand's website says the phonetic spelling was "to keep American tongues from twisting on the Italian pronunciation.") That idea of takeout in a milk bottle spawned an empire, today owned by ConAgra Foods.

One of the leading scholars on international migration and gender and food studies, Donna R. Gabaccia, writes in *History in Focus:* "The American military may have introduced more potential consumers—at home and abroad—to Italian foods than had all the immigrant restaurateurs of Little Italys in American cities."

How could this be? When the United States entered World War II in 1941, the military had 15 million soldiers to feed. It commissioned Chef Boyardee to shift from standard operations for the supermarket industry into 24/7 production to feed the troops.

Meanwhile, several hundred Italian Americans were being interned. (Italy under Mussolini was no longer an ally.) Francesco Panciatichi, for instance, a sixty-four-year-old newspaperman from New York, was sent to Fort Meade, Maryland, to wait out the war. He became the "Italian spokesman" for the ten Italian Americans housed there among mostly German American internees. In a letter to the commander of Fort Meade, Panciatichi wrote:

Although there is no doubt that the food ration for our meals is abundant and of good quality . . . we are compelled to complain once more about the way the food is prepared, cooked and served to us Italian internees by the German cooks. . . . For instance: Germans are showering sugar upon every possible dish and have a marked preference for cakes and sweets, while the Italians soberly prefer simple meals and particularly spaghetti with plenty of bread and butter.

The commander's response was to give the Italian Americans a separate mess hall to cook for themselves.

And by the end of the war, spaghetti and meatballs was a weekly go-to meal for millions of American households.

For the most part, Italians don't eat spaghetti and meatballs. But it became a dish here primarily because one of the first things to be done in adapting Italian food to American life is add meat. *Lots* of meat. According to Warren Belasco, the food scholar, early Italian transplants to the United States followed what he calls the "rule of thumb whenever an immigrant group comes to America": Use "twice as much meat as they used in the Old World." Soon after arriving in the States, immigrant groups notice how much more affordable meat is here, he says. "It's just one huge meat locker. That's really what the American dream is: the ability to access cheap meat."

Though the Italians were not alone in ramping up the meat in their dishes, Belasco says they did it better than others. They took food preparation far more seriously than other immigrant groups did when they arrived (in contrast, say, to the Irish, British, or Germans, who also came to America in large numbers).

In the United States, beef was especially affordable, so it became the animal of choice. The low cost also allowed for larger meatballs, and ones made with a higher density of meat than other ingredients. And where did the idea for meatballs come from? The Swedes have their *köttbullar,* the Turks have their *köfte*, the Brazilians and Portuguese their *almôndegas*, and the Spanish and Mexicans their *albóndigas*. The Italians, they have their *polpette*, made with different types of ground meat, commonly veal and pork, or even fish. But polpette aren't served with spaghetti but rather in a soup or just plain—as the main event. Traditionally, an Italian meatball is made with bread crumbs (using day-old bread) softened with milk and usually some onion and garlic for flavor, some egg for adhesive. It's about equal amounts bread and meat.

The American version, on the other hand, calls for a lot more cow. And you can thank Chicago for that. It was a center for the slaughter, refrigeration, and distribution of cheap beef, and butchers would often sell it ground. It's debatable whether that was to obscure potentially subpar quality and food safety concerns or to make the beef more versatile in American kitchens. But Italian immigrant cooks took the affordable ground beef and molded it into meatballs, topped with tomato sauce poured on piles of spaghetti.

Something similar happened in Argentina, actually, where abundant beef was pounded as veal cutlets had been in Milan, then drowned in canned tomato sauce imported from Naples. The result was a completely new dish called *milanese alla napoletana*.

It's not as if Italian peasants had ever eaten spaghetti and meatballs or *milanese alla napoletana*. These were New World creations. With so many Italians coming to the United States and returning home and coming back, shaped too by American daily life, the cuisine that emerged over time was a stirring, a layering, a kaleidoscopic convergence of influences.

Why Italian American Food
Conquered America

Italian immigrants held on for dear life to the foods they loved, accepting and celebrating that they couldn't be what they had been in the Old World. "Italian" food in America became the flavors of Campania, minus certain cheeses and specialty items, plus way more meat. And more sugar, to appeal to the national sweet tooth Americans had inherited from the British. Then Italians took this food and sold it to as many American customers as they could find.

And we bought a lot of it. But why did Italian American cuisine do so well? Lots of people try to sell lots of things—what *is* it about this food, of all the international foods that have gone mainstream, that Americans just can't get enough of?

Some point to political factors. In World War I, we were allies with Italy. In World War II, although Italy was on the other side, the United States freed the Italian peninsula from the grip of Hitler and Mussolini. In the aftermath, with their country in ruins, we welcomed another 400,000 Italians to U.S. soil. As for the other gastronomic impacts of American foreign relations, I guess falafel has taken off, and the United States supports Israel; on the flip side, you'll notice we don't have that many, say, Russian restaurants. But our roster of enemies is constantly changing, and we eat a hell of a lot of sushi, so that argument doesn't hold up.

Then there's the affordability of Italian dishes, many of which are traditionally meatless. So that's a big sell, as we saw not only during wartime but during the Great Depression and the Great Recession. Regardless of the time period, really, whether you're a budget-strapped college student or a parent trying to feed a family, a pack of ravioli and a jar of sauce is one of the most wallet-friendly crowd-pleasers in the supermarket.

Others argue that the success has to do with Italian American cuisine having the all-star of all-stars any country could have on its culinary team: pizza. Even as recently as 1945, pizza wasn't popular among English-speaking citizens outside of New York and Chicago, or Spanish-speaking citizens outside of Buenos Aires, the cities with some of the largest Italian populations. But that changed in America in the 1950s, in part because of pizza to go in those iconic cardboard boxes. The speed, but also importantly the low price, aligned with other popular fast-food concepts like roadside burgers and fries and hot dog stands.

Pizza satisfies some of the most essential requests of the American food psyche. Food industry analyst Harry Balzer explains: "It's a one-dish meal; it's mostly made by somebody else [80 percent of all pizza eaten in the United States is either frozen or from a restaurant]; it has broad appeal throughout the family; it's relatively inexpensive; it's not meat- but really bread- and plant-based; and at one point it was thought to be good for you."

Pizza has even been called the "perfect food." To be clear, this is not (only) my personal opinion. The data show that the single-greatest difference between what my cohort and I eat as eighteen- to thirty-year-olds, and what our parents ate at our age, is that pizza is a far bigger part of our lives. Here's psychologist Paul Rozin's analysis: "You couldn't design a better dish for anyone's palate: It melts in your mouth—its softness, its crispness. If you took people who had never had anything before [aliens?] and gave them pizza, there wouldn't be anything better than that."

As is true of pasta, there is a universality to pizza. "The appeal of pizza crosses all ethnic, racial and class lines," writes

Ed Levine, the "overlord" of the site Serious Eats, in his book, *Pizza: A Slice of Heaven*. "Everybody, from working class families to college kids to multi-billionaires, loves pizza."

For striking that individualism chord, we also respond favorably to personalizing our pizzas with endless combinations of toppings. Plus, pizza can be regionalized. Both of which make of us feel special. We've got white clam pizza in New Haven, barbecue chicken pizza in Los Angeles, and deep dish in Chicago, of which John F. Mariani writes in his book *How Italian Food Conquered the World*, "The thickness of the dough and the lavish use of disparate ingredients typified the Midwestern idea that making a dish larger is always better." (This is a philosophy apparently applied not only to portion size but also to home design and city planning. Had I a Hummer, I would drive it through the doorway of an average home in the Chicago suburbs and park it in the shoe closet. Had I a fixed-gear bike, aka a fixie, I would overtake one of these home's driveways and declare it a pocket park on behalf of open-space-craving urbanites everywhere.)

Still another argument for why Italian food took hold in America is its inherent mildness. Italian cooking is foreign enough to feel exotic and exciting, but not so "unidentifiable" that it scares off less daring Americans, writes historian Libby O'Connell, in *The American Plate: A Culinary History in 100 Bites*.

From lasagna to pizza, bruschetta to panini, gelato to tiramisu, the flavors are pretty basic. They're mostly combinations of simple sauces and starches. You don't need to build up a tremendous spice tolerance as you do to truly appreciate many other global cuisines.

"If you see in Italy how Italians dress, they're the best dressed people on the planet—effortlessly—and their cuisine is the same," says Clifford A. Wright. "It's very natural . . . It isn't fussy like the French is. It's healthy; it's delicious. But Swedish food is kind of bland; I don't mean to malign the Swedes, and it's very popular among Swedish people. And everyone loves Chinese food, but unless you're Chinese you just can't eat it very day. But Italian food could work its way into the American milieu as everyday food."

The mildness is also a prime reason why children like Italian food so much, why nearly all the items on a typical kids' menu are loosely Italian American. Might adopting a habit of pizza and pasta at a young age be a source of its popularity in our national culture? Wright tells me not to put too much thought into this observation. Kids, he says, aren't the drivers of gastronomic trends.

I'm not so sure. As cereal marketers know, what we eat in the precious window of the first years of our lives shapes our eating habits as adults. It's a basic truth of preference formation. "Psychologists tell us that food and language are the cultural traits humans learn first, and the ones that they change with the greatest reluctance," writes Donna Gabaccia in *Food in the USA*.

Does this mean that later in life we won't jump on board with the idea of a food truck—waltzing up to a former laundry van and trusting that the food made in the little galley might be delicious? No. Does it mean we won't amp up our heat tolerance, our appetite for pork belly, sweetbreads, and blistered *shishito* peppers? Of course not. But it means the foods we like as kids get special status for life.

It's the power of nostalgia that we saw in the previous chapter. Or what you might call comfort food. When you ask what comfort food *means*, different people will likely offer different answers. Perhaps it's something very simple that doesn't set your mouth on fire or upset your stomach. But a common thread will surely relate to what we ate as children. For me, it's things like ginger ale and toast, from days I was sick in bed and my mom took care of me; Top Ramen after running around outside on a winter day; those E.L. Fudge sandwich cookies my dad bought for my school lunch; Rold Gold pretzels from when my brother and I used to stay up late while visiting our grand-parents, biting the pretzels into letters to spell out messages for them to read in the morning.

It may also (though, of course, not always!) be a source of comfort to eat a dish because someone close to you *made* it for you. And you felt loved. Breakfast quesadillas have become a comfort food for me over the past few years because my hus-band makes them on weekend mornings. I never touched an egg between the ages of seven and eighteen; those were the dark ages after my Spit-in-the-Eye* phase in kindergarten, before my egg-white-omelet phase in college. Yet now, nothing hits the spot like a warm, tortilla-wrapped cheesy goo packet. Partly because my husband makes it, and partly because the tastes are simple and soothing.

All of these factors likely have *something* to do with why Italian flavors earned America's favor. But my two cents is this: Most Italian dishes are easy to cook. (Or "make at home," since "cook" may be a bit generous for what it takes to prepare some of the items we've discussed.)

Just about anyone can boil a pot of water, toss in some dried pasta, and swirl it around with sauce from a jar. Lasagna in-volves pretty straightforward layering of a few simple ingredi-ents, yet presents with pizzazz. Pesto from scratch is magic in a blender. (Purists will opt for the mortar and pestle, but that's slightly less magic, slightly more elbow grease.)

Moving up a notch, many Americans have reached the point of even making their own tomato sauce, starting with the garlic

---

* Yes, you can call it Toad in a Hole if you prefer. Or Egg in a Nest. Or Egg in a Basket.

and tomato paste and canned tomatoes, adding herbs and salt as they see fit, and the meditative stirring of a wooden spoon to bring it all together. Others may make their own gnocchi, using potatoes or squash or pumpkin. All of these components and dishes are extremely simple, yet hugely satisfying.

In what is considered the first modern Italian cookbook, *Science in the Kitchen and the Art of Eating Well*, Pellegrino Artusi wrote in 1891, "Don't think I'm pretentious enough to teach you how to make meatballs. This is a dish that everybody can make, starting with the donkey." And the so-called father of Italian cuisine wasn't kidding: Spaghetti and meatballs was the *one* thing my grandpa could cook. An insurance man with seven kids in 1960s Spokane, Washington, he rarely had dinner duty. But when my grandma left him to his own devices, meatballs were the thing that surely saved him. (Clearly they're still saving plenty of us today, as meatballs are among our ten most-searched-for recipes on Google.)

If as a child the first thing you learned to cook on the stove top was Kraft Mac and Cheese, your first encounter with the *inside* of an oven probably involved a frozen pizza. Today, making homemade pizza from scratch is all the rage. I'm willing to bet that Trader Joe's fresh pizza dough for $1.29 has something to do with that. It's in another category entirely from previously available pizza doughs.

So Italian American food's popularity both in *and* outside the home is what truly sets it apart. Italian cuisine has on its side not only easy preparation but also easily accessible ingredients. There's a Chinese restaurant in just about every town in America. But not every household cooks Chinese food at home. I've had *phở* probably eighty times in my life. I've never once made it. Same goes for croissants, pad thai, and miso soup. I'm not saying I couldn't make them. I just . . . haven't. Because they seem, well, hard.

Italian cuisine is less about twenty-one-ingredient sauces or techniques that take years to master. Instead, it's all about the quality of the ingredients. In the past decade or so, we've entered next-gen Italian eating in America—a vastly greater variety of dishes and tastes, the likes of Eataly and restaurants serving the more nuanced cuisines from Italy's distinct regions. But they tend to share this common trait. Take, for instance, the idea that a perfectly grown, perfectly ripe tomato speaks for itself in a Caprese salad, with just the simplest addition of mozzarella, olive oil and vinegar, a sprinkle of salt and pepper, and a few basil leaves. Really good building blocks give an enormous head start. This ethos of Italian cooking makes it easy to wow someone with a home-cooked Italian meal.

The Mainstreaming of Global Cuisines

Italian American cuisine is widely appealing in part because it allowed all of this blending, rather than remaining a strictly authentic, intact cultural import. As we saw, much of its success came at once by leveraging its inherent meatlessness, or meat-as-flavoring-agent, and also adding far more meat to dishes. We put about five times the amount of cold cuts in a "panini" than anyone in Italy would ever use, for example. So what really propelled Italian food to the forefront of our eating is how it merged with just about everything else in the American food environment. From an evolutionary standpoint, to adapt is to flourish.

It's special-occasion food and everyday food. It's family food and solo food, lunch food and dinner food. It hasn't exactly conquered breakfast, but that's another story.

And it's because of blending and iterating rather than siloing and preserving that it has thrived. Now, "Italian" in America can be almost anything to anyone.

Belasco adds, "This interaction between old and new, immigrant and native—which is an American story in so many ways—means instead we have a creole cuisine of mixes of different influences, and that holds up for any ethnic cuisine."

I admit I have a personal connection to Italy, love Italian food, and can't imagine my life without pizza Margherita. But the point of this chapter is not to say that no cuisine rivals Italian in its presence in American food culture. When Americans order takeout and delivery, Chinese, Mexican, and Italian top the list; when we eat at a restaurant, the most popular types of international cuisines are sushi, Thai, Vietnamese, Brazilian/Argentinian, Greek, and Southeast Asian. That's according to a 2015 study conducted on behalf of the National Restaurant Association, entitled "Global Palates: Ethnic Cuisines and Flavors in America."

But historians and food studies experts point to Italian food as the original symbol of a broader phenomenon: the gradual incorporation of foreign cuisines into traditionally bland American palates. Two-thirds of Americans now eat a greater variety of cuisines from around the world than they did just five years ago. The vast majority of us enjoy eating these types of food both at restaurants that serve only that type of food—what you might consider the more authentic experiences—*and* as part of "mainstream menus," as the study called them, at other types of restaurants.

Spaghetti and meatballs is a great case study of our ever-more-daring tastes, and the quests for culinary adventure, that *today* define American appetites. The dish reveals the making of a true fusion cuisine in American culture.

In the culinary community, "fusion" gets a bad rap. It tends

to be taken as meaning the food has no identity. But this is misguided. I'm referring to our cuisine at large.

And when I ask the question, What does our food show
about who we are?, the story of spaghetti and meatballs suddenly isn't just about Italian American food. It's the story of the
melting pot, and the novel, distinctly American cuisine that
bubbles up out of it. Spaghetti and meatballs is merely one of
countless dishes and ways of eating that never existed anywhere else. And collectively, these comprise a national food
culture. One you might call Immigrant American.

Chinese immigrants also found certain dishes that could
appeal to American tastes—General Tso's chicken not least
among them. This adaptation, the mixing and compromising to
create entirely new foods, was much the same. One difference
between Italian food and other immigrant cuisines in America,
though, is the way Italian Americans responded to its Amer-
icanization. Chinese Americans, as Harvey Levenstein writes
in *Food in the USA*, "generally found the concoctions served
in 'chop suey' houses and made-in-Minnesota canned 'chow
mein' to be abominations," while "Italian-Americans generally
shared the native-born WASP's enthusiasm for the Americanized version of their cuisine." They were proud that non-Italian
Americans gave their food recognition.

Not long ago, Levenstein points out, many Americans
"equated tacos and frijoles refritos with stomach cramps and
diarrhea." Consider, for a moment, that by 1991 salsa outsold
ketchup in retail stores. By $40 million. Now, Chipotle is the
envy of every restaurateur in the land.

"In 2009, the dollar share of 'ethnic' frozen meals (Asian,
Mexican, etc.) surpassed the dollar share of traditional American recipes (e.g., beef Stroganoff, Salisbury steak, mac and
cheese, etc.)," reads a presentation slide by the Hartman Group.
Friends: This is a big deal! Hartman also notes that a little fewer

than one in eight adult meals eaten at home involves an "emerging global food," while at a restaurant it's more than one of every five meals.

What's driving the *accelerated* integration of global cuisines into mainstream culture, then, is the increased number of meals we eat outside the home. The greater percentage of the total bites we eat in a given day or week that are made by someone else. Why *not* give lamb adobo a try on your Munchery app? Chicken tikka masala from the Trader Joe's prepared food section looks whirl-worthy. What these and other new food-service models have done from an innovation standpoint, from an industry disruption standpoint, is make foreign dishes more accessible to the masses.

It's the silver lining, if you will, that comes from our not cooking as much anymore.

Two novel business models have dramatically heightened the pace at which—and the fervor with which—American consumers embrace the exotic: food trucks and the Chipotle format of fast-casual dining. Some people are happy committing a whole Saturday night to trying a family-run Himalayan restaurant, or driving to a retail district where they don't recognize the letters on the signs. But some people are not. It's far easier to shift, say, one turkey sandwich you'd normally have for lunch on Tuesday to a kati roll if the food truck is parked right outside your office. The same thinking goes for everything from Indian "nanini" and Filipino pork *sisig* rice bowls to Vietnamese *banh mi* and Austrian schnitzel. The speed and price point of food truck food—you'll be on your way for under ten dollars in under ten minutes—further reduces barriers to consumption.

Fast-casual restaurants with the create-your-own format—also offering that ten-dollar, ten-minute mark—have a similar effect: You start with a base, pick a protein, and add sauces and toppings as you like. Importantly, that cheffing includes tailoring the spiciness and complexity of flavors to your comfort level.

As the author John Hooper notes, there is a crucial distinction between diversity and disunity. We are a country of political, cultural, and ideological diversity, spread across many far-reaching geographic subsections. But there are features that reveal themselves in the foods we eat that characterize us broadly as a people.

Various arguments try to explain why Americans like "foreign" food, such as increased international travel, shifts in immigration policies that have altered our country's demographics, and so on. But it comes down to one uniquely American value: As a people, we are curious, open to the new—the unknown or lesser known. We care about discovery.

All within certain limits of course, because don't forget, all this "mutant mash-up food," as Anthony Bourdain has called it, is happening *alongside* an only deepened popularity of our old standbys: the Five Guys and Shake Shacks selling burgers and milkshakes, except better (apparently), or the craft beer boom with brewpubs selling Reubens and grilled cheese and fries, except with, you know, truffle seasoning. All at a time when the average American still eats three hamburgers a week.

Point being: American fare is far from a thing of the past. It's just a matter of how American fare is defined. So it's not as if we've hopped on another bandwagon entirely—we've welcomed a whole caravan of new wagons into our fleet.

In 2014, *Bon Appétit*'s Andrew Knowlton featured a restaurant in San Antonio, Texas, called Hot Joy, an Asian fusion joint he called "rule-breaking" and "trendsetting." Knowlton writes: "Chef Quealy Watson has never been to Asia. Everything he knows about Chinese, Japanese, Indian, or the rest of that vast region's cuisine he picked up from cookbooks and the Internet. But who cares anymore? Authenticity and rigid adherence to tradition are overrated. Deliciousness is king."

So it turns out that one of our biggest problems as eaters, our unstable food culture, is also one of our greatest strengths: The idea that anything goes—that in throwing it all into the mix something wonderful emerges—is why we have culinary gems you can't find anywhere else.

Korean tacos and naan pizza and California rolls. Some might consider these horrors. Sullied versions of the *true* cultural entities. But not us. In America, collisions are commendable.

CHAPTER 11

What to Make of All This

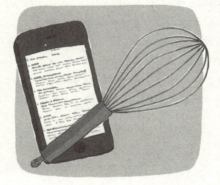

So what to make of all this? From our laid-back approach to wine culture and the unique customs of the Super Bowl to the incredible array of experiences we get to enjoy as part of our Immigrant American cuisine, we've clearly got a lot going for us. Is it so bad that we rely on a steady stream of snacks to get us through each breakneck-paced day?

We now have a greater number of convenient choices than ever before. Greater—and more immediate—access to nearly any food than ever before. And more avenues for having it our way than ever before. Are these really such unfortunate ways to live?

I don't think anyone really knows yet. We're all just making this up as we go—what's healthy, what's "good," what we define as socially reasonable or not.

The ways we're eating today are utterly unprecedented, for

better and for worse. Sure, we're enjoying higher-quality food and a wider range of it than at perhaps any other time in our history. More people seem to be interested in food, thinking about food, and talking about it than ever before.

But we are also regularly bombarded by marketing tactics that can be confounding and concerning. Plus, with everyone eating on a basically constant basis, we seem to have started eating more in total. Gradual, incremental weight gain each year is often difficult to notice, and yet, over many years, it can lead to serious health problems that we'd all probably like to avoid.

Instead of cooking for ourselves, we are outsourcing the making of our food more and more to people who do it for a living. That may be okay for now, but it could be quite a problem if it means losing food literacy altogether—an entire generation that doesn't know how to cook an egg, chop an onion, or, heaven forbid, roast a chicken.

So where do we go from here?

Well, sorry, but I don't have an eight-point plan for a perfect food culture. That was never the idea behind this book. Even if I wanted to, I can't just wave my magic wand and get rid of all the misleading health claims and stressful fad diets. Nor can I snap my fingers and make sure everybody gets three months of vacation. If I believed I could, I would probably . . . run for office. Yikes. I shudder at the thought.

That said, there *are* a few things I wish for us. In the vein of those seven simple words from Michael Pollan—"Eat food. Not too much. Mostly plants"—here are my dozen: Work less and savor more. Make it real and stir the pot.

And to get there, I will leave you with three thoughts on what we might do differently—and one on what we should do the same.

Do differently:

Work less.

When it comes to the state of our eating habits in America, many of us lament that no one cooks anymore. Some of us (writers) stick to lamenting, while others (entrepreneurs) try to fix the problem. They invent apps for personalized eating, meal-assembly kits, grocery-delivery platforms, and other tools to help make dinner easier for the harried worker bee. But people keep struggling to get a handle on the food in their lives.

The problem is, the innovators often forget to look upstream. What is it that's causing people to put food on the back burner in the first place?

To me, it's clear as day: overwork. Stress comes from a variety of places: financial woes, family troubles, medical factors, and so on. All of these have a huge impact on how we eat. And then there's the chronic stress that comes from overwork.

Feeling that there are just never enough hours in the day leads us to some troubling daily conclusions. For instance, we decide we don't have time to cook, exercise, visit with a neighbor, or volunteer at our kids' school—and, more dangerously, some decide they are so busy they can do a digital errand or text while driving. Some of busyness is perception (there is, of course, an important difference between "having" and "making" time), but most of it is reality.

As a country, we simply can't work as many hours as we do and not expect consequences. "Externalities," as they say. So whether it's culinary knowledge, community connectedness, physical activity, the mental-health-boosting power of down-time, or the quality or quantity of sleep or both—some things inevitably fall by the wayside.

The solution starts with employers. Paying people enough

to be *able* to work less would be nice. It's ludicrous to have to work 40 hours a week and still be on public assistance.

For white-collar workers, not giving them ulcers and panic attacks and insomnia would also be nice. That might involve, for instance, establishing office cultures that make it clear that employees won't risk being fired for not working all hours of the day, or for not responding to a midnight e-mail until the next morning.

The federal government could mandate paid time off like the rest of the civilized countries out there so we no longer feel like we have to apologize for taking a vacation.

We can also turn to creative approaches like the communal lunch break at Good Eggs, where employees make a habit of stopping work at the same time each day and eating a real meal together.

Absent an enlightened employer or any nationwide legislation, it might require more grassroots methods of rewriting social norms in your workplace. Turn the extreme working on its head. Instead of "Bravo, Colleague, you're so dedicated," it could be, "Sheesh, Colleague, seen your family lately? Why don't you go take a ceramics class or something?"

A strong work ethic is still—and *should* be—something to be proud of, something to strive for. But, like those kraters of wine, it's the dose that matters.

Savor more.

There are two ways we could savor more. First, we should savor the food we eat more than we typically do.

For this, we can take a tip from the mindfulness movement, which is not just about mindful eating but mindful living. It reminds us to stop watching TV while writing e-mails on our laptops while also scrolling through Facebook on our phones. Instead, we should be present with each individual activity. When you brush your teeth, don't think about your meeting or your to-do list or what you're going to wear that day. Just . . . brush your teeth.

Though mindfulness won't overcome the root cause of being so busy and putting food on the sidelines—overwork— mindfulness is at least a step in the right direction.

So when you eat, before you race to take a picture of your plate or scarf it down to move on to the next activity, instead pay close attention; even engage all five senses around what you're eating—what does it smell like, what is the texture, how does the taste on your tongue change over time, what ingredients do you detect, what taste memories does it remind you of? You don't need to go overboard with this, just slow down enough to focus on the food.

Which brings me to the second way we could savor more: Savor the food *experience*. Find the joy in it—not just the utility.

Take wine, for example. We've made wine our own here in the U.S. of A. We have welcomed labels from all over the world, produced great juice across our own country, and invented all manner of containers to drink it from. We've embraced the value label not as a compromise but as outwitting the show-offs charging $3 a sip instead of $3 a bottle.

But we've got to be careful to keep pleasure in the picture. As we've known for thousands of years, wine is meant to be savored, and it's meant to be fun. Which means we have to keep a level head about wine on the health front and rein in our tendency to take anything that's good for you to the extreme. So enough with the resveratrol pills and the diet booze, reducing wine to a low-calorie vehicle for tipsiness. And check the guilt at the door, please.

It's a little like Denial Dicing. If you're going to eat the donut, just eat the darn donut and *enjoy* it. If you aren't going to enjoy it, then don't bother.

Yes, try to eat mostly whole foods and especially plants. But instead of the more frequent, mindless grazing throughout the day (a cookie here, a handful of M&M's there), when you treat yourself, make it really feel like what it was always meant to be: *a treat*.

One easy way to savor a food experience is to eat with other people. It sounds so simple, and yet it is actually rather profound. Individualism is one of the key traits that sets us apart as Americans. But sometimes we forget that we're also human. We forget that food is social, too.

This is the concern of Steve Case, CEO of investment firm Revolution LLC and cofounder of AOL. In a 2015 article in the tech publication *Re/code,* Case voiced a counterargument to the popularity of Soylent in Silicon Valley. He writes: "The future of food is not a powder mixed with water to create an engineered superfood. It is not a race to consume calories as quickly as possible so as not to disrupt the disrupting. It is not alleviating the 'pain' of having to 'waste time' eating food with friends and family, in order to maximize time building the next app."

Food is more than the efficient delivery of calories, "fuel," as is often said. Which means Soylent marks a step backward, culturally speaking. And brunch signals the way forward.

Americans eat alone more often now than they used to, and that coincides with many of us feeling a loss in connectedness. Luckily, we're doing something about it. Communal tables at restaurants (as well as restaurants where chefs take you along for a culinary adventure that's *anything* but your way) have risen dramatically in recent years. So have community cafés, which often follow a pay-what-you-can model. These cafés allow patrons to volunteer in exchange for a meal, pay the suggested price or less if they can't afford it, or overpay, helping to cover a future diner's meal. Paying it forward, that is.

No one needs to know which category of payer you are; you sit together and share a meal, along with maybe some live music. The café is a neighborhood hub, a way of breaking the ice and relearning how to make eye contact with people. Relearning the art of face-to-face conversation.

Make it real.

The headline of Steve Case's article "The Future of Food Is Food" says it all. Real food, grown responsibly, prepared in fresh, delicious ways, to be enjoyed together. I know, that's a tall order. And I am far from the first to advocate for real food—yet the rapidly flowing river of new (often eye-popping) fake foods that continues to capture our national attention makes it worth repeating.

A good step toward making it real is to reevaluate our relationship with science as the ultimate guide for what to eat. It's a no-brainer that we should continue to care about health and think about it in the context of what we eat. But when we do so, it's time to shift away from our focus on the macronutrients in foods, which too often has led us to look to food companies to formulate food *products* in ways that satisfy our perceived needs and allay our concerns that we're not getting what we need. Instead, we have to start taking a more holistic view.

Wrapped up in eating habits are nearly all the fundamental drives in life: feeling good and looking good, parenting and friendship, family heritage and personal preferences, and the idea of a lifelong "bucket list." Food intersects everything in society: education, the environment, the economy, religion, and politics, to name just a few.

For help finding this more holistic view, we can look at other countries. Brazil, for example, not only pulls the lens out from nutrients—using whole foods as the basis for its national advice about what to eat—but it also looks at *meals* and focuses on the reality of how people actually eat: in a variety of social contexts and within a food environment that, frankly, is more complicated than can be captured by nutrition science. Brazil even tries to help consumers avoid the food industry's misleading marketing ploys. It considers the broader foodscape.

In a groundbreaking move, the 2015 U.S. Dietary Guidelines Advisory Committee's report did call for a shift away from our emphasis on individual macronutrients and instead suggested we pay more attention to whole foods and eating patterns. Granted, they did so in a six-hundred-page report with countless references to individual nutrients, but hey, it's a start.

This kind of shift toward a national *culture* of health related to food can help us regain trust in our instincts. To get there, we will have to take a cue from the history of diet evangelism and recognize that there are no secret elixirs, no quick fixes, no guaranteed results. Instead, we can spot that combination of claims as the tell-tale prescription for a lot of pain, and a lot of time and money we don't deserve to waste.

I'm not suggesting that we stop listening to nutrition science altogether, but that we learn to avoid the rapid swings of the pendulum brought on by every news headline. Nutrition science takes a long time to reach comfortable conclusions. And as complex as it all is, sometimes the reality is disappointingly simple: We just don't know enough yet. Until then, it's safe to stick with the boring but timeless "everything in moderation."

That, and the other boring but timeless adage: Use common sense.

A big part of making it real means *making it*—yes, *you* making it!

There is often a fear that we will invest time in researching a recipe, going to the grocery store, chopping up all the ingredients, and then, after all that, overcook the chicken and ruin the whole meal. By contrast, going out to eat feels like the safe bet. Especially at chain restaurants that deliver reliably consistent tastes at whichever location you visit. Even if you have to stand in line at Chipotle because everyone in your neighborhood, like you, feels like cheffing instead of cooking, you're pretty sure you're going to be happy with the end result.

But we can't simply switch from customizing to cooking from scratch. Many whole foods can be intimidating. Like what on earth do I do with fennel? In order to gain confidence in the kitchen, we need familiarity with ingredients and what flavors go well together and techniques for preparing different dishes.

I am certainly not the cook I'd like to be. I don't have the timing down, the ease, and I'm terribly over-reliant on recipes. It would have been great to start cooking at a young age so it would come more naturally, the way a language does when you learn it as a kid. So to parents, older siblings, babysitters, aunts, uncles, grandparents—anyone who's got a little one they care about—bring kids into the kitchen early on, and make cooking together fun.

Unfortunately, with all the options for not cooking available to us today, we also need incentives for setting out to learn in the first place. The trouble is, while the incentives are there all along, they can be hard to see. In reality, we're inching closer to a time when the only members of our society with even the most basic culinary understanding are professionals in the foodservice industry. And that forecast is not just a cute parable about how we should all go back to home ec. The demise of cooking is about losing our spot in the driver's seat. It's about losing control.

I'm referring not only to control over what we put in our bodies, but control over which growers and retailers we buy from. By extension, that involves having ownership over what kinds of agricultural, environmental, and labor practices we support with our food dollars. Having the power (and taking the time) to make those individual purchasing decisions means actively *shaping* our collective food system, not merely depending on it.

In the same way, cooking means actively shaping our collective food *culture,* not merely existing in it.

While we're busy trying to do these three big things differently—working hard at working less, striving to be exceptionally good at savoring every eating experience, and channeling our desire for continual progress as a society to elevate the pastime of real food eaten in the company of others—we can kick back and do at least one thing exactly the same:

Stir the pot.

To be more specific: *Keep* stirring the pot. The melting pot, that is.

Before we get to that great composite of immigrant cultures, though, first to the stirring: I love living in a country where innovation and creativity reign supreme. If, like countless others, you tend to think our food system is broken, help fix it. Just as innovation drove the development of a massive food processing infrastructure, food safety standards, and industrial scale harvesting and milling and packaging, we can keep applying one of America's greatest values to our current food issues.

That value, of course, is solving problems through science and technology. So we're seeing exciting and new healthy fast-food concepts, payment platforms that make it easier for farmers to sell their produce to nearby restaurants, and on and on.

As we spend our days shaping a better food future, though, all I ask is that we not overlook what's to be learned from the past. It's not that we all have to revert to the routines of our ancestors or pick up farming, though I wholeheartedly applaud those who do. But we shouldn't assume that doing things better automatically means finding new technology to use.

With the resurgence in the popularity of canning, personally killing one's dinner, and making bread and cheese and beer and wine at home, clearly there are many Americans who already recognize that sometimes our newest approaches to food are really a return to our oldest ones. But as such a forward-looking country, we often let a certain crosswalk wisdom slip our minds: We forget to look both ways.

So go ahead—join the disruptors, the "foodpreneurs," as they're called. Challenge the status quo. Do it better. Just don't overlook the foods that come from the ground instead of an R&D lab. The humble peanut. The pumpkin now finally in the latte.

Yet another upside of our food culture's constant churning through new trends and new ways of eating is that we've invented new holidays like the Super Bowl. And on that note, I have another request: When you eat whatever you're going to eat on Super Bowl Sunday, or during the holidays, do it because you want to. Not because an ad warned of its dwindling supply, not because you're afraid it will disappear forever. We live in a land of plenty, with an astonishing number of choices that is both a blessing and a curse. Surely you can find *something* to please your palate that doesn't involve driving yourself crazy in time for kickoff.

Finally, to the pot. The widespread adoption of global cuisines in America—and, yes, the fusion—is not something to hide but to hail. It's the kind of novelty worth cultivating. As long as you make it real—and you make it delicious—I say, bring on the culinary creativity; bring on the converging influences. Because that throw-it-all-into-the-mix mentality is one of the reasons there's *nowhere* else I'd rather be an eater.

So when it comes to cultural coexistence on our plates, let's remember: It's in our roots. It's most certainly the way of the future. And unlike, say, wreathing our pizzas in hot dogs, it's an American food tradition we can be proud of.

Acknowledgments

Years ago, the first person I ever told that one day I wanted to write a book about food in America was my college advisor at the time, the passionate Stanford history professor Carolyn Lougee Chappell. She recommended books for me to read and helped stoke my fascination with food culture that had been sparked as a fourth-grader living in Italy.

When I was in grad school, there were several people who pushed me to take the idea of writing a book from an "if" to a "when": Jen Lachance, whose magic worked not only on me but on every student who has ever walked into her office with either a problem or a goal; each of the 2014 UC Berkeley Center for Health Leadership Fellows; Rebecca Aced-Molina, my life coach, who put up with my squirming throughout the first year at the very *idea* of life coaching; and Bob Klein at Oliveto Restaurant, who agreed to our will-work-for-penne-bolognese arrangement and who planted the seed of my obsession with whole grains (now in full bloom).

This book is what it is because of the unmatched mentorship of Michael Pollan. During his writing seminar and our many sessions talking through my book proposal, he offered patient, thoughtful guidance—and always with a huge smile on his face. What has meant most is that he genuinely *cares*. That's why, beyond the writing, he has patiently and thoughtfully helped me make pretty much all my major life decisions ever since. Michael, I've been trying for years now to find exactly the right words to thank you, and in this case, there simply aren't any. So I'll just say: To think that it all started with a Doritos Locos Taco! And I look forward to what's ahead.

It was also through Michael that I found my fantastic fact checker, Heather Mack. She's a great writer to boot, so I'm sure we'll all be reading her book next.

I would like to acknowledge two editors at *Sunset* magazine who saw potential early on and went out of their way to give me opportunities to grow as a writer: Margo True, who walked me through not only the first book I ever contributed to but the first recipe I ever developed in the test kitchen (veggies for breakfast!), and MacKenzie Huynh, who is also a dear friend, running partner, and constant career cheerleader. Mac, you are such a talented writer, and your work was a huge inspiration on the path to finding my own voice. Speaking of *Sunset,* Haley Bowling's vision for me as an author came so early on that I don't know where to begin with a proper thank-you.

At *The New York Times* Well section, I am grateful to killer editing by Toby Bilanow, and for all the opportunities to bring my story ideas to life; to Tara Parker-Pope for imparting some important journalism lessons that I have taken with me throughout this book project; and to Anahad O'Connor for sharing his own experience as an author, not to mention a great bicoastal friendship. I learned from the many, many outstanding writers at that desk that although we may be writing *about* science, there is still much art in the writing.

At The Culinary Institute of America, I would like to thank Will Rosenzweig—a mentor in every sense of the word—and Christina Adamson and Greg Drescher for their sincere support from day one.

Thank you to all the people who generously gave their time to be interviewed for this book. And to Ciara Gay, the gifted artist behind the beautiful illustrations that open each chapter.

It goes without saying that the book would not have been possible without my editor, Henry Ferris, and everyone at William Morrow: Liate Stehlik, Lynn Grady, Shelby Meizlik, and Leah Carlson-Stanisic. Production editor Rachel Meyers and copy editor Georgia Maas made some great saves, and I'm grateful for the fine teeth on their combs. Henry delivered laser-focused edits and much-appreciated trips to the chopping block. More than anything, thank you for not merely sharing my vision for this project but taking the words right out of my mouth. ("Yes, it's a book about food, but it's not a *food* book. It's a who-we-are book!") It has been a joy to work with someone who so often sees eye-to-eye with me, and at the same time has really good reasons for *not* seeing eye-to-eye with me, which, of course, make everything way better.

I owe much gratitude to my literary agent, Carol Mann, for all her enthusiasm about the topic and for asking the right questions, as well as the tough love from her savvy readers. In particular, I cherish the sound advice she offered at our first meeting to give this thing another year to marinate.

I am grateful for thorough reads by three people who were nice enough to donate their brilliant ideas at no charge: Mollie West, Ashley Baker, and Joe Lyssikatos.

Nailing the right title took some doing. Thank you to my brainstorming task force of Dave Kintz, Keenan Newman, my brother, Casey Egan, and my mom, Joni Balter (Eat's true! Your fungry ideas and smart edits were a great help in getting *across* the finish line, as were your reminders not to eat staples, which aren't as nutritious as they sound). And thanks to Kintzes near and far for the steady stream of thumbs-ups the whole way through. To my dad, Tim Egan, thank you for a lifetime of "book talk" on the deck, far-flung research trips, and an in-house apprenticeship that taught me years' worth of lessons about writing, all in the span of a dark, rainy holiday season. I'm honored to finally be joining you on the shelf.

Last, to my husband, Sam Kintz. It's because of him that I took an evening food-writing class at a time when my day job was turning my brain to mush; it's because of him that I eventually started pouring all my energy into chasing the book dream; and it's because of him that everything else happened in between, so that people can actually be reading these words on this page right now. Sam, thank you for continuing to be what you've always been: my sounding board, my biggest fan, and my best friend.

Glossary

A note on style: Quotation marks indicate that I got the term from someone else. No quotation marks indicates that I coined the term myself or that its use is common enough that I didn't feel it needed quotation marks.

"additivity dominance": The tendency to perceive a food as less natural if something is added to it than if something is removed from it. It comes from a paper in the journal *Judgment and Decision Making* by Paul Rozin, Claude Fischler, and Christy Shields-Argelès.

Artificial Altruism: "Gifts" from coworkers left out on a communal "free table" in an office that are really gifts to the people who left them out—saving them a trip to Goodwill or the guilt of tossing unwanted foods in the garbage, or sparing them the torture of having something around the house that is so irresistible but bad for them. They don't care if *you* get fat on Funfetti frosting, so long as *they* no longer have it lurking in the cupboard. At no time of year is this phenomenon more pronounced than during the week after Halloween. The free table is inevitably overflowing with plastic jack-o'-lanterns full of exclusively lame candy.

"averaging bias": Inaccurately estimating the calories in a meal due to the way we place foods into buckets of "good" or "bad." Used by Alexander Chernev of Northwestern University and David Gal of the University of Illinois at Chicago, this bias is rooted in the human tendency to process information qualitatively: People make value judgments about foods by balancing opposing goals of health and indulgence, virtue and vice.

When eating a healthy food and an indulgent food together, we end up averaging the two in our minds.

brunch: More than just a cross between breakfast and lunch, it signals a meal enjoyed at a slower pace than a weekday "snackfast," as well as the weekly pattern of weekend indulgence versus weekday deprivation. The meal calls for company, often to simmer on the sidewalk with you while you wait for a table. The term hit the United States in 1896; by 1939 Sunday was declared a two-day meal, and evidence of brunching on Saturdays in addition to Sundays has been visible among many Americans since the 1990s.

> **"war on _____":** Objections to the day drinking and lavishness associated with going out for brunch, but really to the gentrification that brunch-going can represent in certain urban areas.

Cheesepocalypse: A fake Velveeta shortage leading up to the 2014 Super Bowl.

"cheffing": Directing your order—adding tomato, subtracting onion, doubling the pepper jack, and so on. Coined by the Stanford engineering professor and innovation consultant Michael Barry. Cheffing happens at the create-your-own meal concept (or assembly-line format) restaurants such as Subway, Chipotle, Blaze Pizza, and countless others. Not only do they not reprimand you for making special requests, they *require* that you be a participant in the process.

cobranding: Crossing two familiar brands rather than inventing something from scratch and having to explain what it is. Preexisting brand recognition and product familiarity go a long way toward getting people to try something that sounds crazy. For example, the marriage of Doritos and Taco Bell, or Oreos and McDonald's. Our desire for novelty is tempered by our need for familiarity.

comfort food: *Definition may include one or more of the following traits:* A dish made for you by a loved one; a dish or food product you ate as a child; an extremely simple, even bland dish or food product. For example, macaroni and cheese.

cooking: Making food at home. In reality, cooking today is often mere *assembly*. For instance, adding frozen peas to a premade soup. Of all our eating occasions, 42 percent involve exclusively prepared foods, and 77 percent involve at least some prepared foods.

"creole cuisine": The description offered by author Warren Belasco for what happens to a cuisine when it arrives in America: the "interaction between old and new, immigrant and native," and the "mixes of different influences." Not only does this apply to the genre we call Italian food in America that is really Italian *American* food, but it "holds up for any ethnic cuisine."

critter labels: The trend of featuring animals on wine-label art, best represented by the playful wallaby from the Yellow Tail label.

Democratization of Wine, the: The many ways that wine has been brought to the masses in the United States; that is, made more available to all people and possible for them to understand.

Denial Dicing: Gradually slicing and slivering little portions of a desirable food that someone brings to work to share with colleagues—often homemade baked goods, bagels, or donuts—while crippled by guilt and yet convinced that the total being eaten isn't all that much, when ultimately it ends up actually being quite a bit.

dessertification of breakfast, the: The blurred lines between the products in the cereal aisle and the products in the cookie aisle of the grocery store, which have largely resulted from decades of breakfast foods gradually turning into morning sugar bombs. It all started in 1906 when Will Keith (W.K.) Kellogg added sugar to corn flakes. Along the way, we've seen products like Cocoa Puffs, Oreo O's, and Smorz. And marshmallows somehow made their way into cereal bowls as reasonable things to eat at 7:00 A.M.

diet evangelism: The predilection for not just latching onto the fad diet of the day but trying to convert friends, family, and the population at large.

digital _____: Preaching the gospel of a certain diet through blogs, podcasts, social media, etc., often as a supplementary tactic to diet books, the traditional and still-much-used platform for diet evangelism.

peer-to-peer _____: As opposed to celebrity → mass of followers, this happens friend → friend, colleague → colleague, hairdresser → client, and so forth. Facebook is a common vehicle for this branch of diet evangelism.

"eating season": The phrase coined by Harry Balzer of the NPD Group to refer to the annual holiday binge-eating pattern in America that extends from Halloween through the Super Bowl.

"edible foodlike substances": The term author Michael Pollan gives to highly processed products that we eat. Unlike whole foods, these products rely on their labels to speak to us as consumers.

"experiential CV": Just as we collect wine corks or shot glasses, coins or seashells, we collect life experiences. In the same way that résumé builders accumulate educational milestones and job experiences, checking off items on our bucket list of personal experiences seems a way of measuring how full a life we're leading. It's also about projecting a self-image of having done a lot of exciting things. And for many people, an important component of that experiential résumé is trying new foods. The phrase comes from Anat Keinan of Harvard Business School and Ran Kivetz of Columbia Business School, who explain that the phenomenon is driven by a **"productivity orientation"** prevalent throughout Western societies and particularly American society—that is, the urge to use time to reach accomplishments and make progress even while engaged in leisure activities.

family dinner, à la carte: Cooking multiple meals or dishes to cater to each family member's highly specific needs and preferences. It's something more than half of families report doing.

fast casual: The Goldilocks of restaurant-going: These chains sell reasonable quantities of reasonable quality food from a menu listing a reasonable number of choices. The food is prepared partly far away and partly on-site to ensure adequate freshness and temperature, sold at decent prices, served within enough time to gather your napkins and beverage and secure a booth. In other words, for many, fast casual is *juuuust* right. (Think Panera Bread, Chipotle, Noodles & Company, Dig Inn, etc.)

food culture: The set of customs, values, and behaviors related to eating and drinking in America.

fridge theft: Stealing your colleagues' food from the office kitchen. Such larceny is so rampant that employees nationwide have adopted all sorts of creative means to combat the issue: labeling their sack lunches as "poison curry" or leaving cat-food sandwiches as traps.

Great Protein Myth, the: The common belief among Americans that we need to consume more protein in a day than we actually do, and that our intake is lower than it actually is. While protein malnutrition is a problem for millions of people around the globe, for most of us eating here in the United States, it's hard *not* to get enough protein on a daily basis.

green guilt: Feeling guilty about one's environmental impact. Americans rank among the lowest according to a Greendex report produced by the National Geographic Society and GlobeScan. Given the total volume of American wine production, the alternative wine-packaging movement and sustainable grape-growing practices represent a potential avenue for improving our overall sustainability standing.

hangry: A combination of hungry + angry. Consider it the adult equivalent of a small child's blood-sugar meltdown: Some men turn sullen, some women turn snippy, and the only way to quell the stirring storm is to shove something into our stomachs—and fast. Hangriness is much more likely to set in not only after a long time without eating any food, but after eating a lot of processed crap.

health halo: The effects that certain labels such as low-fat, gluten-free, reduced-sodium, non-GMO, and so on have on us, causing us to attribute a whole slew of health benefits to foods with those labels.

"hot fudge sundae and the Diet Coke, the": So dubbed by Barb Stuckey of Mattson, this pattern of eating behavior involves having, say, a salad for dinner, but then allowing yourself something indulgent for dessert. This helps explain why even people who mostly eat healthy sometimes still go for stunt foods. It's the same idea as "averaging bias," where we essentially make the calculation that a "good" food and a "bad" food cancel each other out.

Immigrant American: My proposed reframing of the idea of "fusion" cuisine, in celebration of the melting-pot ideal and in recognition that true American fare is a delicious convergence of cuisines from all over the globe. These foods often combine to create never-before-seen culinary delights such as spaghetti and meatballs, among many others.

"index high": As Harry Balzer of the NPD Group explains, this is when consumers collectively eat significantly more of something at a certain point in time compared with how much they eat of that thing most other times of the year. For example, pizza and chicken wings on Super Bowl Sunday compared to most Sundays.

Kind Bar Occupation, the: The rapid sales growth and omnipresence of the energy bar Kind, which emphasizes its high protein content, and what have become known as "clean labels," a short list of recognizable ingredients.

lifehack: A prescription for self-improvement. Or any tip, trick, or nugget of instruction that helps you "get things done more efficiently and effectively," as Lifehack.org explains. For example, following the Paleo diet or doing CrossFit.

mass customization: Taking existing processed foods and delivering them in individual-size portions that meet a wide range of specific demands. Just picture the yogurt section of the grocery store. Or the 500 flavors of coffee or tea capsules available to make in a Keurig machine.

meal: *Traditional definition:* A combination of foods, plated, often eaten at home. *Modern definition may include:* A combination of snacks, portable, each individually packaged.

"nutrification": A word with several meanings. I use it as described by the food scholar Warren Belasco in his book *Appetite for Change*: the strategy in food processing where manufacturers of food products first remove the good stuff, say, the germ and bran from wheat kernels, then add back in fiber and vitamins and minerals that would have been in the whole grain to start with, slap a label on the box of the refined grain product touting these attributes, and charge a bit more.

"Paradox of Choice, the": The situation explained by Swarthmore College psychology professor Barry Schwartz (namely in his book by that title) that having more choices can actually make us feel *less* satisfied. Paralyzed, even.

pizza: Arguably the single most universally loved, perfectly designed food. It's the one dish that satisfies all elements of the American food psyche: quick, cheap, and customizable; usually made by someone else (80 percent of all pizza eaten in the United States is either frozen or from a restaurant); often considered relatively healthy; and consisting of comforting and simple flavors, yet able to be tailored with toppings that are as exotic as one desires.

"privileged" foods: A category identified by Rabobank's Nicholas Fereday that includes all holiday foods, as well as foods associated with happy, fun times, especially those had as children. Nostalgia and the idea of treating ourselves are central, and consumers don't hold these foods and food products to the same health and quality standards as others.

Pumpkin-Flavored Everything Craze, the: The baffling trend whereby Americans consume an ever-growing array of pumpkin-related food products each year despite the fact that very few of them actually contain pumpkin.

Sad Desk Lunch: Instead of taking a lunch break, you eat lunch at your desk while continuing to work at your computer. The entire lunch-at-work paradigm was revolutionized by the invention of two magic-inducing boxes. First, the microwave oven. Second, the desktop computer. Together, they turned white-collar workers into keyboard-clogging victims of early-onset hunchback.

"scientific halo": The tendency to trust the effectiveness or legitimacy of a product or certain information because it is presented in a scientific-looking way (i.e., charts and graphs), as offered by Aner Tal of the Cornell Food and Brand Lab. It stems from our deeply rooted faith in science.

"secular church": In parts of the United States where people aren't as religious, the brunch gathering is the closest substitute for the experience of church: getting out of the house, marking the turn of the calendar, breaking bread together. Perhaps most important, it involves spending time with friends or family, in contrast to rampant solo dining. I borrow the term from Alana Conner of Stanford University.

Selling Absence: The way marketers convince us to buy foods such as fat-free milk, gluten-free pretzel sticks, air-popped snacks, and 100-calorie packs of cookies. We end up purchasing a food not for the crazy reason that it contains worthwhile ingredients—but because of what these items *lack*. (Related term: **"nonundelows,"** dubbed by Emily Green, a writer for the *Los Angeles Times,* for foods whose labels begin with "non-," "un-," "de-" and "low-.")

snack: "Anything small, increasingly nutritional and portable that complements or replaces a meal," as defined by Mike Esterl in *The Wall Street Journal.*

"snackfast": Used by Rabobank, the word means a sequence of morning-oriented food products spread throughout the first half of the day—a Kind bar on our way out the door, a yogurt around 9:30 A.M., and maybe a handful of nuts or a banana to get us across the finish line till lunch.

"stunt foods": Absurdly, unabashedly decadent food innovations, typically produced by fast-food chains and available for a limited time only. The term was first used by Jennifer Wright in *Gourmet,* and it applies to Taco Bell's Doritos Locos Taco, KFC's Double Down, and Burger King's bacon sundae, to name just a few. Collectively they make up what can now be called the **era of "Shock-and-Awe,"** to borrow from Barb Stuckey of Mattson.

Super Bowl Monday (also known as National Sports Day): The name of a proposed new national holiday, the Monday after the Super Bowl.

Superiority Illusion: "The belief that you are better than average in any particular metric," as explained in *Scientific American.* This tendency is especially pronounced in the United States, where being average has always been something of an insult. Few of us want to be pegged as merely "normal"—we want to be extraordinary!

Two-Buck Chuck: Nickname for Charles Shaw wine, available only at Trader Joe's, whose $1.99 price led to record sales and helped reduce the snobbery around wine consumption in America.

Source Notes

Introduction: The American Food Psyche

For insight into customer segmentation and consumer behavior, I talked with Hank Cardello in March 2015.

For the milestone of spending more at restaurants and bars than in grocery stores, I pulled from reports from the Hartman Group on Americans' food attitudes, shopping styles, and spending habits.

The fact that our fast-food consumption is still quite high comes from a Gallup poll, and Doritos Locos Tacos' record-breaking sales were reported in numerous news articles throughout 2012 and 2013.

I looked at the negative effects of the American diet through many reports including ones from the Dietary Guidelines Advisory Committee, the American Medical Association, the Centers for Disease Control and Prevention, the American Heart Association, and the U.S. Department of Agriculture. For a more comprehensive list, see the notes for chapter 4.

My interviews with Harry Balzer provided many of the insights throughout this book, starting here in the introduction with the nuggets of data from his annual report and other NPD Group publications, on what foods have increased in our diets over time and what, how, when, where, and why Americans eat what we do.

Social mores are visible (and audible!) all around us, so much of that discussion is from personal experience. But I made sure I wasn't the only one noticing these particular cultural attributes by sourcing several essays, travel guides, cultural critiques, and news and magazine articles.

Fortunately, I didn't have to count all 42,214 items in a grocery store. The Food Marketing Institute did, and they list all kinds of similar data on their website.

Michael Pollan's take on the American food mentality—built on our multiethnic makeup and our relative newbie status—is conveyed through his many books, speeches, and published interviews. I also had the privilege of doing much of my graduate work under his guidance at the University of California, Berkeley.

My research into the "Muddle of the Modern Meal" and the American work ethic came from sociology texts, reports from the Organisation for Economic Cooperation and Development, Pew Research Center data, and many, many news articles and opinion pieces about overwork. With regard to whom we eat with or don't, how work affects our eating, and much more, the numbers were brought to life with great color thanks to discussions with and presentations by Melissa Abbott of the Hartman Group.

The concept of customization and the definition of a meal were explored through interviews with Michael Barry of Stanford/Quotient Design Research (formerly Point Forward), psychologist Paul Rozin, and Melissa Abbott. Social and behavioral studies are from Swarthmore College and Stanford, Harvard, Columbia, and Cornell Universities; consumer behavior tracking comes from the Food Marketing Institute, Technomic, and other market research firms.

Brunch: A History by Farha Ternikar provided me with plenty of background on brunch, and numerous articles from various news publications further explored the midday meal we line up for in droves. A comprehensive list of brunch sources can be found in the notes for chapter 5.

Stunt foods comes from my reporting on the Doritos Locos Tacos, originally for a piece I wrote for *Wired* magazine in 2013. This involved numerous personal interviews (see chapter 8 source notes) as well as data from the global food company Yum! and marketing research company Datamonitor. Information about individual stunt foods comes from each of the items' public debut, which was heavily publicized in media and advertising.

Pew Research Center supplied evidence of Americans' love affair with science and technology, which provided a foundation of our philosophy that innovation is king. This often translates into our excitement about food hacks such as the drinkable gruel that is Soylent, whose information is derived from 2014 news articles and by reading its company website that spring. Data from the U.S. Department of Agriculture (USDA) told me that so many new food products are released every year.

Chapter 1: The Muddle of the Modern Meal

"Gobble, gulp, and go," is based on a combination of *Revolution at the Table: The Transformation of the American Diet* by Harvey Levenstein and *What's Cooking? The History of American Food* by Sylvia Whitman.

Market research on snacking as well as ease of preparation and consumption as the main drivers of food purchases comes from the Hartman and NPD Groups.

The increase of individual-size coffee and other beverages is from industry publications such as *Food Processing* as well as company websites. Prepared foods' increased prominence is from my weekly reading of restaurant and retail industry newsletters, and the stat on single-family households is from the U.S. Census Bureau paired with *The Washington Post* and CBS News analysis of its data.

I interviewed Harry Balzer of the NPD Group and Melissa Abbott of the Hartman Group to discuss eating patterns, mainly focusing on how snacks are becoming meals.

Food and Work

Americans work a lot, as per data from the Organisation for Economic Co-Operation and Development. The 2014 Pew Global Attitudes survey and numerous news articles indicate that we have strong feelings that we *should* work a lot, as well as the fact that we don't have federally mandated parental leave or hardly any vacation time. Comparisons to Scandinavian countries come from a 2014 *Fast Company* piece, and *karoshi* material is a combination of the *Washington Post* piece and a case study from the International Labour Organization.

Vacation time stat is from the U.S. Travel Association. Amazon's now-infamous workplace policies were described in an August 2015 *New York Times* article and other media coverage.

For the section on productivity, I drew from a June 2010 paper in the journal *Human Relations* by Kimberly D. Elsbach, of the University of California, Davis Graduate School of Management, and Jeffrey Sherman, of the UC Davis Department of Psychology, for insights on people's perception of time in the office, reliability, and so on; productivity drops and errors and the importance of breaks come from summaries of various related findings from the psychology literature in *Psychology Today, Fast Company,* and *Financial Times.*

World's smelliest food is from a study reported by Scandinavian publishing firm Pinetribe.

What Is a Meal?

I drew from interviews with Michael Barry of Stanford/Quotient Design Research on how consumers define a meal and with Harry Balzer about packaged food versus meals and the rise of snacking.

Supplementary snacking data, including key comparisons between what a snack used to mean to what it means today, came from consumer research firm the Hartman Group, and my interview and discussion of their data with their vice president of Consumer Insights, Melissa Abbott.

I also found information on snacking behavior from a large report by the consumer research firm Nielsen, which conducted a global survey of snacking in 2014 that polled over 30,000 consumers in sixty countries.

Figures on percent increase in calories consumed from snacks versus other meals are from a 2012 review, by Pierre Chandon of INSEAD and Brian Wansink of Cornell, of food marketing's influence on food intake published in *Nutrition Reviews*. The stats on increased daily calorie intake between 1970 and 2010 are from the USDA.

Protein Can Do No Wrong

The firm Nielsen found that Americans bought $16 billion worth of products with protein claims, and this was reported in the spring of 2015 in *The Wall Street Journal*. Numerous consumer research firms including Hartman have found that consumers are actively looking to increase their protein intake.

For the section on the science of protein and how much we eat compared to how much we need (what I'm calling the Great Protein Myth), I drew from personal communication with Christopher Gardner, professor at Stanford Medical School, who has studied this for decades, National Institutes of Health research, CDC nutrition data, as well as publications from the Harvard T. H. Chan School of Public Health.

My assessment of protein and snacks and their related trends and products like Kind bars and yogurt is based in part on popular media such as *Fortune, The Wall Street Journal,* and *Fast Company* but also largely from insights from trade media including *Food Processing, Food Business News, Nation's Restaurant News,* and *QSR* magazine. Yogurt information specifically is from NPD Group data, as well as New York State law. Snack bars as one of the fastest-growing items is from an interview with NPD's Harry Balzer.

For the section on breakfast and cereal, I read reports from Dutch bank Rabobank and talked to the company's Nicholas Fereday for information about snacks' replacing breakfast. I studied how breakfast came to be with *Breakfast: A History* by Heather Arndt Anderson, reports from the Hartman Group, and Michael Moss's *Salt Sugar Fat*. These cover cereal's rise to the top; recent data on cereal came from Rabobank and Nicholas Fereday, the Environmental Working Group, Euromonitor, and the NPD Group. What children from around the world eat is derived in part from a great 2014 *New York Times Magazine* piece by Malia Wollan.

Instant Gratification

I used data from the Organisation for Economic Co-operation and Development to find how much time Americans spend cooking compared to people in other nations, as well as how much cooking has declined over the years. The rise of delivery and ready-made foods in a variety of locations like Walgreens is from industry and business publications.

When Is a Meal?

Michael Barry and I spoke about how frequently people are eating, and I've spoken with not only Barry and Melissa Abbott but numerous professionals in my field about the widespread acceptance among Americans to eat anywhere and everywhere. People make healthier food choices when others are around per a 2013 study published in the journal *Appetite* by researchers at Maastricht University, the Netherlands; George Washington University; and the Amsterdam School of Communication Research. Analysis from *Food Processing* and numerous reports by food marketing experts show that this may only be the beginning of our snacking obsession.

Chapter 2: Food at Work

I attended Vitality Institute's Food@Work conference on April 17, 2014, at San Francisco's Ferry Building. I worked as a note taker and writer for the event, so those details are drawn from my personal experience. The number of working hours compared with 1970 comes from Juliet Schor's YouTube video on the Plenitude Economy, from the Center for a New American Dream. An alternative figure comes from Michael Pollan's article in *The New York Times:* 167 additional hours compared with 1967. Figures on lunch breaks and eating at desks are from a 2012 Right Management Survey and ConAgra/American Dietetic Association.

For information on Google, I drew from the *Fortune* best companies ranking list, as well as articles in *Business Insider* and *The Atlantic*. The analysis of Google and food comes from an interview with Marion Nestle, her blog *Food Politics,* a 2012 *Gourmet* article on Google food, as well as details on healthy Google food offerings described in many presentations by the Google Food team at The Culinary Institute of America's food industry leadership conferences, such as the 2015 Menus of Change leadership summit.

The University of Illinois at Urbana–Champaign study on chocolates in the office and visibility and convenience was published in *Appetite* in 2002. I know the implications of studies like this and many others for healthy behaviors from both personal interviews on habit formation with lead author Brian Wansink (now at Cornell), from my master's work on health and social behavior at UC Berkeley including a course on applying design thinking to food-related challenges, and from working with health behavior and foodservice professionals.

Food You Bring Yourself

The backstory on lunch (and bringing it to work) comes from *Lunch: A History* by Megan Elias. The book also covers trends like salads.

Percy Spencer and microwave history is from the book *Eating History: Thirty Points in the Making of American Cuisine* by Andrew F. Smith. Pew Research Center found that the microwave is viewed as a necessity.

The details on the rise of frozen entrées come from interviews with Harry Balzer and Richard Wilk. Figures on the frozen food industry come from the American Frozen Food Institute and articles from *Food Business News, Bloomberg News,* and *Food Processing.* Specific information on frozen food brands comes from the company websites.

Thirty-four percent not in the workforce comes from a Gallup poll.

Food You Get from Colleagues

Stories of people doing insane things for food are from viral headlines.

Habits around eating in the office and candy in the workplace are my own assessment based on anecdotes and personal experience. An official definition of sensory-specific satiety is from *Nutrition and Metabolism,* edited by Susan A. Lanham-New, Ian A. Macdonald, and Helen M. Roche.

The figures on American workers who are not engaged with work are from a Gallup report.

Food Employers Provide

A Glassdoor survey of employees showed food is second only to money as an appreciated form of recognition.

The history of drinking at work comes from *The Alcoholic Republic: An American Tradition; Lunch: A History;* and *The Empire of Tea* by Alan McFarlane and Iris MacFarlane. Office-party data came from executive research firm Battalia Winston.

Happiness and work productivity comes from a study by University of Warwick researchers published in 2015 in the *Journal of Labor Economics.*

I learned about the value of food in tech from personal experience living in the Bay Area, as well as media coverage and tech companies' highly publicized interest and investment in local food. Charlie Ayers's history is from his personal website and media coverage.

The need to work less—but the flattening of wages—comes from a *Mother Jones* report citing the Bureau of Labor Statistics, the Congressional Budget Office, the Economic Policy Institute, the U.S. Census Bureau, the Center for American Progress, the McGill Institute for Health and Social Policy, and the Pew Internet and American Life Project.

Chapter 3: Having It Our Way

Dialogue is from *I Am Sam*. Super Bowl research on food shortages and the ensuing mayhem over novelty was from interviews with Richard Wilk, Harry Balzer, and Nicholas Fereday. Figures on the most popular food items come from the NPD Group and those on work productivity from Glassdoor; examples of shortages, advertising, and hype come from media coverage, company websites, and press releases. The bragging rights of each customizable item are from each company's website and advertising campaign, although Starbucks has never given anyone a straight answer on just how they calculated that 87,000 figure.

Having It Our Way, *At a Restaurant*

"Have It Your Way" history and descriptions are from Burger King's website and old video of the commercial on YouTube.

The study on the American preference for uniqueness (and pen choice) by Heejung Kim and Hazel Rose Markus was published in 1999 in the *Journal of Personality and Social Psychology*. Variations by social class are from a study by Markus, Nicole M. Stephens, and Sarah S. M. Townsend published in 2007 in the *Journal of Personality and Social Psychology*.

Superiority Illusion and examples of it come from a summary of findings from the psychology literature in *Live Science* and *Scientific American*. The Warren Belasco quote about resisting standardization and homogeneity is from his book *Food: The Key Concepts*.

Having It Our Way, *At a Restaurant 2.0: Fast Casual*

Paul Rozin material is from a personal interview. Traffic growth in fast casual is from the NPD Group and *Forbes*. The number of items on a McDonald's menu is from the company website. For more on the "Paradox of Choice," see the book by that name and the TED Talk by Barry Schwartz.

Harry Balzer and I talked in an interview about how there are more customized options available now than ever. Specific customization options come from those company's websites.

Starbucks proximity is from the 2014 *Time* magazine Answers Issue, and Starbucks gift cards is from *Fortune* in January 2015. Michael Barry and the idea of "cheffing" and customization are from a personal interview.

Having It Our Way, *Thanks to Technology*
Customization is from personal experience and each company's website.

Melissa Abbott and I talked about half of eating occasions being alone, user technology, smartphones as shopping tools, and how Americans prefer to catch up on social media by eating alone, but many of those findings have been written about at length in popular news outlets, and I supported this section with information from FoodNavigator-USA.

Shifts in grocery behavior, primary shoppers, less frequent visits, and planned meals are from Food Marketing Institute research. Millennials' driving much of this change, such as payment platforms, is also from the Food Marketing Institute, a 2014 Hartman Group report, and media coverage.

Having It Our Way, *At Home*
Gallup data show 53 percent of American adults with children under eighteen eat dinner together six or seven nights per week.

Pew Research data revealed Americans' preference for individualism. The puzzle study and children is from "Rethinking the Value of Choice: A Cultural Perspective on Intrinsic Motivation" by Sheena S. Iyengar and Mark R. Lepper, as described by Hazel Rose Markus and Barry Schwartz in a paper on freedom, choice, and well-being published in 2010 in the *Journal of Consumer Research*. Oldsmobile ads are from *Advertising Age* and the GM website, and numerous other cautionary tales in advertising.

Cost of Keurig versus drip coffee is based on a variety of calculations summarized in a March 2015 *Money* magazine article, though various business publications have found different ratios based on when their calculations were done and how people define a "cup" of coffee.

Studies from the Organisation for Economic Co-operation and Development show Americans spend less time cooking and eating than do people in other countries.

Chapter 4: Selling Absence
The concept of averaging bias and Americans' being off target in gauging the healthfulness of certain foods is from a 2010 Northwestern University study published in the *Journal of Marketing Research*.

Health halos have been written about extensively, but I drew specifically from a 2013 study out of Ulster University in Northern Ireland, published in the *International Journal of Obesity,* as well as the 2012 food marketing review by Pierre Chandon of INSEAD and Brian Wansink of Cornell published in *Nutrition Reviews*.

Marion Nestle's quote is from personal communication. Ancel Keys and the history of low-fat advice are drawn from a variety of sources including news coverage by NPR and *Time* as well as a paper about the lipid hypothesis by Jason Andrade of the University of British Columbia et al. published in 2009 in the *British Columbia Medical Journal*. Foods with health claims on the rise since 2002 is from the USDA Economic Research Service.

Michael Pollan's idea of "edible foodlike substances" is from *In Defense of Food*. The figure on impulse buys is from a 2008 research article in the *American Journal of Health Education* by Randy Page et al. of Brigham Young University.

"Low-Fat"

The M&M's study on university students and their families was done by Brian Wansink and Pierre Chandon, published in 2006 in the *Journal of Marketing Research*. This study also covered how people serve themselves more than the recommended serving size of most foods, and the fact that products labeled low-fat actually contain about the same number of calories as regular versions on average.

Consumer preference for items that are "free-from X" is from the 2014 Food & Health Survey from the International Food Information Council Foundation.

Irony of unhealthfulness of replacements is from numerous sources including statements and articles by Mark Bittman, Andrew Weil, and Walter Willett. New products with claims to be gluten-free, 0 trans fat, etc. is from USDA data and *Food Processing News*. Reviewing fat is from the 2015 Dietary Guidelines Advisory Committee report as well as interpretations from Gallup polls, and the 2009 *British Columbia Medical Journal* article.

Agreement among the medical community, including the Center for Science in the Public Interest, on the heart disease–related dangers of trans fat is widespread. Overviews on types of fat come from the Harvard T. H. Chan School of Public Health's Nutrition Source, and additional details on trans fat labeling and urging the American public to avoid it come from the Food and Drug Administration. Information about heart disease in America is pulled from CDC data and combined with U.S. Census figures.

Saturated fat avoidance and the examples of milk and cheese are from the 2012 paper by Brian Wansink and Pierre Chandon, which also provided the statistic that a lower percentage of our calories now come from fat but that is just because we have consumed so much of everything else, confirmed with data from the CDC.

Paula Deen and Kraft as dynamic duo is from Food Network and company advertising.

Getting sicker even in spite of "nonundelow" foods, increases in obesity and diabetes rates since 1980, and leading causes of death are from the CDC and the Harvard T. H. Chan School of Public Health. Changes in caloric intake over time is from CDC data, USDA data, and the *American Journal of Clinical Nutrition,* which also supplied information about fat and satiety signaling, supplemented with information from the Cleveland Clinic.

"Natural"

The Warren Belasco information is from his book *Appetite for Change* and a personal interview, and the Paul Rozin information is from a personal interview and several of his journal publications. "Natural" as the leading claim of all new food products is from data from the research firm Mintel. The survey in which Europeans and Americans were asked to define the word "natural" is from *Consumer Reports*. Preference for natural over artificial and other insights on how people perceive the meaning of "natural" are from research by Rozin et al. at the University of Pennsylvania and the Rand Corporation published in the journal *Appetite* in 2004.

"Gluten-Free"

Value and projections of gluten-free industry are from a report by research firm MarketsandMarkets. For statistics on celiac and explanations of gluten and avoidance of it, I drew from the Mayo Clinic, WebMD, Celiac Disease Foundation website, and the great 2014 *New Yorker* article by Michael Specter, "Against the Grain."

The healthfulness of whole grains is from National Health and Nutritional Examination Survey and the 2015 Dietary Guidelines Committee's report. Gluten product ingredients are from package labeling. The style in which people are going gluten-free, and the irony of its having been started as a way to eat less processed food, is from the Hartman Group.

100-Calorie Packs

Sales data and shopping behavior after the advent of 100-calorie packs come from Brian Wansink's *Slim by Design: Mindless Eating Solutions for Everyday Life* and Michael Moss's *Salt Sugar Fat*.

Air-Popped

The 20,000 figure for new food products is from the USDA. Sales for snacks on the rise is from the NPD Group and Rabobank.

Celebrity investors in air-popped snacks is from the company websites and articles in *Forbes* and *Serious Eats*.

"Lesser Evil" and other specific labeling figures were pulled from the labels themselves and company websites.

Empty Promises (and Often Empty Calories)

Non-GMO Cheerios statement and history is from the General Mills website, and the information about GMO corn versus oats has been written about widely, but I drew from an article in *Modern Farmer.*

Labeling of milk and eggs comes from NPR coverage sourcing from the American Humane Society, the Coalition for Sustainable Egg Supply, the USDA, and the Cornucopia Institute.

Majority of American-consumed salt from processed foods is from a 1991 study in the *Journal of the American College of Nutrition,* conducted by Monell Chemical Senses Center in Philadelphia, which found that three-quarters of the salt consumed among participants—who, like most Americans, bought most of their food from supermarkets—came from processed foods. Crave-ability, sodium intake, cholesterol warnings, and the rise of food processing and convenience products are all from *Salt Sugar Fat* by Michael Moss. The educational material produced by The Culinary Institute of America and Harvard T. H. Chan School of Public Health is called "Tasting Success with Cutting Salt," and was released in 2010. Package labeling of specific foods is from their labels and company websites.

Chapter 5: Secular Church

Brian Wansink information is from his Cornell study on weight and his book *Mindless Eating: Why We Eat More Than We Think.*

The increase of brunch in America is from Google search trends, and Saturday in addition to Sunday brunching is from a 2015 *Washington Post* piece by Roberto A. Ferdman and Christopher Ingraham; that the popularity of brunch has grown and is also in our roots is from *Brunch: A History* by Farha Ternikar. The vast majority of the analysis in this chapter, though, is from my own experiences and interpretation of this trend and the coverage of it.

The Meaning of Brunch

Guy Beringer quote and essay excerpt are from *Breakfast: A History* by Heather Arndt Anderson. The history of brunch is from *Brunch: A History* by Farha Ternikar; this includes when brunch began to be referenced in cookbooks and etiquette guides, the New Orleans versus New York question, cocktails and Prohibition, its British origins, its global popularity, what types of dishes people cooked, and its always having been for busy people who didn't have time to host on weekdays. Further detail and the stigma about women's drinking during the day and hiding it with fruits is from the *Washington Post* piece, and the hotel connection is from an article in *Smithsonian* magazine. All this was supplemented by news coverage of blue laws' lingering effects as well as websites of restaurants known for their brunch.

Our Omelets, Ourselves
Figures on more people living in cities is from 2012 Census data.

Sunday Service
I pulled from a few different surveys from Pew Research Center to get a pulse on how religion fits into the lives of people around the world and how America stands out. Walter Willett's insight about replacement is based on having worked with him personally and observed that he makes a point of emphasizing this during interviews, presentations, and writings. Quotes from Alana Conner are from a personal interview I conducted with her during the spring of 2014.

The "War on Brunch" is from a few different proposed bans on serving on a sidewalk before noon in New York, along with New York State laws and copious media coverage. I got information about blue laws from the online *Encyclopedia Britannica, The Christian Science Monitor,* and *Smithsonian* magazine. The Georgia Brunch Bill is from the state legislation database, and its economic impact is from coverage in *Atlanta* magazine.

Time
Americans' work ethic as a global standout is from Pew Research Center data, and I was inspired by the idea of a digital Sabbath and taking control (as well as information on how addicted we are to technology) from NPR coverage as well as personal conversations with Matt Richtel, author of the book *A Deadly Wandering: A Tale of Tragedy and Redemption in the Age of Attention,* who has written extensively about our relationship to our devices. "Exhaustion as a status symbol" comes from a *Washington Post* interview with Brene Brown (and her professional website) and, as background, her TED Talk on vulnerability.

The Meaning of Breakfast
Skipping breakfast, and statistics on breakfast habits, as well as those specifically about young people (millennials and Gen Z'ers) are from USDA analysis, commentary in *Food Business,* and Technomic's Consumer Trend Report. The ousting of cereal as a breakfast mainstay is from Nicholas Fereday's report with Rabobank. This report also covers the rise of the

breakfast sandwich as the number one food item, which has also been written about in several trade publications. I found the figure about 72 percent of the population preferring breakfast food all day from global research firm Mintel. Breakfast sandwiches abound in the marketplace, as evidenced from company websites, advertisements, and media coverage. Clifford A. Wright quotes are from a personal interview conducted during the spring of 2015.

The Psychology of Line Waiting

The overarching mentality of how humans deal with waiting in line is from David Maister's 1985 "Psychology of Waiting Lines." I supplemented with analysis from Gretchen Rubin in a blog she wrote for *Psych Central;* the stat about people wishing breakfast foods were served all day came from National Restaurant Association research, as reported by the Philadelphia Media Network (Philly.com). The World War II anecdote about elevator mirrors was from a 2012 op-ed in *The New York Times* about why waiting in line is torturous. Traffic figures per city come from Texas A&M's Annual Mobility Study, published in 2013. The rise of "snackfast" is from Rabobank data and reports.

The Meaning of Brunch, Continued

The stats on ice cream are from the July/August 2015 issue of *Food Network* magazine, from a poll conducted on Americans' ice cream habits. I heard about the naysayers of "conspicuous consumption" from news articles and opinion pieces as well as the book *Brunch: A History* by Farha Ternikar.

Feeling guilty for not being productive is from Pew Research data, as well as supporting evidence from NPD and Hartman Groups. Clifford A. Wright quotes about our fixation on dietetics and superfoods over cuisine are from a personal interview.

The long meal traditions of other cultures are from personal experience (ciao down, Italy!) as well as perusing travel websites and culinary blogs. The quote from the *Chicago Tribune* comes from *Brunch: A History.*

Chapter 6: Diet Evangelism

Information on Soylent is from the company's own website, YouTube videos, and copious media coverage in places like *The New Yorker* and *Grist.* Information on Blue Zones is from the Blue Zones website and a *New York Times Magazine* article by Dan Buettner with the great title "The Island Where People Forget to Die."

Global and American obesity figures, as well as the most common tactics for losing weight, come from the Nielsen Global Health and Wellness Survey, the World Health Organization, Gallup polls, and articles in *The Lancet*. Differences by gender come from Louise Foxcroft's *Calories and Corsets: A History of Dieting over 2,000 Years* and a personal interview with her. Regarding the differences between ideal and actual weight, note that underreporting is common with self-reported weights so if actual weights are higher than those provided by respondents in the Gallup poll, the difference between ideal and actual could be even higher.

A Brief History of Weight-Loss Programs and Products

Jean Anthelme Brillat-Savarin and his book *Physiology of Taste,* along with the history of dieting, are from Louise Foxcroft's *Calories and Corsets: A History of Dieting over 2,000 Years*. Additional information on fad diets like Fletcherism and vulcanized rubber come from a BBC story.

The Modern Diet Landscape

Dieting as big business is from Marketdata Enterprises, with further support from financial publications such as *Business Week* and business sections of news outlets including CBS, ABC, and *US News & World Report*, which also provided information on celebrity endorsements, supplemented with sourcing from the National Weight Control Registry; the American Society for Metabolic and Bariatric Surgery; Jo Piazza, author of *Celebrity Inc.: How Famous People Make Money*. Halloween and pet industry stats are from NBC. Information on 22 Days Nutrition is pulled from articles in *Business Insider, Vanity Fair,* and *The New York Times*. What to do about fraud because of no regulation comes from the FDA website.

Eating Season

Harry Balzer quotes and insights on eating season habits are from a personal interview and his research with the NPD Group. Additional stats about holiday and Super Bowl–specific eating habits are from studies by Cornell University Food and Brand Lab researchers, namely their report entitled "New Year's Res-Illusions: Food Shopping in the New Year Competes with Healthy Intentions."

Paleo

CrossFit numbers, descriptions, and contests come from the brand's website, motivational and personal training blogs, as well as widespread media coverage, plus devotees in major urban areas whom you just can't seem to avoid. Growth in gym memberships and athletic wear comes from market analysis in *The Washington Post* and *Fortune*.

Spreading the Good Word

A note on "chemists" in the 1600s: Long before this time, alchemists had been mixing various things together and hoping something interesting would happen, but Robert Boyle is credited in the 1600s with helping distinguish *chemistry* from alchemy by applying actual hypotheses. Traci Mann quotes are from a personal interview. I found the number of diet books and cookbooks by searching Amazon. Louise Foxcroft quotes are from a personal interview.

The evolution of the ideal body size and shape—full-figured to slim, comes from referencing *How to Be Plump, Calories and Corsets,* interviews with Foxcroft, *Fat History: Bodies and Beauty in the Modern West* by Peter N. Stearns, and the everyday onslaught of messages from ads and entertainment. The concept of food as fashion is from an interview with Harry Balzer. On failing our diets is from Brian Wansink at Cornell, Traci Mann at the University of Minnesota, and UCLA researchers' meta-analysis of thirty-one diets.

Why Evangelize?

Sermonizing as social reinforcement and dieting's relationship to religion are from personal interviews with Louise Foxcroft, Traci Mann, and Marion Nestle, as well as my own observations of social media and dieting blogs and *The Gospel of Food: Everything You Think You Know About Food Is Wrong* by Barry Glassner.

Making Sense of It All

Michael Pollan quote is from *In Defense of Food*. The Epictetus quote is from Goodreads.

Chapter 7: The Democratization of Wine

The opening anecdote is from a personal interview with Joe Coulombe, which was originally for a *Sunset* magazine article on the life-changing foods of select luminaries in the food world. The history and current data on Trader Joe's are from a combination of the company's website and *The Trader Joe's Adventure: Turning a Unique Approach to Business into a Retail and Cultural Phenomenon* by Len Lewis.

Our increased wine consumption, purchasing, and production is pulled from Wine Institute research, the National Association of American Wineries, the International Organisation of Wine and Vine, and research firm Technomic, Inc. Data on our growing wine industry is from the U.S. Department of Commerce. There are wine appellations in all fifty states, according to the Alcohol and Tobacco Tax and Trade Bureau.

Robert Smiley told me personally about how millennials are changing wine consumption. Information on Gary Vaynerchuck is from his website, various media coverage, and a New York event of his I attended in 2013.

Here's My Two Bucks

Evolution of the California wine industry and Charles Shaw's rise to the top is from *The Trader Joe's Adventure*, the Wine Institute, Bronco Wine Company data, and coverage in *Business Insider, The New Yorker, Time, The New York Times,* and *Wine Enthusiast*. Yes, I actually calculated just how much wine it would take to fill an Olympic-size swimming pool. Costco as America's favorite and largest wine store is from *The Wine Economist*. Wine corks for centuries is from *Inventing Wine: A New History of One of the World's Most Ancient Pleasures* by Paul Lukacs.

The assessment of Yellow Tail as America's favorite imported wine is from *The New York Times* coverage sourcing from *The Wine Market Report* and California wine industry consultants, plus a U.S. Drinks Conference report on beverage trends. Women's preference for wine (and men's for beer) is from a Gallup poll. Skinnygirl information is from the company website and labels.

The relationship between health and wine is a combination of *The Atlantic*'s reporting by James Hamblin, research from the Harvard T. H. Chan School of Public Health and Brigham and Women's Hospital, WebMD, and research published in the journal *Nutrients* by University of Barcelona researchers.

Quotes from Richard Wilk are from a personal interview. Quotes from Warren Belasco are from a personal interview. The quote from Eric Rimm is from his 2015 presentation at the Healthy Kitchens, Healthy Lives conference at The Culinary Institute of America.

I came to understand trickle-down theory from *The Advanced Dictionary of Marketing: Putting Theory to Use* and from my conversations with Richard Wilk. Robert Parker's statement that our open-mindedness is an advantage is from an article in *The Los Angeles Times*, with additional details on his relative influence from coverage by *Slate* and CBS.

What Sets Us Apart

Our history of drinking is from *The Alcoholic Republic: An American Tradition* by W. J. Rorabaugh. I learned how we rank as drinkers by pulling information from the Wine Institute of California wine map of 2012, the data presented at the 2013 Unified Wine and Grape Symposium, and *Bloomberg News* and *Business Insider* coverage.

Our willingness to try new things (like slumming with Two-Buck Chuck) is from a Nielsen survey, a *New York Times* article examining our entrepreneurial economy, and countless food industry reports I read about experimentation and millennials in particular. Millennials and American adults' wine consumption habits and what type of wine we buy comes from my interview as well as a presentation by Robert Smiley, plus data from the Wine Market Council.

Wine and the Environment
What we drink out of (Bandit, Underwood, Turn 4, Copa di Vino, Bota Box) is from the companies' websites, my own experience with all of these new types of packaging, and *Bon Appétit*.

Americans and the Environment
That we are more likely to recycle (and have "green guilt"), along with the other data on sustainability, are from multiple stories in *National Geographic*. Sixty percent of wine consumption and 90 percent of wine production from California is from Wine Institute data. National drinking culture is exemplified by trends presented at the US Drinks Conference, along with the aforementioned numbers on our consumption polls, and my personal experience and analysis.

Chapter 8: The Age of Stunt Foods
The genesis of the Doritos Locos Taco comes from interviews with employees from Taco Bell corporate: Steven Gomez, Erin Peffly, Stephanie Perdue, Kat Garcia, and Greg Creed. The description of Taco Bell headquarters, the LEED-certified "Restaurant Support Center," comes from my personal visit there. Sales and stats including new jobs and comparison to McDonald's come from company press releases and news coverage about its success. All information provided by Barb Stuckey comes from a personal interview with her in the fall of 2012.

I learned about stunt foods—Burger King bacon sundae, Baskin Robbins "nachos," Cinnabon pizza rolls, Del Taco Chili Cheese Fry Burritos, Carl's Jr. ice cream sandwiches, Dunkin Donuts bacon-egg donut sandwiches, Pizza Hut cheeseburger wreaths, hot dog crust, and "Stuffed Italiano"—from company website information, food and business media coverage, and the ubiquitous advertising surrounding their debuts.

KFC Double Down as the granddaddy of stunt foods is from company press releases and media coverage, nutrition facts are from the company website, and the sodium levels are from U.S. Dietary Guidelines. Calories and nutrition facts on Burger King's bacon sundae, the Starbucks Mocha Cookie Crumble Frappuccino, and Snickers bars are from company websites.

Inside the World of Fast-Food Menu R&D

Twice as many items on menus as the 1990s is according to data by the NPD Group. From interviews at Taco Bell headquarters with Stephanie Perdue, Erin Peffly, Kat Garcia, and Greg Creed, I learned about the union of Frito-Lay and Taco Bell in early 2009, the "ideation session," the innovation forum, concept ratings, challenges and development, and consumer insights from focus groups from interviews. The takeover by Yum!, the relationship with PepsiCo, social media, and brand partnership information are from a wide variety of popular business publications. Yum! figures are from the company website. Information from Harry Balzer is from a personal interview. Quotes and information from Steven Gomez on the failure of the first Doritos Locos Taco is from personal communication, as are quotes from Mike Salem (formerly of Del Taco), Dominique Vitry (of Pizza Hut), and Brad Haley (of Carl's Jr.), about the challenges of executing stunt foods.

The number of calories in the Oreo shake is from nutrition facts listed on the company website. The Argentinian "DestapaBanana" gadget was created in 2011. KFC UK edible coffee cup is from company website and food media coverage. American food chains' influence on the rest of the world (including France and fast-food receipts) is from coverage in *The Seattle Times, Forbes,* and *Fast Company.*

Stunts and Social Media

The social media campaign from DLT was described in numerous articles along with interviews with Perdue, Creed, and Garcia, as were social media campaigns by the representatives from the other fast-food companies I interviewed about the R&D behind each menu item.

The Health-Food Agitprop Rejectionist Movement

Lyfe Kitchen information is from the company website. Hank Cardello quotes are from a personal interview. The Fried S'mOreo at the Texas Rangers stadium was the brainchild of Delaware North Food Companies, which operate the concessions at the stadium. Pulled Pork Parfait at Milwaukee Brewers' stadium speaks for itself: It has its own Twitter feed. The extra stunts like Church's Chicken Oreo Biscuit Bites, Little Caesars Bacon Pizza, Olive Garden's $100 Never Ending Pasta Pass, Jack in the Box Munchie Meal, and Papa John's Frito Chili Pizza were likewise aggressively marketed and talked about on social media and in food industry media coverage. Guiltless Grill is a part of Chili's menu, as shown on the company's website and in restaurants.

Why Do They Work?

The anecdote about Natalie Jones—which is a pseudonym—and her students is from an interview I conducted with her during the fall of 2012. Eat, Drink & Be Merrys is from Hank Cardello interview and presentation slides. The stat on fast-food consumption is from Gallup polling. Information on our craving new experiences is from Anat Keinan and Ran Kivetz of Harvard Business School and Columbia Business School, respectively, published in 2011 in the *Journal of Consumer Research*.

More from the Stunt-Food Kingpins

Doritos just won't stop: From the original Doritos to the DLT to DLT Chips, then 7-Eleven's Doritos Loaded and Dewitos, these moves were chronicled in company press releases, social media, and business media coverage. Pizza Hut cannons were documented in *Time* magazine. Stunt foods aren't going away any time soon per a Datamonitor consumer report calling "mash-up mania" a top-ten trend of 2015.

Chapter 9: Cheesepocalypse

"Indexing high," from pizza to carrots, are from NPD Group research; quotes on the subject are from personal interviews with Harry Balzer. Chicken-wing and pizza sales are from the National Restaurant Association. Figures on Americans calling in sick after Super Bowl is from research gathered in a survey by workforce consultants Kronos.

The Super Bowl in American Culture

History of the Super Bowl is from *The Ultimate Super Bowl Book* by Bob McGinn and *The Billion Dollar Game: Behind the Scenes of the Greatest Day in American Sport—Super Bowl Sunday* by Allen St. John. How it came to dominate entertainment and TV companies comes from *Entertaining from Ancient Rome to the Super Bowl: An Encyclopedia*, edited by Melitta Weiss Adamson and Francine Segan, along with viewership data (comparing to M*A*S*H, awards shows, and *Seinfeld*) pulled from *Time* magazine, *Money* on CNN, *Forbes, Los Angeles Times,* and *International Business Times*. Other ratings are from Nielsen. The ever-increasing advertising prices comes from 2012 research from University of Wisconsin–Eau Claire, 2007 research out of the University of Colorado Boulder, and coverage from *The Wall Street Journal, Forbes, The Atlantic,* and *USA Today*. "Worst play in history" has been widely cited by *Sports Illustrated, ESPN, The Washington Post,* YouTube, NPR . . . you name it. 110.7 million gallons of beer is a widely quoted stat, namely from Fox News.

The Super Bowl's Most Iconic Foods

Indexing high is from an interview with Harry Balzer, second-highest day of consumption is from the USDA, chicken-wing stats such as production, eating trends, dips, and consumer profiles (plus data used to show the fake shortages) are from the National Chicken Council, and coverage from *The Christian Science Monitor, Smithsonian,* and *Bloomberg Monitor.* Super Bowl as second-biggest grilling weekend is from Fox Sports News coverage.

Prices of tickets, plus history, comes from *The New York Times.* I learned from a study by the INSEAD business school in France (published in the *Journal of Psychological Science* in 2013) that people stress eat when their team does poorly, consuming more unhealthy food.

The Super Bowl as National Holiday

The number of male patient ER visits during sports events is from a 2009 University of Maryland study, plus several local news headlines.

Fake Shortages

Quotes from Richard Wilk are from a personal interview. Avocado data is from the Hass Avocado Board, the Avocados From Mexico campaign, and coverage in *Smithsonian* magazine, and *The Christian Science Monitor, The Packer, Dallas News,* and *The Pittsburgh Post-Gazette.* Velveeta and Cheesepocalypse were explored in articles by *Advertising Age* and NPR. Size of stadiums is from each NFL team's website. Data on higher corn and feed prices are from an article in *Scientific American.*

Foods of Privilege

Quotes from Nicholas Fereday are from a personal interview. The "snack-adium" trend is alive and well on several social media and DIY websites. Velveeta and Cheesepocalypse captured headlines in *Advertising Age, The Washington Post,* and CBS, mainly because the company did such a good job advertising its shortage. Nostalgia and the ways that children are shaped by foods they eat early on in their lives and by advertisements they see as children have been studied extensively, namely by Paul M. Connell, Merrie Brucks, and Jesper H. Nielsen in their 2014 paper in the *Journal of Consumer Research*; by Randy Page, Katie Montgomery, Andrea Ponder, and Amanda Richard in their 2008 paper in the *American Journal of Health Education;* and Kaye Mehta et al. in their 2012 paper in *Public Health Nutrition.*

Limited Time Only

Quotes from Hank Cardello are from my personal interview with him. All limited-time offer products were well marketed through traditional advertising, social media, company press releases, and media coverage. The figures on our spending on pumpkin-flavored products are from Nielsen data; increased pumpkin prices are from the USDA. Starbucks also states that the PSL is its most popular seasonal of all time on its website. Number of Trader Joe's pumpkin products is from Gothamist. Pop-Tart pumpkin ingredients are from package labeling and website nutrition information.

Chapter 10: The Story of Spaghetti

Fort Missoula history is from the Fort Missoula Museum's website. "Do you think this is a concentration camp?," the photo of the pasta, and the details from Fort Missoula are from *The Lifestyle of Italian Internees at Fort Missoula Montana, 1941–1943 Bella Vista,* by Umberto Benedetti. Jerre Mangione quote is from his chapter, "Concentration Camps—American Style" in *Una Storia Segreta: The Secret History of Italian American Evacuation and Internment during World War II,* edited by Lawrence DiStasi. "Peet-za" is from John F. Mariani's *How Italian Food Conquered the World.* The top three of Mexican, Italian, and Chinese is from *Nation's Restaurant News.* More restaurants serving Italian food than any other international cuisine in the United States is from Andrew F. Smith's *Food and Drink in American History.*

An Abbreviated History of Pasta

I found information on dispelling the rumor of Marco Polo as our pasta padre, the origin of pasta, what it is made from and how, theories of how it came west, Thomas Jefferson and his refined palate, and pasta's designation as comfort food on PBS, *The History Kitchen,* "Uncover the History of Pasta," an *Atlantic* article published in 2010, and *Food Processing: Recent Developments,* edited by Anilkumar G. Gaonkar.

What can be said about Jefferson, "macaroni" as the early general term for pasta, and historical records showing that a basic baked macaroni dish with Parmesan cheese was served at Monticello are from Monticello's website; *The Founding Foodies: How Washington, Jefferson, and Franklin Revolutionized American Cuisine* by Dave DeWitt; *Pasta: The Story of a Universal Food* by Silvano Serventi and Françoise Sabban; and *The American Plate: A Culinary History in 100 Bites* by Libby H. O'Connell.

Types of pasta is from the Italian food website Eataly plus the International Pasta Organisation. Information about Russia and wheat is from the Imperial War Museum's website and *Globalization: Encyclopedia of Trade, Labor, and Politics,* volume 1, by Ashish K. Vaidya. For that I also drew from *Pasta: The Story of a Universal Food* by Silvano Serventi and Françoise Sabban, which provided the story about Zerega and Brooklyn's first pasta factory.

The Evolution of Italian Food in America

Donna R. Gabaccia from the University of Minnesota provided a comprehensive guide with her *History in Focus* article "Pasta and Red Sauce: Italian or American?" Gabaccia touched on migration patterns, climate, and the food staples of the Americas and Europe.

I got my history of Italian immigration during the 1880s and early 1900s and the difference between Northerners and Southerners from Harvey Levenstein's chapter 7, "The American Response to Italian Food, 1880–1930" in *Food in the USA: A Reader,* edited by Carole M. Counihan, as well as Gabaccia's "What Do We Eat?" chapter in that same book.

The availability of ingredients (and lack of traditional ones), regional varieties, and the shift toward Americanized versions of Italian food (hey, mac and cheese), sugar and Worcestershire sauce in marinara recipes, plus Franco-American styles and Campbell's and Heinz are from the same Harvey Levenstein chapter in *Food in the USA: A Reader.*

More information about the cultural identity and impact of newly arrived Italians on America, the lack of a national language, and the formation of Italian identity is from *The Essence of Italian Culture and the Challenge of a Global Age,* edited by Paolo Janni and George F. McLean, chapter 4, "Italian Cultural Identity and Migration: Italian Communities Abroad and Italian Cultural Identity through Time" by Maddalena Tirabassi (also for the point that by the 1920s Italian food had gained some popularity for its healthfulness).

Distrust of Italian ingredients like garlic is from *Revolution at the Table: The Transformation of the American Diet* by Harvey Levenstein. Fear of tomatoes as poisonous (before we understood it was the pewter plates they were being served on) is from *Smithsonian* magazine.

Origins of Meatless Monday and Wheatless Wednesday can be found on the USDA website. The story of the history and career trajectory of Chef Boyardee is from an NPR feature, plus the company's website. A 1986 article in *The Atlantic* discussed the following: the Campania influence on Italian food; how it was Americanized by the elements of added meat—but fewer types of vegetables and cheeses were available; the advent of cooking classes; hospitals serving pasta; the proliferation of spaghetti houses; cafeterias; and the Kraft parmesan cheese "kit."

Worldwide rankings of pasta consumption in 2012 are from the International Pasta Organisation. The difference between diversity and disunity and poverty as the main driver of emigration to the United States from southern Italy in the 1880s are from *The Italians* by John Hooper.

Unification of Italy in 1961 is from Hooper's book and the USDA website. Note that unification was a gradual process that took place over many years, but 1861 was the year the new Kingdom of Italy was announced and the year that the United States officially recognized Italian independence.

The first canned tomatoes is from *The Oxford Encyclopedia of Food and Drink in America,* edited by Andrew F. Smith. The anecdote and excerpt of the letter from Francesco Panciatichi come from archival research I conducted at the National Archives in College Park, Maryland, from RG 389—Records of the Office of the Provost Marshal General, 1920–1975, Records Relating to Italian Civilian Internees During World War II, 1941–1946, Box 15, Italians in U.S. Custody, Pagano-Picco.

Warren Belasco quotes on the difference in American versus foreign meat consumption are from a personal interview. History of U.S. beef production is from the Environmental Protection Agency's website. History and different types of meatballs are from *Smithsonian* magazine. Clifford A. Wright quotes are from a personal interview.

Why Italian American Food Conquered America

What we eat as kids stays with us for life. I know this from a 2007 Pennsylvania State University study by Leann Birch, Jennifer S. Savage, and Alison Venture as well as numerous other studies I learned about during my graduate studies at UC Berkeley on health and social behavior.

The rising popularity of pizza is from *How Italian Food Conquered the World* by John F. Mariani, who describes pizza margherita, Naples street food, the first pizzeria in the United States, pizza's popularity, regional types of pizza around the country, plus the rise in popularity of Mediterranean food as healthy. Harry Balzer quotes on pizza are from a personal interview. Paul Rozin pizza quotes are from a personal interview. The everything in Chicago is big is from personal experience.

Meatballs among our top searched recipes is from *Bon Appétit.*

The Mainstreaming of Global Cuisines

Quotes from Warren Belasco are from a personal interview. Salsa outselling ketchup stat is from a *Food Network* magazine article called "Know It All: Ketchup." Remaining facts come from the National Restaurant Association, Hartman Group, and the publications referenced in the chapter.

Bibliography

Books

Anderson, Heather Arndt. *Breakfast: A History*. Lanham, MD: Rowman & Littlefield, 2013.

Belasco, Warren. *Food: The Key Concepts*. New York: Berg, 2008.

Benedetti, Umberto. *The Lifestyle of Italian Internees at Fort Missoula, Montana, 1941–1943, Bella Vista*. Missoula, MT: Umberto Benedetti, 1986.

Brym, Robert J., and John Lie. *Sociology: Your Compass for a New World*. 2nd ed. Mason, OH: Cengage Learning, 2010.

Counihan, Carole M. *Food in the USA: A Reader*. New York: Routledge, 2002.

Dacko, Scott G. *The Advanced Dictionary of Marketing: Putting Theory to Use*. New York: Oxford University Press, 2008.

DeWitt, David. *The Founding Foodies: How Washington, Jefferson, and Franklin Revolutionized American Cuisine*. Naperville, IL: Sourcebooks, 2010.

DiStasi, Lawrence, and Sandra Gilbert. *Una Storia Segreta: The Secret History of Italian American Internment During World War II*. Berkeley, CA: Heyday, 2001.

Duncan, Thomas Cation. *How to Be Plump, Or, Talks on Physiological Feeding*. Chicago: Duncan Brothers, 1878.

Elias, Megan. *Lunch: A History*. Lanham, MD: Rowman & Littlefield, 2014.

Foxcroft, Louise. *Calories and Corsets: A History of Dieting over Two Thousand Years*. London: Profile Books, 2012.

Gaonkar, Anilkumar. *Food Processing: Recent Developments*. New York: Elsevier Science, 1995.

Glassner, Barry. *The Gospel of Food: Why We Should Stop Worrying and Enjoy What We Eat*. New York: HarperCollins, 2007.

Grayson, Robert. *The U.S. Industrial Revolution*. Edina, MN: Abdo Publishing, 2010.

Janni, Paolo, and George McClean, eds. *The Essence of Italian Culture and the Challenge of A Global Age*. Washington, DC: Council for Research in Values and Philosophy, 2003.

Kamp, David. *The United States of Arugula: How We Became a Gourmet Nation*. New York: Broadway Books, 2006.

Kaufman, Frederick. *A Short History of the American Stomach*. Orlando, FL: Mariner Books, 2009.

Levenstein, Harvey. *Paradox of Plenty: A Social History of Eating in Modern America*. Berkeley: University of California Press, 2003.

———. *Revolution at the Table: The Transformation of the American Diet*. Berkeley: University of California Press, 2003.

Lewis, Len. *The Trader Joe's Adventure: Turning a Unique Approach to Business into a Retail and Cultural Phenomenon*. Chicago: Dearborn Trade Publishing, 2005.

Lukacs, Paul. *Inventing Wine: A New History of One of the World's Most Ancient Pleasures*. New York: W. W. Norton, 2012.

Macfarlane, Alan and Iris. *The Empire of Tea: The Remarkable Story of a Plant That Took Over the World*. New York: Overlook Press, 2004.

Mariani, John F. *How Italian Food Conquered the World*. New York: Palgrave MacMillan, 2011.

Moss, Michael. *Salt Sugar Fat: How the Food Giants Hooked Us*. New York: Random House, 2013.

Nestle, Marion. *Food Politics: How the Food Industry Influences Nutrition and Health*. Rev. ed. Berkeley: University of California Press, 2007.

O'Connell, Libby H. *The American Plate: A Culinary History in 100 Bites*. Naperville, IL: Sourcebooks, 2014

Pollan, Michael. *In Defense of Food: An Eater's Manifesto*. New York: Penguin, 2008

———. *The Omnivore's Dilemma: A Natural History of Four Meals*. New York: Penguin, 2006.

Popkin, Barry. *The World Is Fat: The Fads, Trends, Policies, and Products That Are Fattening the Human Race*. New York: Avery, 2009.

Robinson, Jancis, and Julia Harding. *The Oxford Companion to Wine*. New York: Oxford University Press, 1994.

Rorabaugh, W. J. *The Alcoholic Republic: An American Tradition*. New York: Oxford University Press, 1979.

Serventi, Silvano, and Françoise Sabban. *Pasta: The Story of a Universal Food*. New York: Columbia University Press, 2000.

Smith, Andrew F. *Eating History: Thirty Turning Points in the Making of American Cuisine*. New York: Columbia University Press, 2009.

————. *Food and Drink in American History: A "Full Course" Encyclopedia*. Santa Barbara, CA: ABC-CLIO, 2013.

————. *The Oxford Companion to American Food and Drink*. New York: Oxford University Press, 2007.

Standage, Tom. *A History of the World in 6 Glasses*. New York: Bloomsbury, 2006.

Starr, Chester G. *A History of the Ancient World*. 4th ed. New York: Oxford University Press, 1991.

St. John, Allen. *The Billion Dollar Game: Behind the Scenes of the Greatest Day in American Sport; Super Bowl Sunday*. New York: Anchor Books, 2012.

Ternikar, Farha. *Brunch: A History*. Lanham, MD: Rowman & Littlefield, 2014.

Wansink, Brian. *Slim By Design: Mindless Eating Solutions for Everyday Life*. New York: HarperCollins, 2014.

Weiss Adamson, Melitta, and Francine Segan, eds. *Entertaining from Ancient Rome to the Superbowl: An Encyclopedia*. Westport, CT: Greenwood Press, 2008.

Whitman, Sylvia. *What's Cooking? The History of American Food*. Minneapolis, MN: Lerner Publications, 2001.

Reports and Presentations

Abbott, Melissa. "Defining the 'New Healthy' in Today's Modern Food Culture." Presented at The Culinary Institute of America's Latin Flavors, American Kitchens conference in San Antonio, on October 2, 2014.

Balzer, Harry. "The NPD Group's 29th Annual Report on Eating Patterns in America." Presented at The Culinary Institute of America's Greystone Flavor Summit in St. Helena, California, on March 12, 2015.

Cardello, Hank. "The Financial Impact of Offering Lower-Calorie Foods & Beverages." Presented at The Culinary Institute of America–Harvard T. H. Chan School of Public Health's Worlds of Healthy Flavors invitational leadership retreat in St. Helena, California, on January 23, 2015.

Coote, Anna, Jane Franklin, and Andrew Simms. "21 Hours." New Economics Foundation, London, February 13, 2010.

Datamonitor. "10 Trends to Watch in Fast-Moving Consumer Goods in 2015." Datamonitor Research Store overview and highlights, December 17, 2014.

————. "Personalization Trends in Food and Drinks: From Customization to Nutrigenomics." Datamonitor Research Store overview and highlights, November 30, 2014.

Fereday, Nicholas. "The Cereal Killers: Five Trends Revolutionizing the American Breakfast." Rabobank Industry Note # 378, Rabobank International, The Netherlands, April 2013.

————. "Consumer Foods Talking Points." Rabobank International, New York, from Consumer Analyst Group of New York's Annual Conference, February 25, 2015.

————. "More Bankers than Hippies: Natural Foods Come of Age." Rabobank International, from Natural Products Expo West, March 2015.

————. "The Popcorn Blockbuster: What the Snack's Comeback Means for the Future of the U.S. Food Industry." Rabobank Industry Note # 472, Rabobank International, The Netherlands, January 2015.

Food Chain Workers Alliance. "The Hands That Feed Us: Challenges and Opportunities for Workers Along the Food Chain." Los Angeles, June 6, 2012.

Food Marketing Institute. "U.S. Grocery Shopper Trends 2015: Executive Summary." Arlington, VA, 2015.

Gardner, Christopher. "Protein: Plant Forward: Science, Policy, and the Next Culinary Approach." Presented at The Culinary Institute of America–Harvard T. H. Chan School of Public Health's Menus of Change Leadership Summit in Hyde Park, New York, June 18, 2015.

The Hartman Group. "Food Shopping in America." Bellevue, WA, 2014.

————. "Modern Eating: Cultural Roots, Daily Behaviors." Hartman Group Syndicated Study, Bellevue, WA, 2013.

————. "Outlook on the Millennial Consumer 2014 Report." Bellevue, WA, 2014.

Hoyert, Donna L. "75 Years of Mortality in the United States, 1935–2010," National Center for Health Statistics Data Brief, No. 88, Hyattsville, MD, March 2012.

International Pasta Organisation. "The World Pasta Industry Status Report 2012." Rome, 2013.

Kirin Holdings. "Kirin Beer University Report." Kirin Holdings, Tokyo, January 8, 2014.

MarketsandMarkets. "Gluten-Free Products Market by Type: Global Trends and Forecast to 2020." Pune, India, September 2015.

Mayo Clinic. "Calorie and Protein Content of Common Foods." Mayo Foundation for Medical Education and Research, Rochester, Minnesota, 2012.

The Nielsen Company. "Snack Attack: What Consumers Are Reaching For Around the World." Nielsen Company, New York and Dieman, The Netherlands, September 2014.

The Nielson Global Health and Wellness Report. "We Are What We Eat: Healthy Eating Trends Around the World." Nielson Company, New York and Dieman, The Netherlands, 2015.

Pestano, Paul, Etan Yeshya, and Jane Houlian. "Children's Cereals: Popular Brands Back More Sugar Than Snack Cakes and Cookies." Environmental Working Group, Washington, DC, December 2011.

Rimm, Eric. "Of Ethanol and Phytochemicals: A Guided Tasting of California Wine." Presented at The Culinary Institute of America–Harvard T. H. Chan School of Public Health–Samueli Institute's Healthy Kitchens, Healthy Lives gathering in St. Helena, California, on February 7, 2015.

Taylor, Paul, Cary Funk, and April Clark. "Luxury or Necessity? Things We Can't Live Without: The List Has Grown in the Past Decade." Pew Research Center, Washington, DC, 2010.

Technomic. "Breakfast Consumer Trend Report." Chicago, accessed September 24, 2015.

———. "Food Industry Transformation: The Next Decade." Chicago, May 2015.

U.S. Census Bureau. "The 15 Most Populous Cities: July 1, 2013," Washington, DC, May 2014.

U.S. Department of Agriculture, Agricultural Research Service. "Breakfast: Percentages of Selected Nutrients Contributed by Food and Beverages Consumed at Breakfast, by Gender and Age. *What We Eat in America*, NHANES 2011–2012," Washington, DC, 2014.

U.S. Department of Agriculture and U.S. Department of Health & Human Services. "Scientific Report of the 2015 Dietary Guidelines Advisory Committee." Washington, DC, February 2015.

U.S. Food and Drug Administration. "Code of Federal Regulations Title 21." Silver Spring, Maryland, updated April 1, 2015.

———. "Guidance for Industry: A Food Labeling Guide (9. Appendix A: Definitions of Nutrient Content Claims). Silver Spring, Maryland, January 2013.

Vaynerchuk, Gary, "The State of the Union in Social Media." The New York Times Building, New York, July 2013.

Vespa, Jonathan, Jamie M. Lewis, and Rose M. Kreider. "America's Families and Living Arrangements: 2012." U.S. Census Bureau, Washington, DC, August 2013.

White House Council of Economic Advisers. "15 Economic Facts about Millennials," Washington, DC, October 2014.

Wine Institute. "California Wine Profile 201." San Francisco, 2014.

———. "Per Capita Wine Consumption by Country, 2009–2012 and % Change 2012/2009 Liters per Capita." Sacramento and San Francisco and Washington, DC, 2012.

———. "World Wine Production by Country 2010–2013 and % Change 2013/2010 (Liters 000)." Sacramento and San Francisco and Washington, DC, 2013.

Surveys

Brager, Danny. "Generations on Tap: Beverage Alcohol Purchases Vary by Age Group," Nielsen Survey from September 16–October 2, 2013.

Consumer Reports National Research Center. "Food Labels Survey," *Consumer Reports*, Princeton, New Jersey, 2014.

Gallup. "Americans' Effort to Lose Weight Still Trails Desire." Gallup Poll, November 26, 2014.

———. "Americans Not Avoiding Fat and Salt as Much," Gallup Poll, July 8–12, 2015.

———. Consumption Habits Survey from July 7–10, 2014.

———. "Most Families Still Dine Together Regularly at Home," Gallup Poll, December 5–8, 2013.

———. U.S. Employee Engagement Survey, January–December 2014.

———. U.S. Payroll to Population Survey, March 2011–December 2013.

Gallup Healthways. Gallup Poll, January–December 2012.

Glassdoor. "Employee Appreciation Survey," Glassdoor Survey, Sausalito, California, November 13, 2013.

Pew Research Center. "America's Changing Religious Landscape," Washington, DC, May 2015.

———. "Emerging and Developing Economies Much More Optimistic than Rich Countries About the Future," Washington, DC, October 9, 2014.

———. "On Pay Gap, Millennial Women Near Parity—For Now," Washington, DC, December 11, 2013.

Personal Interviews

Abbott, Melissa. Phone, October 20, 2014.

Balzer, Harry. Phone, September 26, 2012 for *Wired* magazine article "Stunt Foods," published September 2013; Phone, March 11, 2014; E-mail, March 3, 2014; Phone, March 27, 2014.

Barry, Michael. Phone, March 18, 2014.

Belasco, Warren. Phone, March 7, 2014.

Cardello, Hank. Phone, March 17, 2015.

Caruso, Barbara. E-mail, May 22, 2013, for *Wired* magazine article "Stunt Foods," published September 2013.

Chillingworth, Noah, and Mike Salem. Phone, May 24, 2013, for *Wired* magazine article "Stunt Foods," published September 2013.

Conner, Alana. Phone, March 6, 2014.

Coulombe, Joe. Phone, March 2011, for *Sunset* magazine article "What Food Changed Your Life?" published July 2011; E-mail, November 17–18, 2014.

Creed, Greg. In person, Taco Bell Headquarters, Irvine, CA. February 1, 2013 for *Wired* magazine article "Stunt Foods," published September 2013.

Fereday, Nicholas. Phone, April 2, 2015.

Foxcroft, Louise. Phone, February 2, 2015.

Garcia, Kat, Erin Peffly, and Stephanie Perdue. In person, Taco Bell Head-quarters, Irvine, CA, February 1, 2013, for *Wired* magazine article "Stunt Foods," published September 2013.

Gardea, Heather. E-mail, May 14, 2013, via Eniko Bolivar of ZENO Group; Phone, May 23, 2013, for *Wired* magazine article "Stunt Foods," published September 2013.

Gardner, Christopher. E-mail, August 9–21, 2015.

Gomez, Steve. Phone, November 14, 2012, for *Wired* magazine article "Stunt Foods," published September 2013.

Haley, Brad. E-mail, May 13–14, 2013; June 28, 2013; July 3, 2013; August 9, 2013; August 22, 2013; and September 3, 2013 for *Wired* magazine article "Stunt Foods," published September 2013.

Mann, Traci. Phone, January 16, 2015.

Nestle, Marion. E-mail, March 6, 2014; In person, Food@Work event, Ferry Building, San Francisco, CA, April 17, 2014.

Peffly, Erin. Phone, March 11, 2013 for *Wired* magazine article "Stunt Foods," published September 2013.

Rozin, Paul. Phone, March 2014.

Smiley, Robert. Phone, March 2014.

Stuckey, Barb. Phone, 2012, for *Wired* magazine article "Stunt Foods," published September 2013.

Vitry, Dominique. E-mail, May 14, 2013–August 23, 2013, via Doug Ter-fehr, for *Wired* magazine article "Stunt Foods," published September 2013.

Wilk, Richard. Phone, March 2014.

Wright, Clifford. Phone, May 21, 2015.

Archival Material

Box 15, Italians in U.S. Custody Pagano-Picco, Record Group (RG) 389 Records of the Office of Provost Marshal General (1920–1975). Records Relating to Italian Civilian Internees during World War II, 1941–1946. National Archives and Records Administration (NARA), College Park, Maryland.

Academic Papers and Journal Articles

Andrade, J., A. Mohamed, J. Frohlich, and A. Ignaszewski. "Ancel Keys and the Lipid Hypothesis: From Early Breakthroughs to Current Management of Dyslipidemia." *British Columbia Medical Journal* 51, no. 2 (March 2009): 66–72.

Birch, L., J. S. Savage, and A. Ventura. "Influences on the Development of Children's Eating Behaviours: From Infancy to Adolescence." *Canadian Journal of Dietetic Practice and Research* 68, no. 1 (2007): s1–s56.

Chandon, P., and B. Wansink. "Does Food Marketing Need to Make Us Fat? A Review and Solutions." *Nutrition Reviews* 70, no. 10 (October 2012): 571–593.

Chernev, A., and D. Gal. "Categorization Effects in Value Judgments: Averaging Bias in Evaluating Combinations of Vices and Virtues." *Journal of Marketing Research* 47, no. 4 (August 2010): 738–747.

Chowdhury, R. et al. "Association of Dietary, Circulating, and Supplement Fatty Acids with Coronary Risk: A Systematic Review and Meta-analysis." *Annals of Internal Medicine* 160, no. 6 (March 2014): 398–406.

Colby, S. E., L. Johnson, A. Scheett, and B. Hoverson. "Nutrition Marketing on Food Labels." *Journal of Nutrition Education and Behavior* 42, no. 2 (March–April 2010): 92–98.

Connell, P. M., M. Brucks, and J. H. Nielsen. "How Childhood Advertising Exposure Can Create Biased Product Evaluations That Persist Into Adulthood." *Journal of Consumer Research* 41, no. 1 (June 2014): 119–134.

Cornil, Y., and P. Chandon. "From Fan to Fat? Vicarious Losing Increases Unhealthy Eating, but Self-Affirmation Is an Effective Remedy." *Psychological Science* 24, no. 10 (October 2013): 1936–1946.

DeAngelis, T. "Why We Overestimate Our Competence." *American Psychological Association* 34, no. 2 (February 2003): 60.

Drewnowski, A., H. Moskowitz, M. Reisner, and B. Krieger. "Testing Consumer Perception of Nutrient Content Claims Using Conjoint Analysis." *Public Health Nutrition* 13, no. 5 (May 2010): 688–694.

Dunning, D., C. Heath, and J. M. Suls. "Flawed Self-Assessment." *Psychological Science in the Public Interest* 5, no. 3 (May 2005): 69–106.

Ford, E. S., and W. H. Dietz. "Trends in Energy Intake among Adults in the United States: Findings from NHANES." *American Journal of Clinical Nutrition* 97, no. 4 (February 2013): 848–853.

Groesz, L. M., S. McCoy, J. Carl, L. Saslow, J. Stewart, N. Adler, B. Laraia, and E. Epel. "What Is Eating You? Stress and the Drive to Eat." *Appetite* 58, no. 2 (April 2012): 717–721.

Grosso, G. et al. "Mediterranean Diet and Cancer: Epidemiological Evidence and Mechanism of Selected Aspects." *BioMed Central Surgery* 13, suppl. 2 (October 2013): S14.

Iyengar, S. S., and M. R. Lepper. "Rethinking the Value of Choice: A Cultural Perspective on Intrinsic Motivation." *Journal of Personality and Social Psychology* 76, no. 3 (March 1999): 349–366.

Jacobs Jr., D. R. and L. C. Tapsell. "Food Synergy: The Key to a Healthy Diet." *Proceedings of the Nutrition Society* (June 2012), Plenary Lecture II at the Conference on Translating Nutrition: Integrating Research, Practice and Policy.

Jerrard, D. A. "Male Patient Visits to the Emergency Department Decline During the Play of Major Sporting Events." *Western Journal of Emergency Medicine* 10, no. 2 (May 2009): 101–103.

Johnson, R. K. et al. "Dietary Sugars Intake and Cardiovascular Health: A Scientific Statement from the American Heart Association." *Circulation* 120 (August 2009): 1011–1020.

Keinan, A., and R. Kivetz. "Productivity Orientation and the Consumption of Collectable Experiences." *Journal of Consumer Research* 37, no. 6 (April 2011): 935–950.

Kim, H., and H. R. Markus. "Deviance or Uniqueness, Harmony or Conformity? A Cultural Analysis." *Journal of Personality and Social Psychology* 77, no. 4 (October 1999): 785–800.

Lee, J. H., J. Hwang, and A. Mustapha. "Popular Ethnic Foods in the United States: A Historical and Safety Perspective." *Comprehensive Reviews in Food Science and Food Safety* 13, no. 1 (January 2014): 1–17.

Liem, D. G., F. Miremadi, E. H. Zandstra, and R. S. Keast. "Health Labelling Can Influence Taste Perception and Use of Table Salt for Reduced-Sodium Products." *Public Health Nutrition* 15, no. 12 (December 2012): 2340–2347.

Maister, D. "Psychology of Waiting Lines." In *The Service Encounter: Managing Employee/Customer Interaction in Service Businesses,* edited by John A. Czepiel, Michael R. Solomon, and Carol Suprenant. Lexington, MA: Lexington Books, 1985.

Mann, T., A. J. Tomiyama, E. Westling, A.-M. Lew, B. Samuels, and J. Chatman. "Medicare's Search for Effective Obesity Treatments: Diets

Are Not the Answer." *American Psychologist* 62, no. 3 (April 2007): 220–233.

Markus, H. R., and B. Schwartz. "Does Choice Mean Freedom and Well-Being?" *Journal of Consumer Research* 37, no. 2 (August 2010): 344–355.

Mehta, K., C. Phillips, P. R. Ward, J. Coveney, E. Handsley, and P. Carter. "Marketing Foods to Children through Product Packaging: Prolific, Unhealthy and Misleading." *Public Health Nutrition* 15, no. 9 (May 2012): 1–8.

Meier, A., and K. Musick. "Variation in Associations between Family Dinners and Adolescent Well-Being." *Journal of Marriage and Family* 76, no. 1 (February 2014): 13–23.

Oswald, A. J., E. Proto, and D. Sgroi. "Happiness and Productivity." *Journal of Labor Economics* 33, no. 4 (October 2015): 789–822.

Page, R., K. Montgomery, A. Ponder, and A. Richard. "Targeting Children in the Cereal Aisle: Promotional Techniques and Content Features on Ready-to-Eat Cereal Product Packaging." *American Journal of Health Education* 39, no. 5 (September/October 2008): 272–282.

Painter, J. E., B. Wansink, and J. B. Hieggelke. "How Visibility and Convenience Influence Candy Consumption." *Appetite* 38, no. 3 (June 2002): 237–238.

Peloza, J., C. Ye, and W. J. Montford. "When Companies Do Good, Are Their Products Good for You? How Corporate Social Responsibility Creates a Health Halo." *Journal of Public Policy & Marketing* 34, no. 1 (Spring 2015): 19–31.

Pope, L., A. S. Hanks, D. R. Just, and B. Wansink. "New Year's Res-Illusions: Food Shopping in the New Year Competes with Healthy Intentions." *PLOS ONE* 9, no. 12 (December 2014): e110561

Provencher, V., J. Polivy, and P. C. Herman. "Perceived Healthiness of Food. If It's Healthy, You Can Eat More!" *Appetite* 52, no. 2 (April 2009): 340–344.

Rozin, P., C. Fischler, and C. Shields-Argelès. "Additivity Dominance: Additives Are More Potent and More Often Lexicalized Across Languages Than Are 'Subtractives.'" *Judgment and Decision Making* 4, no. 5 (August 2009): 475–478.

———. "European and American Perspectives of the Meaning of Natural.," *Appetite* 59, no. 2 (October 2012): 448–455.

Rozin, P. et al. "Preference for Natural: Instrumental and Ideational/Moral Motivations, and the Contrast between Foods and Medicines." *Appetite* 43, no. 2 (October 2004): 147–154.

Schatzkin, A. et al. "Dietary Fiber and Whole-Grain Consumption in Relation to Colorectal Cancer in the NIH-AARP Diet and Health Study." *American Journal of Clinical Nutrition* 85, no. 5 (May 2007): 1353–1360.

Steffen, L. M., D. R. Jacobs Jr., J. Stevens, E. Shahar, T. Carithers, and A. R. Folsom. "Associations of Whole-Grain, Refined-Grain, and Fruit and Vegetable Consumption with Risks of All-Cause Mortality and Incident Coronary Artery Disease and Ischemic Stroke: the Atherosclerosis Risk in Communities (ARIC) Study." *American Journal of Clinical Nutrition* 78, no. 3 (September 2003): 383–390.

Stephens, N. M., H. R. Markus, and S. S. M. Townsend. "Choice as an Act of Meaning: The Case of Social Class." *Journal of Personality and Social Psychology* 93, no. 5 (November 2007): 814–830.

Tighe, P. et al. "Effect of Increased Consumption of Whole-Grain Foods on Blood Pressure and Other Cardiovascular Risk Markers in Healthy Middle-Aged Persons: A Randomized Controlled Trial." *American Journal of Clinical Nutrition* 92, no. 4 (October 2010): 733–740.

Venn, B. J., and J. I. Mann. "Cereal Grains, Legumes and Diabetes." *European Journal of Clinical Nutrition* 58 (November 2004): 1443–1461.

Wansink, B., and P. Chandon. "Can 'Low-Fat' Nutrition Labels Lead to Obesity?" *Journal of Marketing Research* 43 (November 2006): 605–617.

Yelker, R., C. Tomkovick, and P. Traczyk. "Super Bowl Advertising Effectiveness: Hollywood Finds the Games Golden." *Journal of Advertising Research* 44, no. (March 2004): 143–159.

News Articles, Blogs, and Web Content

Adams, Noah. "As Bourbon Booms, Demand for Barrels Is Overflowing." NPR, December 29, 2014.

Adcock, Siobhan, and Genevieve Tsai. "Dim Sum Dos and Don'ts." *Epicurious,* accessed September 23, 2015.

AFP Relax. "Paleo Cookbooks Are Having Their Moment." *Yahoo News,* July 19, 2013.

Alexander, Karen. "From Google to Noodles: A Chef Strikes Out on His Own." *New York Times,* September 20, 2005.

Ali, Muhammad, and Simone Weichselbaum. "CityBike Black Hole in Black Hat Williamsburg." *New York Daily News,* May 22, 2013.

Allen, Cooper. "Dewitos? Pepsi Tests Doritos-Flavored Mountain Dew." *USA Today,* November 10, 2014.

"America's Most Promising Companies." *Forbes,* accessed September 23, 2015.

"Americans Now Drink More Wine Than the French as Sales Surge." *Daily Mail,* June 2, 2011.

Amidor, Toby. "The Health Benefits of Greek Yogurt." *U.S. News & World Report,* May 5, 2014.

"The Approval Matrix." *New York Magazine,* accessed June through September 2015.

Aristotle Munarriz, Rick. "Cap'n Crunch Enlisted to Boost Taco Bell's Breakfast Sales," *Daily Finance,* March 3, 2015.

Arnold, Eric. "The Whine Critics," *Forbes,* April 23, 2009.

Arthur, Rachel. "Prosecco Raises a Glass to US Export Leap: How Much Further Can the Market Grow?" BeverageDaily.com, October 3, 2014.

Asimov, Eric. "Europeans Stray from the Vine." *New York Times,* November 21, 2013.

———. "Pop Goes the Critic." *New York Times,* September 8, 2009.

———. "Red Wine Is the Drink of Choice on 'Scandal' and 'The Good Wife.'" *New York Times,* October 28, 2014.

AskReddit. "What Is Your Favorite Product That Has Been Discontinued?" Reddit, Archived post, Accessed September 24, 2015.

Atchley, Charlotte. "Tracking Breakfast Ingredient Trends." *Food Business News,* February 9, 2015

Aubrey, Allison, "Cutting Back on Carbs, Not Fat, May Lead to More Weight Loss," NPR, September 1, 2014.

Avey, Tori. "Uncover the History of Pasta," PBS, July 26, 2012.

Bajekal, Naina. "Olive Garden Introduces the 'Never-Ending' Pasta Pass." *Time,* September 8, 2014.

Barakat, Zena and Roopa Vasudevan. "Super Bowl XLVII, by the Numbers." *New York Times,* January 27, 2014.

Barclay, Eliza. "Eating to Break 100: Longevity Diet Tips from the Blue Zones." NPR, April 11, 2015.

Barlow, Tom. "Americans Cook the Least, Eat the Fastest." *Forbes,* April 15, 2011.

Barry, Donna. "Protein Achieves 'Superfood' Status," *Food Business News,* September 29, 2014.

Batali, Mario. "Secrets of a Tender Meatball." *Chicago Tribune,* January 31, 2013.

Bates, Martha. "The Italian Sunday Lunch." *A Path to Lunch* blog, accessed September 23, 2015.

Battaglio, Stephen. "With 114.4 Million Viewers, Super Bowl XLIX Is Most-Watched TV Show Ever." *Los Angeles Times,* February 2, 2015.

"Belly up to the Bar: Alcohol Sales Expected to Improve Modestly in 2015." *Fast Casual,* December 4, 2014.

Berger, Joseph. "As Greenpoint Gentrifies, Sunday Rituals Clash: Outdoor Cafes vs. Churchgoers." *New York Times,* May 10, 2012.

Beth Cooper, Belle. "8 Reasons Why You Should Definitely Take That Lunch Break," *Fast Company,* March 12, 2014.

Bhushan, Ratna. "India Emerges as Domino's Biggest Market outside U.S." *Economic Times,* December 1, 2014.

Bialik, Carl. "Starbucks Stays Mum on Drink Math." *Wall Street Journal,* April 2, 2008.

Bittman, Mark. "Butter Is Back." *New York Times,* March 25, 2014.

Blain, Glenn. "Yogurt Rules New York's Snack World." *New York Daily News,* October 15, 2014.

Blodget, Henry. "Inside Apple. They Don't Even Serve Free Food!" *Business Insider,* January 20, 2012.

"Blue-collar Red and White Get Starter Wine." Today.com, May 22, 2013.

"Blue Law: American History." Brittanica.com, updated July 21, 2014.

Bonné, Jon. "10 More Foods That Make America Great." *Today,* July 7, 2006.

Borelli, Christopher. "Enduring Love." *Chicago Tribune,* April 20, 2011.

Bradford, Harry. "Here Is the Most Disproportionately Popular Cuisine in Each State." Huffington Post, January 19, 2015.

Brandau, Mark. "NPD: Fast-Casual Restaurants Lead Traffic Growth Again in 2013." *Nation's Restaurant News,* February 5, 2014.

Braun, Adee. "Alone Together: The Return of Communal Restaurant Tables." *Atlantic,* March 31, 2014.

Brennan, Morgan. "America's Most Expensive Zip Codes," *Forbes,* October 12, 2011.

Brooks, Chad. "You Are What You Eat . . . Even at Work." *Business News Daily,* January 8, 2013.

Brownlee, John. "Oscar Mayer Rebrands Lunchables for Adults." *Fast Company,* March 4, 2014.

Burger King. "Our Story." BK.com, accessed September 23, 2015.

Burritobox Website. TastetheBurritoBox.com, accessed September 23, 2015.

Cantor, Stuart. "Snack Trends 2013: Health and Indulgence Square Off." *Food Processing,* February 28, 2013.

Carroll, Abigail. "Cheese and Crackers: A Meal for the Ages." *Boston Globe,* September 14, 2014.

Castillo, Michelle. "Americans Will Spend More than $60 Million on Their Pets This Year." NBC News, July 12, 2015.

CBS Videos. "The Nose." *60 Minutes,* October 9, 2008.

Centers for Disease Control and Prevention. "Heart Disease Facts." CDC.gov, updated August 10, 2015.

———. "Leading Causes of Death." CDC.gov, updated August 21, 2015.

Centers for Disease Control and Prevention Diabetes Public Health Resource. "Crude and Age-Adjusted Rate per 100 of Civilian, Noninstitutionalized Population with Diagnosed Diabetes, United States, 1980–2011." CDC.gov, updated September 5, 2014.

Centers for Disease Control and Prevention Website, Nutrition Section. CDC.gov/nutrition, accessed September 23, 2015.

Chase, Chris. "Super Bowl Monday? Petition Asks White House for Day Off after Big Game." *USA Today*, January 25, 2013.

Chillag, Ian. "Sandwich Monday: Papa John's Frito Chili Pizza." NPR, November 17, 2014.

"The Cigarette Diet." DietsinReview.com, accessed September 23, 2015.

"Confounded by Fast-Casual." *QSR* magazine, accessed September 23, 2015.

Connolly, Ellen. "The Biggest Food Trends of 2014." *Guardian*, December 29, 2014.

Cook, James. "The IRS Is Auditing the Free Food Tech Employees Get in Silicon Valley Cafeterias." *Business Insider*, September 2, 2014.

Coote, Anna. "10 Reasons for a Shorter Working Week." NEF blog, July 29, 2014.

Corporate Profiles. "Frozen Meals." *Food Business News*, October 1, 2012.

Crane, Emily. "The Superfood Shortage: Hipsters Have Made Kale So Popular That Farmers Are Struggling to Meet Demand." *Daily Mail*, July 23, 2014.

CrossFit. "CrossFit Games Purse Grows in 2015." Games.CrossFit.com, January 7, 2015.

———. "What is CrossFit?" CrossFit.com, accessed September 23, 2015.

Crouch, Bob. "How Will Generation Z Disrupt the Workplace?" *Fortune*, May 22, 2015.

Crucchiola, Jordan. "A Taco Company is #Cheeseblasting Unsuspecting Twitter Users." *Wired*, August 12, 2014.

Crudele, John. "Burger King's Revamped 'Be Your Way' Slogan Isn't Meaty Enough." *New York Post*, May 21, 2014.

Cuda, Amanda. "Bowled Over: ERs Busy Day after Big Game." *Connecticut Post*, February 2, 2014.

Cunningham, Lillian. "Exhaustion Is Not a Status Symbol." *Washington Post*, October 3, 2012.

Dan, Avi. "The Real Reason That Super Bowl Ads Are Worth the Money." *Forbes*, January 28, 2013.

Dawsey, Josh. "Now Legal—10 a.m. Brunch." *Wall Street Journal*, August 4, 2013.

Dean, Jeremy. "Why Do People Watch Scary Movies, Stay in Ice Hotels or Eat Bacon-Flavoured Ice Cream?" PsyBlog, April 30, 2009.

"Declare the Monday Following the Super Bowl a National Holiday." Petitions.whitehouse.gov, accessed September 24, 2015.

De La Hamaide, Sybille. "China Wine Growers Beat France into Second Place." Reuters, April 27, 2015

De Rosa, Anthony. "The Social Media Sommelier." *Mediaite,* July 28, 2009.

Donna Gabaccia Professional Website. Utsc.utoronto.ca, accessed September 24, 2015.

Douglas-Gabriel, Danielle. "The Fitness Trends That Will Rule in 2015." *Washington Post,* January 27, 2015.

Downey, David. "SUPER BOWL: Avocados Are the Star of the Snack Table." Press Enterprise, January 29, 2015.

Dumenco, Simon. "In the Wake of the Velveeta Shortage, Are We Now Running Out of Froot Loops?" *Advertising Age,* January 21, 2014.

Eataly. "Pasta di Gragnano," Eataly.com, accessed September 24, 2015.

Eber, Hailey. "Why 'Diet Booze' Leaves a Bad Taste in Our Mouths." *New York Post,* December 26, 2013.

Empson, Rip. "Gary Vaynerchuk, 'The Sommelier of Social Media,' Partners with Consumr." *Tech Crunch,* July 25, 2011.

Endolyn, Osayi. "Brunch Bill Aims to Start Sunday Alcohol Sales at 10:30 am," *Atlanta Magazine,* March 10, 2015.

"Enjoy Life Foods Grows Free-Form Food Category through Mobile and Social Technology." *Business Wire,* March 5, 2014.

Esposito, Shaylyn. "Is Spaghetti and Meatballs Italian?" *Smithsonian,* June 6, 2013.

Esterl, Mike. "Forget Dinner. It's Always Snack Time in America." *Wall Street Journal*, July 2, 2014.

Etiquette Hell Website. EtiquetteHell.com, accessed September 23, 2015.

European Food Information Council. "Parental Influence on Children's Food Preferences and Energy Intake." *Food Today,* September 2012.

Eveleth, Rose. "Americans Buy So Many Wings, They're Now the Most Expensive Part of the Chicken." *Smithsonian,* January 31, 2013.

"Experts Who Reviewed the Diets." *U.S. News & World Report,* Health .USNews.com, accessed September 23, 2015.

"Factbox: Corn Plant and Products Made from Corn." Reuters, September 29, 2010.

Fainaru-Wada, Mark. "CrossFit's Big Growth Fuels Concerns," ESPN, July 27, 2014.

Fairchild, Caroline. "Why Kind Bars Are Suddenly Everywhere." *Fortune,* February 10, 2014.

Fears, Danika. "Horrifying or Heavenly? Taste Testing the New Pecan Pie Pringles." *Today,* November 19, 2013.

Feloni, Richard. "How 3 Diehard Fans Convinced Coca-Cola to Bring Back Surge Soda." *Business Insider,* September 16, 2014.

Ferdman, Roberto A. "Americans Are Tired of Long Restaurant Menus." *Washington Post,* September 18, 2014.

———. "The Definitive Guide to How People Around the World Snack." *Washington Post,* September 30, 2014.

———. "How the World Drinks Whiskey—Visualized." *Atlantic,* January 13, 2014.

———. "The Rise of the Avocado: America's New Favorite Fruit." *Washington Post,* January 1, 2015.

———. "The Slow Death of the Home-Cooked Meal." *Washington Post,* March 5, 2015.

———. "The Slow Death of the Microwave." *Quartz,* March 19, 2014.

———. "So Much for New Year's Resolutions: People Eat Even More after the Holidays." *Washington Post,* January 6, 2015.

———. "Surge, Everyone's Favorite '90s Soda, Is Back, and It's Already Selling Like Crazy." *Washington Post,* September 16, 2014.

Ferdman, Roberto A., and Christopher Ingraham. "How Brunch Became the Most Delicious—and Divisive—Meal in America." *Washington Post,* April 10, 2015.

Fermino, Jennifer. "City Council Moves to Abolish Law Banning Brunch before Noon on Sunday." *New York Daily News,* May 7, 2013.

Filloon, Whitney. "Are McDonald's Plans for All-Day Breakfast A Moot Point?" *Eater,* July 29, 2015.

"Find the Best Diet for You." *U.S. News & World Report,* Health.USNews.com, accessed September 23, 2015.

Flannery, Tim. "We're Living on Corn!" *New York Review of Books,* June 28, 2007.

Fletcher, Miles. "Watch 48 Years of Classic Super Bowl Ads." *Slate,* January 29, 2015.

Flint, Joe. "Saints' Super Bowl Win Nips 'MASH' Finale for Most-Watched Show Ever." *Los Angeles Times,* February 8, 2010.

Foley, Jonathan. "It's Time to Rethink America's Corn System." *Scientific American,* March 5, 2013.

Food Marketing Institute. "Supermarket Facts." FMI.org, accessed September 23, 2015.

Forgrieve, Janet. "How California's Wineries Are Leading the U.S. in Sustainable Wine." *SmartBlog* on Food & Beverage, July 31, 2015.

Forsythe, Tom. "The One and Only Cheerios." *Taste of General Mills* blog, January 2, 2014.

Friend, Tad. "V-Va-Va-Voom." *New Yorker,* June 7, 2010.

Frizell, Sam. "The New American Dream Is Living in a City, Not Owning a House in the Suburbs." *Time,* April 25, 2014.

————. "The World's Second-Richest Man Thinks You Should Work Only 3 Days a Week." *Time,* July 19, 2014.

Frost, Peter. "Can Custom Burgers Fire Up McD's Sales?" *Crain's Chicago Business,* October 21, 2014.

Gabaccia, Donna. "Pizza, Pasta and Red Sauce: Italian or American?" *History in Focus,* 2006.

Gale, Hannah. "DestapaBanana Will Fulfill All Your Fruit-Based Fantasies—It Inserts Liquid Caramel and Chocolate into Your Banana." *Metro,* August 14, 2014.

Gambino, Megan. "The 50 Best Food Trucks in Every State." *Smithsonian,* February 23, 2012.

Gao, George. "How Do Americans Stand Out from the Rest of the World?" Pew Research Center, Washington, DC, March 12, 2015.

Gary Vaynerchuk Personal Website. GaryVaynerchuk.com, accessed September 23, 2015.

Gasparro, Annie, and Mike Esterl. "Keurig Reels In Dr Pepper for Its Coming Soda Machine." *Wall Street Journal*, January 7, 2015.

Georgescu, Paul. "Capitalists, Arise: We Need to Deal With Income Inequality." *New York Times,* August 7, 2015.

Ghose, Tia. "Why We're All above Average." *Live Science,* February 6, 2013.

Gilson, Dave. "Overworked America: 12 Charts That Will Make Your Blood Boil." *Mother Jones,* July/August 2011.

"Girl Scout Cookies Taken: Mercer Island Police Log." *Mercer Island Patch,* March 16, 2013.

"Giving Email a Holiday." Editorial. *New York Times,* August 22, 2014.

Goff, Brian. "A Look into 50 Years of Super Bowl Viewership." *Forbes,* January 29, 2015.

Goldfarb, Alan. "Meet the Real 'Two Buck Chuck'—Charles Shaw." *Weekly Calistogan,* October 9, 2003.

Goodyear, Dana. "Drink Up." *New Yorker,* May 18, 2009.

Green, Elizabeth. "Why Do Americans Stink at Math?" *New York Times,* July 23, 2014.

Greenaway, Twilight. "How Did Avocados Become the Official Super Bowl Food?" *Smithsonian,* January 30, 2013.

Greenhouse, Steven. "How Costco Became the Anti-Wal-Mart." *New York Times,* July 17, 2005.

Gross, Daniel. "Can This Taco Save America?" *The Daily Beast,* March 12, 2013.

Gray, Melissa, and Joe Sterling. "Hungry Patron Delivers Knuckle Sandwich, with a Side of Pickles." CNN News, May 13, 2013.

Guttman, Amy. "Italy's Chocolate Easter Eggs: Big, Bold and Full of Bling." NPR, March 31, 2013.

Hairopoulos, Kate. "Debunking Super Bowl Myths about Avocados, Bathroom Sewer Backups and Hangovers." *Dallas Morning News,* February 6, 2011.

Halzack, Sarah. "How We Shop for Food Is Changing, in Three Charts." *Washington Post,* August 28, 2014.

Hamblin, James. "Lucky Charms, the New Superfood." *Atlantic,* June 23, 2015.

———. "Wine and Exercise: A Promising Combination." *Atlantic,* September 3, 2014.

Hamblin, James, Katherine Wells, and Paul Rosenfeld. "Wine Is Healthy—Isn't It? It Is—No?" *Atlantic,* July 11, 2014.

Hamedy, Saba. "Grammys Drop in TV Ratings; West Coast Twitter Users Gripe about Delay." *Los Angeles Times,* February 9, 2015.

Hansen, Kristine. "Wines By the Glass." *FSR* magazine, June 2015.

Harden, Blaine. "Japan's Killer Work Ethic." *Washington Post,* July 13, 2008.

Harmon Jenkins, Nancy. "From Italy, the Truth about Pasta; The Italians Know That Less Is More: A Call to Return to Basics." *New York Times,* September 17, 1997.

Harris, Jenn. "Burrito Box: A Hot and Melty Burrito from a Gas Station Vending Machine." *Los Angeles Times,* January 7, 2014.

———. "A McDonald's in a Church? McMass Wants to Build One." *Los Angeles Times,* November 27, 2014.

———. "New Caramel Apple Oreos at Target: Will You Bite?" *Los Angeles Times,* August 22, 2014.

Harrison-Dunn, Annie-Rose. "Corporate Responsibility Programmes May Create a 'Health Halo.'" FoodNavigator.com, November 12, 2014.

Hartman Group. "The Cultural Transformation of the American Breakfast." *Hartbeat Newsletter,* July 30, 2014.

———. "Gluten Free Eating Returns to Its Whole-Grain Roots." *Hartbeat Newsletter,* December 16, 2014.

———. "Snacks Become Mini-Meals: How Food Companies Can Keep Up." *Hartbeat Newsletter,* January 28, 2014.

Harvard T. H. Chan School of Public Health. "Alcohol: Balancing Risks and Benefits." The Nutrition Source, accessed September 23, 2015.

———. "Ask the Expert: Healthy Fats." The Nutrition Source, accessed June 21, 2012.

———. "Protein." The Nutrition Source, accessed September 24, 2015.

Hayden, Kathy. "Breakfast Wars Reverse." *QSR* magazine, August 2014.

Hellmich, Nanci. "Pass the Super Bowl Sunday Plate: Chips, Pizza, Veggies." *USA Today,* January 22, 2014.

Hibberd, James. "Golden Globes Ratings Dip 11%." *Time,* January 12, 2015.

Higgins, Kevin T., and David Fusaro. "2014 Food and Beverage Industry Outlook," *Food Processing,* January 14, 2014.

Hinnant, Lori. "Fast Food Is Front-Runner in France." *Seattle Times,* August 7, 2013.

Hirsch, J. M. "Avocado Consumption During Super Bowl Has Grown Significantly in the Past Decade." Huffington Post, January 31, 2013.

Historic American Cookbook Project. "The Virginia Housewife, by Mary Randolph," Michigan State University Digital Library, "Feeding America" Collection, accessed September 23, 2015.

Historical Museum of Fort Missoula. "Fort Missoula History," Fortmissoula museum.org, accessed September 24, 2015.

Ho, Erica. "Trader Joe's Two-Buck-Chuck Gets a Price Hike." *Time,* January 25, 2013.

Hoffman, Jan. "When Teams Lose, Fans Tackle Fatty Foods." *New York Times,* September 16, 2013.

Holahan, Catherine. "Gary Vaynerchuk Is Thirsty." *Bloomberg Businessweek,* May 20, 2008.

Horovitz, Bruce. "Americans Snack Differently Than Other Nations." *USA Today,* September 29, 2014.

———. "Cheesy Doritos Loaded to Roll Out at 7-Eleven." *USA Today,* July 1, 2014.

———. "Dunkin': Croissant Donut Permanent." *USA Today,* February 11, 2015.

———. "Food Marketers Score with Portion-Controlled Snacks." *USA Today,* April 13, 2006.

———. "Little Caesars Tries Bacon-Wrapped Crust Pizza." *USA Today,* February 18, 2015.

———. "Oreo Biscuits to Roll Out at Church's." *USA Today,* November 19, 2014.

———. "Taco Bell Tests Cheese-Stuffed Shell." *USA Today,* February 6, 2015.

"How Italian Food Became a Global Sensation." *Fresh Food,* NPR, March 24, 2011.

Jamrisko, Michelle. "Americans' Spending on Dining Out Just Overtook Grocery Sales for the First Time Ever." *Bloomberg News,* April 14, 2015.

Jennings, Lisa. "Latest Restaurant Promotions Highlight Health, Not Calories." *Nation's Restaurant News,* January 9, 2015.

———. "Survey: Human Touch Still Vital in Restaurants." *Nation's Restaurant News,* November 10, 2014.

————. "Taco Bell Updates Menu to Focus on Protein." *Nation's Restaurant News,* July 10, 2014.

Jessop, Alicia. "Americans Will Consume Billions of Chicken Wings and Millions of Pizza Slices on Super Bowl Sunday." *Forbes,* February 3, 2013.

"Jimmy Kimmel Asks, 'What Is Gluten?'" ABC News, accessed September 23, 2015.

Juli. "Fashion Fridays." *PaleOMG* blog, February 6, 2015.

J. S. and G. D. "High Spirits: Who Drinks Most Vodka, Gin, Whiskey and Rum?" *The Economist,* June 17, 2013.

Kalin, Curtis. "McRage: Woman Sets Car on Fire After Man Refuses to Buy McFlurry," CNS News, March 18, 2014.

Kantor, Jodi, and David Streitfeld. "Inside Amazon: Wrestling Big Ideas in a Bruising Workplace." *New York Times,* August 15, 2015.

Kaplan, Melanie D. G. "Nonprofit Pay-What-You-Can Cafes Let Diners Pay It Forward." *Washington Post,* June 18, 2015.

Kell, John. "Athletic Apparel: Outperforming the Competition in 2014." *Fortune,* December 25, 2014.

————. "Nearly 46 Million Americans Received Starbucks Gift Cards This Holiday." *Fortune,* January 5, 2015.

Kelto, Anders. "Farm Fresh? Natural? Eggs Not Always What They're Cracked Up to Be." NPR, December 23, 2014.

Kettlebell Kitchen. "Why Paleo?" KettlebellKitchen.com, accessed September 23, 2015.

Kiersz, Andy. "Here Are the Countries That Drink the Most Hard Liquor." *Business Insider,* February 10, 2014.

Kjerulf, Alexander. "5 Simple Office Policies That Make Danish Workers Way More Happy Than Americans," *Fast Company,* April 15, 2014.

"Know It All: Ketchup." *Food Network Magazine,* July/August 2015.

Kowitt, Beth. "Inside the Secret World of Trader Joe's—Full Version." *Fortune,* August 23, 2010.

————. "The War on Big Food." *Fortune,* May 21, 2015.

Krader, Kate. "Best and Worst Food Trends of 2013." *First Coast News,* December 27, 2013.

Kuang, Cliff. "In the Cafeteria, Google Gets Healthy." *Fast Company,* March 19, 2012.

Kurtzleben, Danielle. "Lots of Other Countries Mandate Paid Leave. Why Not the U.S.?" NPR, July 15, 2015.

Lam, Francis. "The Curious History of General Tso's Chicken." *Salon,* January 6, 2010.

Lambert, Lisa. "More Americans Move to Cities in Past Decade—Census." Reuters, March 26, 2012.

LaRue, Landon. "How to Speak Crossfit: Viewer's Guide." ESPN, July 30, 2014.

Levit, Alexandra. "Make Way for Generation Z." *New York Times,* March 28, 2015.

Lifehack. Assorted headlines, Lifehack.org, accessed February 12, 2015

Li, Shan. "Office Holiday Parties Are Fewer and Less Elaborate." *Los Angeles Times,* December 14, 2010.

Litman, Laken. "Texas Rangers Unveil Groundbreaking S'mOreo Dessert and Bacon Beer." *USA Today,* March 18, 2015.

Little, Katie. "Taco Bell Meets Cap'n Crunch in New Dessert." CNBC, February 27, 2015.

Lorenz, Taylor. "Beyoncé Launches Vegan Meal Delivery." *Business Insider,* February 2, 2015.

Long, Heather. "The Sunday Blues: Some US States Don't Seem to Realize Prohibition Is Over." *Guardian,* March 3, 2013.

Lowry, Brian. "'Seinfeld's Finale Ends Up in Sixth Place of All Time." *Los Angeles Times,* May 16, 1998.

Luckerson, Victor. "Is Lunch a Waste of Time—or a Productivity Booster?" *Time,* July 16, 2012.

Lukovitz, Karlene. "Avocados from Mexico: A Fresh Super Bowl Entry." *MediaPost,* January 7, 2015.

Luscombe, Belinda. "Online Dating That Matches As You Do, Not As You Say." *Time,* July 31, 2014.

Lutz, Ashley. "Costco's Unorthodox Strategy to Survive the Big Box Apocalypse." *Business Insider,* March 7, 2013.

"Luxury for Less." CNBC, April 25, 2012.

Lyons, Will. "Who's Driving World Wine Consumption?" *Wall Street Journal,* January 28, 2015.

Mabrey, Vicki, and Meredith Blake. "'Two Buck Chuck' Wine Aims for Both Quality and Quantity." ABC News, August 13, 2009.

Madarang, Charisma. "The 17 Most Popular Items at Trader Joe's." *Foodbeast,* May 7, 2014.

———. "Jack in the Box Has a Cheeseburger Topped with a Grilled Cheese Sandwich & More Munchie Monstrosities." *Foodbeast,* September 24, 2013.

Madhani, Aamer. "'Evenings' at Starbucks: Coffee Shop to Sell Wine, Craft Beer, Small Plates." *USA Today,* August 18, 2015.

"Make Way for the Critters; ACNielsen Data Show Wine Labels with 'Critters' Have an Increasingly Positive Impact on Wine Sales." *Business Wire,* March 20, 2006.

"Man Breaks into Home Dressed as a Teletubby, Steals Leftover Chinese Food." *People,* October 30, 2014.

"The Man, the Can: Recipes of the Real Chef Boyardee." *All Things Considered,* NPR, May 17, 2011.

Mann, Court. "The Tastiest Gauntlet." *Daily Herald,* December 18, 2014.

Marks, Gene. "How to Forever Avoid the Line at Starbucks." *Forbes,* September 13, 2013.

Martin, Hugo. "More than Half of Americans Have Gone 12 Months without a Vacation." *Los Angeles Times,* August 13, 2015.

Martinez, Stephen. "Obesity and Other Health Concerns Lead Food Companies to Step Up Health and Nutrient Claims." USDA.gov, July 1, 2013.

Maslin, Janet. "Caught Amid Life's Own Sly Tricks." *New York Times,* June 20, 2012.

Matthews, Christopher. "The 3 Best and 3 Worst States in America for Drinking." *Time,* December 5, 2013.

———. "Americans Are Painfully Aware of How Broke They Are." *Time,* January 28, 2014.

Mayo Clinic Staff. "Gluten-Free Diet." Mayoclinic.org, accessed September 24, 2015.

McCarthy, Michael. "Burger King Tries Old Slogan Again." *USA Today,* May 23, 2005.

McConnell Schaarsmith, Amy. "Big Dipper: Suit up for the Super Bowl with These Game-Day Tips." *Pittsburgh Post-Gazette,* January 18, 2007.

McDermott, Nicole. "Low Calorie Wine Sounds Great, but It's an Awful Idea." Greatist.com, November 22, 2013.

McNamara, Melissa. "Diet Industry Is Big Business." CBS News, December 1, 2006.

Merrill, Laurie. "Super Bowl: Burgers, Merchandise by the Numbers." *Arizona Republic,* January 27, 2015.

Miller, Julie. "In Defense of Beyoncé's Controversial Vegan Week." *Vanity Fair,* June 11, 2015.

Miller, Sara B. "In Battle for Sunday, the 'Blue Laws' Are Falling." *Christian Science Monitor,* December 5, 2003.

Miller Llana, Sara. "Super Bowl Success Story: Mexico's Avocados." *Christian Science Monitor,* January 31, 2009.

Milliken, Mary Sue, Susan Feniger, and Helene Siegel. "Huevos Rancheros," Dummies.com, accessed September 23, 2015.

Milman, Louis. "Taco Bell Says It Has Sold One Billion Doritos Locos Tacos." ABC News, December 12, 2014.

Mitchell, Dan. "The Hazelnut News Frenzy Continues." *Modern Farmer,* September 24, 2014.

Modha, Sanjana. "30 Crazy Meals from McDonald's Menus Around the World." Food Network, accessed September 22, 2015.

Mojadad, Ida. "Super Bowl 2015: Ad Revenue by the Millions and Chicken Wings by the Billions." *SF Weekly,* January 26, 2015.

Mooney, Kate. "Why NYC Men Are Falling (Rock) Hard for the Paleo Diet." *New York Observer,* July 24, 2014.

Morrison, Maureen. "Burger King Launches New Tagline: 'Be Your Way.'" *Advertising Age,* May 19, 2014.

Moye, Jay. "Meet the Three Guys Behind the Movement to Bring Back SURGE." The Coca-Cola Company blog, September 18, 2014.

Moynihan, Sandi. "#Cheesepocalypse: Surviving the Super Bowl without Velveeta." *Washington Post,* February 1, 2014.

Mulvany, Lydia. "The Super Bowl Wings Will Be Fat, Yes, but Pricey Too." *Bloomberg News,* January 23, 2015.

Nassauer, Sarah. "From Kale to Acai: Plot the Arc of a Food Fad." *Wall Street Journal,* April 15, 2015.

The National Association of American Wineries. "About the United States Wine and Grape Industry (General Industry Stats 2014)." Wineamerica .org, accessed September 24, 2015.

National Chicken Council. "Americans to Eat 1.23 Billion Chicken Wings Super Bowl Weekend." Nationalchickencouncil.org, January 22, 2013.

National Geographic. "Increased Fears about Environment, but Little Change in Consumer Behavior, According to New National Geographic/GlobeScan Study." National Geographic Press Release, September 26, 2014.

National League of Cities. "The 30 Most Populous Cities," Nlc.org, accessed September 23, 2015.

National Restaurant Association. "New Research Finds Americans Embrace Global Cuisine." National Restaurant Association News & Research, August 19, 2015.

Nelson, Andy. "Record Avocado Volumes Expected for Super Bowl." *The Packer,* January 8, 2015.

"Nestle Lean Cuisine Sales Drop as Shoppers Shun Freezer." *Bloomberg News,* March 13, 2014.

Nestle, Marion. "Google's Impressive Healthy Food Program." *Food Politics* blog, July 13, 2011.

————. "What Google's Famous Cafeterias Can Teach Us about Health." *Atlantic,* July 13, 2011.

Nisen, Max. "All Hail King Whiskey." *Atlantic,* October 15, 2014.

Noguchi, Yuki. "Stop, Thief! When Colleagues Steal from the Office Fridge." NPR, April 2, 2014.

Notopoulos, Katie. "Definitive List of Best And Worst Halloween Candy." BuzzFeed, October 29, 2012.

NPR Staff. "A Journey through the History of American Food in 100 Bites." NPR, November 15, 2014.

————. "Marketers Turn to Memories of Sweeter Times to Sell Cereal." NPR, January 3, 2015.

Nunes, Keith. "Mintel: Gluten Free Will Hit $8.8 Billion in Sales in 2014." *Food Business News,* November 18, 2014.

Oaklander, Mandy. "We're More Concerned with Nutrients than Actual Foods." *Time,* June 10, 2015.

"100 Million Dieters, $20 Billion: The Weight-Loss Industry by the Numbers." ABC News, May 8, 2012.

Organisation for Economic Co-operation and Development. "About." Oecd.org, accessed September 23, 2015.

————. "Average Annual Hours Actually Worked per Worker." Stats .oecd.org, accessed September 24, 2015.

The Paleo Mom. *The Paleo Mom* blog, accessed September 23, 2015.

Pallotta, Frank. "Emmys Ratings Were Lowest Ever." CNNMoney, September 21, 2015.

————. "Super Bowl XLIX Posts the Largest Audience in TV History." CNNMoney, February 2, 2015.

Parmley, Suzette. "The New 'Breakfast Club.'" Philly.com, June 21, 2015.

"PepsiCo Confirms Doritos-Flavored Mountain Dew Is Real." Fox News, November 10, 2014.

Pepitone, Julianne, and Stacy Cowley. "Facebook's First Big Investor, Peter Thiel, Cashes Out." CNNMoney, August 20, 2012.

"Percentage of Americans Who Drink Wine," WineMarketCouncil.com, accessed September 23, 2015.

Peterson, Hayley. "Why Trader Joe's Wine Is So Cheap." *Business Insider,* December 19, 2014.

Peterson, Kim. "12 Things about Costco That May Surprise You." CBS News, July 16, 2014.

Phillips, David. "Are Frozen Foods on Thin Ice?" *Food Processing,* June 3, 2013.

Picchi, Aimee. "Kraft Could Face a Cheesy Meltdown with Velveeta Shortage." CBS News, January 7, 2014.

Pinsker, Joe. "The Man Who Kept Trader Joe's Whimsical." *Atlantic,* November 11, 2014

———. "The Psychology behind Costco's Free Samples." *Atlantic,* October 1, 2014.

Pollan, Michael. "Out of the Kitchen, Onto the Couch." *New York Times Magazine,* July 29, 2009.

"Possible Chicken Wing Shortage Looms Ahead of Super Bowl." Fox News, January 23, 2012.

Prial, Frank J. "The Wallaby That Roared across the Wine Industry." *New York Times,* April 23, 2006.

Quagliani, Diane. "Who Is the 'Free-From' Shopper?" *Progressive Grocer,* April 1, 2015.

Rai, Saritha. "How Domino's Reinvented Itself to Win in India." *Fast Company,* February 2015.

Reisner, Rebecca. "The Diet Industry: A Big Fat Lie." *Bloomberg Businessweek,* January 2008.

Rhodes, Jesse. "The Birth of Brunch: Where Did This Meal Come from Anyway?" *Smithsonian,* May 6, 2011.

Riccobono, Anthony. "Super Bowl 2014 Ratings: How Many People Watched the Seattle Seahawks vs. Denver Broncos?" *International Business Times,* February 3, 2014.

Right Management. "Just One-in-Five Employees Take Actual Lunch Break." Thoughtwire at Right.com, October 6, 2012.

Rijkhoff, Babette. "Issue 12: Millennials." *Food Inspiration Magazine,* June 9, 2015.

Robinson, Jancis, and Linda Murphy. "Time to Widen View of U.S. Wine Scene." Huffington Post, June 9, 2013.

Rocha, Isai. "KFC's Breakthrough Edible Coffee Cup Taste[s] Like Cookies." *Foodbeast,* February 25, 201.

Rose, Brent. "The Beef-Jerky-Potato Chip Hybrid Is Real, and We Taste-Tested It." *Gizmodo,* August 19, 2014.

Rosenthal, Elizabeth. "Our Fix-It Faith and the Oil Spill." *New York Times,* May 29, 2010.

Rubin, Courtney. "Jay-Z and Beyoncé Want to Put You in a Vegan State of Mind." *New York Times,* May 7, 2015.

Rubin, Gretchen. "The Psychology of Waiting: 8 Factors That Make the Wait Seem Longer." Psych Central, accessed September 22, 2015.

Russell, Mallory. "How Burger King Went from McDonald's Greatest Rival to Total Trainwreck." *Business Insider,* April 15, 2012.

Sanger-Katz, Margot. "Americans Are Finally Eating Less." *New York Times,* July 24, 2015.

Saval, Nikil. "The Secret History of Life-Hacking." *Pacific Standard,* April 22, 2014.

Scott-Thomas, Caroline. "The 'Health Halo' Effect: Nutrition Claims May Lead to Bigger Portions." FoodNavigator.com, May 20, 2013.

Seifer, Darren. "Do I Need to Eat This Snack Bar?" *The NPD Group Blog,* February 20, 2014.

———. "Main Meal, Snack Foods Cross the Lines." *The NPD Group Blog,* accessed September 22, 2015.

———. " 'What Can I Bring?' " *The NPD Group Blog,* January 31, 2014.

Shaftel, David. "Brunch Is for Jerks." *New York Times,* October 10, 2014.

Shah, Khushbu. "McDonald's Franchise Owners Hope New CEO Will Slash the Chain's Menu." *Eater,* January 30, 2015.

"Shocking Super Bowl Facts." Fox News, accessed September 24, 2015.

Shute, Nancy. "Frozen Food Gets Ready For Its Image Upgrade," NPR, April 19, 2013

Silver, Marc. " 'American Hustle' Didn't Get Its Microwave Facts Straight." *National Geographic,* January 9, 2014.

Skerrett, Patrick J. "Resveratrol—the Hype Continues." *Harvard Health Publications,* February 3, 2012.

"Slideshow: New Products from General Mills, Campbell, Taco Bell." *Food Business News,* August 6, 2013.

Smith, K. Annabelle. "Why the Tomato Was Feared in Europe for More Than 200 Years." *Smithsonian,* June 18, 2013.

Smith, Ned. "Super Bowl Crisis? Chicken-Wings Shortage Looms." *Christian Science Monitor,* January 24, 2013.

Souza, Dan. "How Popchips Are Made, Why They're So Popular." *Serious Eats,* August 7, 2012.

Sort This Out Cellars. Description of 2008 Elvira Macabrenet. SortThis OutCellars.com, accessed September 23, 2015.

Specter, Michael. "Against the Grain." *New Yorker,* November 3, 2014.

Stampler, Laura. "80 Reasons Why Drinking Alcohol Is Great." *Time,* December 4, 2013.

———. "Pizza Hut Built a Giant, Real-Life Teenage Mutant Ninja Turtle Pizza Thrower." *Time,* July 23, 2014.

———. "TV Viewers Deserted the Oscars This Year," *Time,* February 23, 2015.

Steel, Tanya. "Inside Google's Kitchens." *Gourmet,* March 7, 2012.

Steinberger, Michael. "The Great and Powerful Shnoz." *Slate,* June 17, 2002.

Stewart, James. "A Fearless Culture Fuels U.S. Tech Giants." *New York Times,* June 18, 2015.

Stewart, Jocelyn Y. "California Chef Pioneered Gourmet Pizza Revolution." *Los Angeles Times,* January 4, 2008.

Stone, Alex. "Why Waiting Is Torture." *New York Times,* August 18, 2012.

Stone, Dan. "You're Eating Too Many Avocados." *National Geographic,* October 14, 2014.

Strom, Stephanie. "Cereals Begin to Lose Their Snap, Crackle and Pop." *New York Times,* September 10, 2014.

"Super Bowl Sunday: What We're Eating." Fox Sports News, February 1, 2012.

Sussner Rodgers, Fran. "Who Owns Your Overtime?" *New York Times,* June 22, 2015.

Swanson, Ana. "What Super Bowl Manvertising Says about Men's New Role in America." *Washington Post,* February 2, 2015.

Swindell, Bill. "Influential Costco Executive Discusses Wine Business in Q&A." *Santa Rosa Press Democrat,* October 12, 2014.

Sytsma, Alan. "Watch John Oliver Trash Pumpkin Spice Lattes, 'the Coffee That Tastes Like a Candle.'" *Grub Street,* October 13, 2014.

Taibi, Catherine. "Jon Stewart Calls Out Fox News for Overhyping Super Bowl 'Velveeta Shortage.'" Huffington Post, January 25, 2014.

Taylor, Paul, and Wendy Wang. "The Fading Glory of the Television and Telephone." Pew Research Center, Washington, DC, August 19, 2010.

Think Splendid and Kelly Ashworth Design. "How Millennials Eat" infographic. ThinkSplendid.com, March 7, 2012.

Team, Trefis. "How the Fast Casual Segment Is Gaining Market Share in the Restaurant Industry." *Forbes,* June 23, 2014.

———. "Taco Bell and Starbucks Challenge McDonald's Morning Dominance with New Breakfast Menu." *Forbes,* February 28, 2014.

Thorn, Bret. "Top 5 Ethnic Food Trends for 2015." *Nation's Restaurant News,* February 27, 2015.

Tice, Carol. "The American Fast Food the World Loves: Top Global Brands." *Forbes,* March 11, 2013.

Tilak, Visi R. "The Great Lure of Indian Fast Food." *Wall Street Journal,* April 9, 2013.

Tita, Bob. "Super Bowl Challenge for Box Makers: 12.5 Million Pizzas." *Wall Street Journal,* January 29, 2015.

"Tracking Consumer Purchase Behavior on Health and Wellness Products." *Food Processing,* October 1, 2006.

Traverso, Amy. "Celebrate Pesto's Premiere." *Sunset,* accessed September 24, 2015.

Tuder, Stefanie. "Papa John's Debuts a Fritos Chili Pizza." ABC News, October 29, 2014.

Tunks, Jane. "Super Bowl Save—Grocers Avert Guacamole Shortage." *San Francisco Chronicle*, February 1, 2009.

University of California, Davis. "UC Davis Study Finds Telecommuting Can Be Hazardous to Your Career." *UC Davis News and Information*, June 9, 2010.

U.S. Census Bureau. "State and County Quick Facts." Quickfacts.census .gov, updated August 31, 2015.

———. "U.S. and World Population Clock." Census.gov, accessed September 24, 2015.

U.S. Department of Agriculture's Economic Research Service. "New Product Introduction of Consumer Packaged Goods, 1992–2010." Ers.USDA .gov, updated October 30, 2014.

U.S. Food and Drug Administration. "Beware of Products Promising Miracle Weight Loss." FDA Consumer Updates at FDA.gov, accessed September 23, 2015.

———. "Dietary Supplements." FDA.gov, accessed September 23, 2015.

———. "The FDA Takes Step to Remove Artificial Trans Fats in Processed Foods." FDA News Release, June 16, 2015.

U.S. National Library of Medicine. "Protein in Diet." Medline Plus, updated April 30, 2013.

Virbila, S. Irene. "Robert Parker Goes Toe-to-Toe with His Critics." *Los Angeles Times*, February 27, 2014.

Voight, Joan. "Unpretentious Millennials Are Changing the Way We Drink Wine, Barefoot's CMO Says." *Adweek*, January 12, 2015.

Walker, Rob. "Animal Pragmatism." *New York Times Magazine*, April 23, 2006.

Wallace, Gregory. "French Toast Crunch Cereal Is Back." CNNMoney, December 8, 2014.

Watson, Elaine. "Eating Alone, Continuous Snacking and the Slow Death of the Primary Shopper: 10 Things You Need to Know about the Changing American Consumer." *FoodNavigator-USA*, August 11, 2015.

———. "Non-GMO, Kosher, Vegan, All-Natural . . . What Can We Learn from Claims Made on New Products in the US in 2014?" *FoodNavigator-USA*, December 15, 2014.

Webber, Katrina. "Woman Busted for Stealing Sausage Worth $6,400." KSAT News, November 26, 2014.

Wehrum, Kasey. "Super Bowl Hangover." *Inc.*, January 27, 2006.

Weil, Andrew. "Fat-Free Half-and-Half?" Huffington Post, May 8, 2012.

Weise, Elizabeth. "66% of Consumers Wrongly Think 'Natural' Means Something." *USA Today*, June 17, 2014.

Weissmann, Jordan. "Why Super Bowl Ads Keep Getting More Expensive." *Atlantic*, January 3, 2012.

Wells, Jane. "The Really Big Ruckus over 'Two Buck Chuck.'" CNBC, August 11, 2014.

Werbach, Adam. "The American Commuter Spends 38 Hours a Year Stuck in Traffic." *Atlantic,* February 6, 2013.

"What's the Story behind Cheerios?" Cheerios.com, accessed September 23, 2015.

White, Martha C. "6 Tips for Surviving the Office Holiday Party." *Time,* December 2, 2013.

———. "Snack Bar Sales Soar on Hunger for Productivity, Convenience." NBC News, February 18, 2014.

———. "Why Super Bowl's 'Hangover Monday' Is Worse than Usual This Year." *Today,* February 4, 2013.

Who Made America? "Charles Goodyear," PBS.org, accessed September 23, 2015.

"The Why Behind the Dine." *International Food Inspiration Magazine,* accessed September 23, 2015.

"20 Regional Chains We Wish Would Go National." Zagat.com, January 21, 2014.

"Why You Should Buy Your Next Bottle of Wine at Costco." *Esquire,* June 16, 2015.

Widdicombe, Lizzie. "The End of Food." *New Yorker,* May 12, 2014.

Wild Flavors, Inc. "Women: Trends & Health Ingredients," *Food Processing,* accessed September 23, 2015.

Willett, Megan. "The Most Talked-About Food in Every State." *Business Insider,* September 23, 2014.

Williams, Geoff. "The Heavy Price of Losing Weight." *U.S. News & World Report,* January 2, 2013.

Williams, Ray. "Slowing Down Can Increase Productivity and Happiness," part 1. *Psychology Today,* June 17, 2014.

"Wine Consumption in the U.S." Wineinstitute.org, August 26, 2015.

Witherington, Laurence. "Which Country Drinks the Most Alcohol?" *Wall Street Journal,* August 22, 2014.

Wolf, Robb. "Revolutionary Solutions to Modern Life." RobbWolf.com, accessed September 23, 2015.

Wollan, Malia. "Rise and Shine: What Kids Around the World Eat for Breakfast." *New York Times Magazine,* October 8, 2014.

Wong, Elaine. "100-Calorie Packs Pack It In." *Adweek,* May 26, 2009.

Wong, Venessa. "America's Biggest Beer Drinkers." *Bloomberg Businessweek,* June 27, 2011.

———. "Doritos-Flavored Mountain Dew and the Genius of PepsiCo's Gross-Out Marketing." *Bloomberg Businessweek,* November 13, 2014.

———. "General Mills Has Plans to Spark a Breakfast Cereal Revival." *Bloomberg Businessweek,* July 9, 2014.

The World Bank. "Population, Total." Data.worldbank.org, accessed September 23, 2015.

World Health Organization. "Cardiovascular Diseases (CVDs) Fact Sheet N° 317." WHO.int, updated January 2015.

Wright, Lawrence. "Slim's Time." *New Yorker,* June 1, 2009.

Zelman, Kathleen M. "6 Best Foods You're Not Eating." WebMD.com, July 18, 2011.

Index

About the Author

Sophie Egan is the director of programs and culinary nutrition for the Strategic Initiatives Group at The Culinary Institute of America. Based in San Francisco, Egan is a contributor to *The New York Times*'s Well blog, and has written about food and health for KQED, *Wired,* and *Sunset* magazine, where she worked on *The* Sunset *Cookbook* and *The One-Block Feast* book. She holds a master of public health from University of California, Berkeley, with a focus on health and social behavior, and a bachelor of arts with honors in history from Stanford University.